Theories and techniques of oral implantology

VOLUME TWO

Theories and techniques of oral implantology

Leonard I. Linkow, B.S., D.D.S., F.A.G.D.

Attending Associate Chief of Oral Implantology, Jewish Memorial Hospital, New York, N. Y.; Chief of Implantology, Haifa Center for Continuing Dental Education, Haifa, Israel; Consultant, Tel-Aviv University, Tel-Aviv, Israel; Visiting Lecturer, Brookdale Hospital, Brooklyn, N. Y.; Lariboisière Hospital, Paris; Royal Society of Medicine, London; Postgraduate Instructor and Clinician, Institute for Graduate Dentists, New York, N. Y.; University of Detroit, Detroit, Mich.; Washington University, St. Louis, Mo.; State University of New York at Buffalo School of Dentistry, Buffalo, N. Y.; Loyola University School of Dentistry, Maywood, Ill.; Visiting Faculty, Temple University School of Dentistry, Philadelphia, Pa.; Oregon University School of Dentistry, Portland, Ore.; Guest Lecturer on Implantology, University of Maryland, College Park, Md.; Tufts University, Boston, Mass.; Ohio State University School of Dentistry, Columbus, Ohio

Raphael Cherchève, STOMATOLOGIST

Paris, France

Edited and illustrated by
Maureen Jones

With 2,234 illustrations

The C. V. Mosby Company

Saint Louis 1970

Distributed in Great Britain by
HENRY KIMPTON
205 Great Portland Street, London, W.1.

Printed in the United States of America
Standard Book Number 8016-3018-5
Library of Congress Catalog Card Number 70-124051
Distributed in Great Britain by Henry Kimpton, London

Dedicated to all the pioneers

Because of my several years' association with Dr. Raphael Cherchève and my great respect and admiration for his pioneering work in the field of implantology, I feel it only fitting that, in addition to the above distinction, Dr. Cherchève be included as a co-author of this book.

Leonard I. Linkow

There is a space between man's imagination and man's attainments that may only be traversed by his longing.

Kahlil Gibran, from Sand and Foam, Alfred A. Knopf, Inc.

PROLOGUE

The author is particularly well qualified for the preparation of this book. He has spent the greater part of his research and clinical practice in the field of implantology. He has lectured widely, written extensively, and taught numerous graduate classes. This book bears the imprint of the vigor and excitement of the author for his field of endeavor.

This book represents an important contribution to the literature in a discipline that, up to now, has been vague and confusing, while at the same time controversial. Implantology still remains for most of us at the border of the "twilight zone."

Those among us who have implanted natural teeth realized that in a relatively short time the root was resorbed. From these observations came the concept of using some foreign substance. Today the purity of the material used in implants is not as important as its toleration by the tissues.

At the present time we are transplanting entire human organs, among which are hearts, kidneys, and even lungs. What is feared and far from being entirely understood is the rejection by the body of these so-called foreign substances. In dental implants we are faced in a similar manner with the process of rejection. It is the hope of the author that successful answers will be found so that implantology will be on a firmer foundation.

When any technique, dental or otherwise, reaches the magnitude of being used by a growing number of practitioners who are experienced in their fields, serious consideration must be given the technical point of view, even though some practitioners may feel it is ahead of its time. This resolute treatise by an innovator, using accepted scientific principles and documentary evidence of trial and error—success and failure—decrees that one must respect the innovator and the experimentation. The results of the work of Leonard I. Linkow comes under such an aegis, and his book *Theories and Techniques of Oral Implantology* is evidence of such forward-looking activity.

All forms of experimentations in any field have always been attempted with confidence; an assurance of success is an integral part of the desires of the experimenter.

This book comes to us with the confidence and enthusiasm of the author and his feeling that the techniques described herein, with careful consideration and under the proper circumstances, can be successfully implemented.

At no time has he insisted that his ideas are the only ones to be considered, that his recommendations are the panacea of widespread problems, or that past good practices should be sidetracked; rather, he has taken the direct opposite stand and submits the results of his labors so that the worth of his points of practice may be analyzed within the framework of the reader's practice background and in the light of his own needs.

Commendation for such pioneering must be high, for without the "inner gleam" reaching for improvement, little real progress can ever be made. This author has that inner gleam, and his devotion to it has produced this profound and dedicated study. In the field where the future has no limiting boundaries, growth must be shown, for nothing is really impossible.

The author wishes to look forward without forsaking the traditions and essential aspects of the past. The text represents the boldness and judgment of a single individual. It comes at a time when research in oral diseases has reached a new and elevated degree of sophistication. Regardless of the fact that the field of implantology has been the object of unremitting controversy and that he is unquestionably an easy man to disagree with, he has opposed unyielding rigidity in thinking and his contributions are vigorous and unique. He has challenged not only the established policies but even his own preconceived opinions. His is a form of empiricism restrained by reason. It permits the discordant facts to sing for themselves.

This book is the most profound treatise of its kind to date and represents a tremendous effort to place the various aspects of this fragmented discipline in their proper relationship.

I salute the author.

Jerome M. Schweitzer, B.S., D.D.S.

INTRODUCTION

It is both refreshing and gratifying to push the vistas of human knowledge and its benefits forward. Yet the transplanting of ideas presupposes mental readiness on the part of a profession and its practitioners to assimilate ideas and incorporate them into practice. This is particularly so with regard to dentistry and its implications for the well-being of society.

Since professional advance, like human progress, is slow, there is the further implication that inertia is overcome only with great effort. There is, of course, intellectual curiosity aimed at higher levels of knowledge and achievement which must be interspersed with scientific caution, but hopefully geared to human service.

Implantology has certainly seized the imagination of our profession. It has also, unfortunately, created temptation for some of our colleagues to proclaim proficiency after attending short introductory courses or several lectures. We must be cognizant of the fact that great scientific spurts contain negative counterparts and possible dangers.

Implantology further sharpens our focus on the responsibility of our profession to preserve natural teeth, minimal as they may be, and at any cost in effort, knowledge, and skill. The signs of omission and commission of the dental profession with regard to adequate care and safeguards for the restorative facets of dentistry are well reflected in the reception now afforded in this new modality of implantology.

It is my strong feeling that dental progress has been brought forward by a combination of professional integrity, thoughtful proficiency, imagination, and courageous innovative skills. Because of my esteem and admiration for Dr. Leonard Linkow, I am delighted to express my commendation for his contribution in this specialty. This text should do much to clear the confusion and augurs well for the future of implantology and the benefit to the health and comfort of our patients.

I. Franklin Miller, B.S., M.A., D.D.S., F.I.C.D., F.A.G.D.

FOREWORD

What can anyone say about Dr. Leonard Linkow that is not already known? His inventiveness, his unusual vitality, and, of course, his thorough experience are widely known.

I felt really elated and quite happy when Dr. Linkow asked me to write the foreword to his book. The problem is that the few lines usually allowed in a foreword are not adequate.

Dr. Linkow's practice of implantology goes back several years and to this he has dedicated all his energy and exceptional resourcefulness. After having built up a sizable following in general stomatology (in addition to many articles, in 1962 he published *Full Arch Fixed Oral Reconstruction*), Dr. Linkow expanded his knowledge of implantology from subperiosteal implants (which were his starting point and still bear the mark of his individuality) to the endosseous implants which, during the last several years, have been his main object of interest and scientific application.

The present volume, which no doubt will attain its merited success, is unique in its field; it is surely the most complete, as it reviews all the principal techniques in use and gives a detailed description of Dr. Linkow's own techniques, made more interesting by a great number of photographs.

In this book the author's main idea is clearly revealed: *Implantology is an important as well as a difficult undertaking.* In order to be successful, one must keep abreast of all the various techniques, for not all cases can be treated by just one method. A well-prepared operator must be able to judge correctly when to use a subperiosteal or an endosseous implant and must be able to select the method best suited to a particular case and a particular area.

Dr. Linkow has presented his material with great clarity and authority in a manner consistent with his professional commitment to implantology.

In the future, I earnestly hope that this field will attract other colleagues, who, like Dr. Linkow, will continue to develop new techniques and skills leading to the further success and acceptance of implantology.

Professor Giordano Muratori
President, Italian Society of Implant Dentistry
Affiliate Member, A.A.I.D.

PREFACE

The history of dentistry resembles that of other areas of medicine. Many researchers and practitioners contribute to the growth and depth of the field. The field expands in numerous, sometimes seemingly unrelated, directions, and then scattered bits of evidence crystallize into a concept that becomes a tremendously important and exciting landmark in the field. For some time now, investigators working in various areas of specialization have been developing their ideas and making small but important contributions to the field of implantology. Now comes a unifying concept—the endosseous implant.

The endosseous implant is the most exciting idea in modern dentistry. It is the herald of a new era that can benefit esthetically, psychologically, and physically most of the partially and many of the totally edentulous patients. The idea is to put into bone an implant designed to complement the natural forces operating in the health and welfare of the jaws. The implant is accepted by the tissues in which it has been set and is tightly bound there, providing a tenacious abutment to which a permanent or a temporary prosthesis may be attached. This gives the patient a prosthesis that is closer to the look and feel of natural teeth than any other artificial appliance to date. It is radically different in concept and totally exciting in its potential benefits.

The history of dentistry has also been plagued by the needlessly slow recognition and acceptance of a startlingly different idea. Despite ample proof that a new technique will immeasurably benefit a patient, there is a tendency to stick to traditional methods. This is understandable, for many operators prefer to repeat familiar techniques with predictable results rather than to experiment with the unfamiliar. However, this attitude should be objectively evaluated.

The ultimate goal in dentistry is maximum benefit to the patient, not the continuance of merely adequate methods for the convenience of an operator. Granted, the procedures involved in implantation are more radical than current procedures for providing removable dental prostheses. Granted, the techniques require a great deal more clinical skill on the part of the operator than do current conventional approaches. Yet the benefits to the patient are so much greater that the ethics of dentistry demand that a new technique be carefully judged and evaluated in terms of its inherent merits.

Of course an endosseous implant technique cannot be performed on all patients. Because the implant must be set in alveolar bone, those patients with extensive bone resorption are not suitable candidates. However, they may be candidates for a subperiosteal implant. Some patients, because of overall poor health—such as those with uncontrolled diabetes—can never be candidates for any kind of implant intervention. Others, such as a patient with a temporary condition, may be restored to good health and become candidates. Of all presenting patients, from 70% to 85% may be candidates for some type of implant intervention, either endosseous or subperiosteal.

To date, I have treated well over 1,200 cases involving endosseous implant interventions, and together with those cases completed by my co-author, Dr. Raphael Cherchève, the figure exceeds 2,000. Although many of the early attempts were unsuccessful—primarily as a result of inappropriately designed implants and lack of experience in placing the implant—the majority of our later attempts have been successful. In those later cases where failure resulted, it was not because of basic flaws in the concept of an endosseous implant procedure but because of overenthusiasm in attempting an intervention. But from our mistakes, we have learned.

This book is a synthesis of my experiences in the field of implantology. It describes several techniques that are successful because they have been carefully designed to be compatible with the laws of nature. It explores the reasons why an implant succeeds or fails, from both operatory and physiologic viewpoints. It prepares the reader for the kind of experience that can be gained only through actual clinical work. It tells the individual operator why the procedures *should* work; his own experiences based on a thorough understanding of the factors involved will finally prove that they *do* work.

I sincerely feel that this book is important because the information herein explores what an ever-increasing number of operators is proving is the modern miracle in dentistry.

I wish to express my appreciation to all those people who contributed so unselfishly in one way or another to the preparation of this volume by providing information, suggestions, and constructive criticism. I also wish to express my gratitude and sincere appreciation to all those who gave me my start in the field of oral implantology by allowing me to bring forth my acquired knowledge in the field.

I wish, therefore, to give special thanks to Dr. Myron M. Lieb, Director of the Institute for Graduate Dentists, for expressing faith in me by allowing me to teach implantology while it was still in its early development. Many thanks to Dr. Harry M. Worth and Dr. Surindar N. Bhaskar for unselfishly contributing numerous roentgenograms on bone diseases, which are so important for the added success of this book. To Dr. George Greene, Jr., I extend my appreciation for his reading of and constructive comments on the histology chapter.

To Dr. Al Edelman, for his early cooperation and hard work in manufacturing my various-shaped prototype vent-plants and screws and the various instruments necessary for their insertion, I give my gratitude. I wish to thank Mr. Al Taylor for processing according to my specifications the many photographs that appear in this book. To Jack Wimmer and Abe Liwerent of Park Dental Research, I extend thanks for their cooperation in maintaining the designs and quality of blade implants at the highest standards. To Eric Bausch of Howmedica, sincere thanks for his pioneering efforts from the very beginning in the field of oral implantology.

To Dr. Jack Leonard Weiss, who has been a friend and advisor in so many ways, I wish to express my deep gratitude. His knowledge in many facets of dentistry has enlightened me considerably. To my dear friends, Dr. Giordano Muratori, Dr. Paul Glassman, Dr. Norman Mulnick, Dr. Ronald Cullen, and Dr. Hans Graffelmann, thanks for having enough faith and confidence in me during many frustrating years, and for listening to what I had to say.

To Dr. Frank Celenza, a true friend in need, who placed his own highly regarded reputation of dental gnathology on the line to back up my principles and philosophies in front of many outstanding dental organizations, thanks from the bottom of my heart.

To my staff of wonderful and hard-working nurses, Phyllis Athenson, Virginia Edwards, Yetta Goldberg, Karen Fishman, Nancy Levene, and Marilyn Berger, I wish to also express my thanks for cooperating with me during the hard times I gave them.

A very special thanks to my secretary and Girl Friday, Evelyn Gruber, whose hard work enabled the publication of this volume. The typing of the manuscript and correspondence with countless numbers of contributing dentists, companies, and so on could not have been done without her.

I wish to thank Bob Bosworth and Joe Andino, my two dental technologists who have been devoted to me for the past 5 years, from the bottom of my heart for helping me pioneer the field of implantology. Without them and their wonderful work it could not have been as easy.

To Maureen Jones, for the excellent work in editing my manuscript which required revision and condensation to make it readily understood, I am eternally grateful.

Last, but certainly not least, to my family; my mother and father, thanks for being such wonderful and understanding parents, and for those fruitful years of teaching me right from wrong. To my wife, Jean, who typed countless numbers of the earlier drafts of the book over and over again and who had to cooperate and sacrifice according to my many moods during the 5½ long years of preparation for this book, thank you. To my wonderful daughters Robin, Sheree, and Shelley I want to say, stay as sweet as you are.

Leonard I. Linkow, B.S., D.D.S., F.A.G.D.

CONTENTS

Theories and techniques of oral implantology

CHAPTER 9 Mandibular endosseous implant interventions

A great range of endosseous implant techniques can be used in the mandible. Not only may the type of implant itself vary, but the method of insertion and fabrication of a restoration may differ considerably from case to case.

Assuming that the patient's health is good, the prime consideration when contemplating an endosseous implant is the amount of alveolar bone, its shape, and its condition. When a good amount of alveolar bone exists between the alveolar crest and an anatomic landmark, post type implants can be used. Pin implants are most beneficial when used to circumvent various anatomic landmarks, where less bone structure is available. Knife-edge ridges require either narrow ridge implants or the newly designed blade-vent. Because the blade-vent implant has an even wider range of application, it will be dealt with in a separate chapter.

The material presented here shows the various situations in which vent-plants, spiral-shaft implants, triplants, and some of the other more common endosseous implants can be used.

UNILATERAL RESTORATIONS

To evaluate a unilateral edentulous area, intraoral, periapical radiographs are taken of the intended implant sites. These studies should include the entire edentulous free-end saddle area; a fairly clear picture of the mandibular canal, especially its superior wall; the two anterior teeth closest to the edentulous area intended as natural tooth abutments; and the mental foramen, if it is included in the edentulous area. If implants are to be used in the area of the mandibular canal, a Panorex or a lateral plate roentgenogram should also be taken to determine the outline of the canal.

Case 1
Unilateral posterior free-end saddle restoration using vent-plants and a temporary splint

In this first case two implants and two natural teeth constituted the supports for a four-unit fixed partial denture. The type of implant used, the Linkow vent-plant, is a modified post with an opening at its base through which bone can possibly grow (Fig. 9-1). This implant, like any other post implant, must be used only when there is sufficient alveolar bone in which to bury the implant's spirals and a good portion of its narrower shaft. Because the implant comes in several lengths with a variable number of spirals, it has a wide range of applications.

The two anterior tooth abutments were prepared for full coverage restorations (Fig. 9-2). Modeling compound in copper tube impressions, as well as a wax bite, were taken. In addition, an alginate impression was taken of the two prepared natural tooth abutments along with the edentulous spaces and of the opposing jaw. These impressions were used to fabricate two veneer castings and a temporary acrylic splint to cover the prepared natural teeth and implant abutments. Such a splint is used immediately after implant insertions to help stabilize them and to protect the tongue, cheeks, and lips from laceration by the sharp line angles of the protruding implant posts (Fig. 9-3).

At the beginning of the second visit, just prior to inserting the implants, the castings were fitted over the natural tooth abutments (Fig. 9-4). Their gingival

335

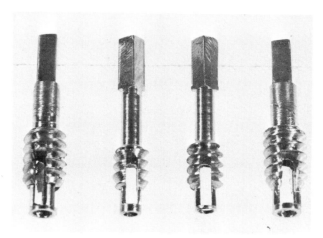

Fig. 9-1. Various sized vent-plants. (From Linkow, L. I.: Prefabricated mandibular prostheses for intraosseous implants, J. Prosth. Dent., 20:367-375, 1968.)

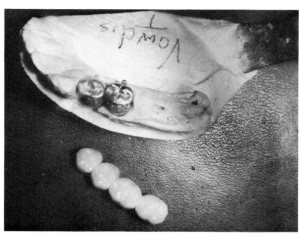

Fig. 9-3. A temporary acrylic splint and two bicuspid veneer castings are fabricated. (From Linkow, L. I.: The radiographic role in endosseous implant interventions, Chron. Omaha Dent. Soc. 29[10]:304-311, 1966.)

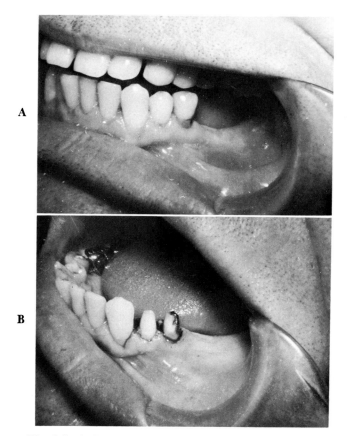

A

B

Fig. 9-2. A, The two bicuspid teeth before preparation. B, The teeth are prepared for full crown restorations. (From Linkow, L. I.: The radiographic role in endosseous implant interventions, Chron. Omaha Dent. Soc. 29[10]: 304-311, 1966.)

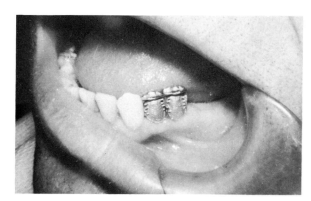

Fig. 9-4. The castings are fitted.

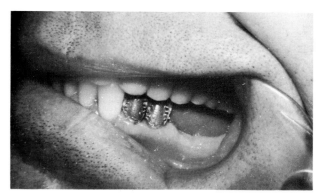

Fig. 9-5. The occlusion is carefully equilibrated. (From Linkow, L. I.: The radiographic role in endosseous implant interventions, Chron. Omaha Dent. Soc. 29[10]: 304-311, 1966.)

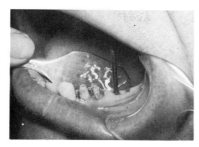

Fig. 9-6. A round bur is drilled through the crest of the ridge and into the underlying alveolar bone. (From Linkow, L. I.: The radiographic role in endosseous implant interventions, Chron. Omaha Dent. Soc. **29**[10]: 304-311, 1966.)

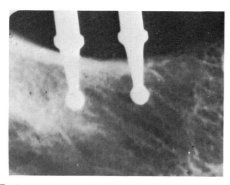

Fig. 9-7. An x-ray revealing two No. 6 round burs parallel to each other. (From Linkow, L. I.: The radiographic role in endosseous implant interventions, Chron. Omaha Dent. Soc. **29**[10]:304-311, 1966.)

margins and occlusal relationships were checked and adjusted as necessary (Fig. 9-5). The tissue-bearing surface of the temporary acrylic splint was hollowed out. The splint was tried in position and ground into proper occlusion.

To insert the first vent-plant, a No. 6 round bur, placed in a slow running contra-angle with a water spray attachment, was positioned over the center of the alveolar crest and drilled directly through the mucoperiosteum into the underlying osseous tissues until stopped by the built-in "stop guard" on the bur shaft. The bur was left in position (Fig. 9-6) and radiographed. The x-ray reveals its proximity to the mandibular canal and its degree of parallelism to the previously prepared natural tooth abutments.

Leaving the first bur in the alveolus as a parallel guide, a second round bur was drilled into the bone about 4 mm. behind the first and radiographed (Fig. 9-7).

Leaving one of the round burs in position, the other was removed, and a helical bone bur was inserted through its vacated hole. This was driven deeper into the bone, making sure that it was parallel both mesiodistally and buccolingually with the prepared teeth and with the extended shaft of the round bur (Fig. 9-8). Another x-ray was taken to determine the depth of the helical bur, its proximity to the mandibular canal, and its degree of parallelism with the prepared teeth and round bur shaft. Leaving the helical bur in the bone as a parallel guide, the remaining round bur was removed and the second helical bur driven into its site parallel to the shaft of the first helical bur and deeper than the hole created

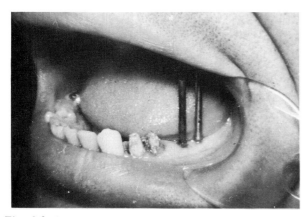

Fig. 9-8. Two helical burs are then drilled into the bone deeper than the previously removed round burs. (From Linkow, L. I.: The radiographic role in endosseous implant interventions, Chron. Omaha Dent. Soc. **29**[10]:304-311, 1966.)

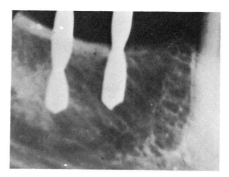

Fig. 9-9. An x-ray showing both helical burs in position. (From Linkow, L. I.: The radiographic role in endosseous implant interventions, Chron. Omaha Dent. Soc. **29**[10]: 304-311, 1966.)

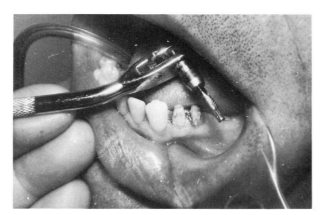

Fig. 9-10. The first vent-plant is then screwed into position using a ratchet. (From Linkow, L. I.: The radiographic role in endosseous implant interventions, Chron. Omaha Dent. Soc. **29**[10]:304-311, 1966.)

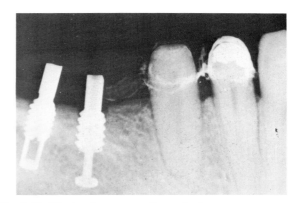

Fig. 9-12. The implants are radiographed.

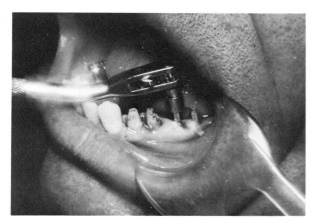

Fig. 9-11. The second vent-plant is inserted. (From Linkow, L. I.: The radiographic role in endosseous implant interventions, Chron. Omaha Dent. Soc. **29**[10]:304-311, 1966.)

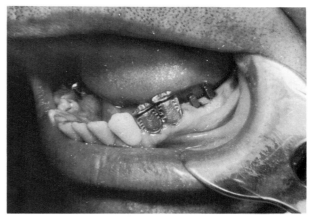

Fig. 9-13. The veneer castings are fitted over both bicuspid teeth. (From Linkow, L. I.: The radiographic role in endosseous implant interventions, Chron. Omaha Dent. Soc. **29**[10]:304-311, 1966.)

by the preceding round bur. Another x-ray was taken (Fig. 9-9).

One of the helical burs was then removed, and in its place a helical bur of a larger diameter was inserted. The diameter of this second helical bur corresponded to that of the desired vent-plant. This bur was drilled into the bone parallel to the remaining helical bur and to the prepared crowns and x-rayed. The purpose of this x-ray, as well as others taken at different levels during the insertion of the taps and burs, was to ensure accurate placement. The remaining smaller helical bur was replaced by one of a larger diameter, and another roentgenogram was taken.

The appropriate vent-plant was then ready for insertion. One of the helical burs was removed, and

the first vent-plant was screwed into its hole (Fig. 9-10) and x-rayed. The remaining bur was then removed and the second vent-plant inserted (Fig. 9-11). Both implants were radiographed (Fig. 9-12).

The castings were fitted over the prepared teeth (Fig. 9-13), and copings of some sort—in this case gold, although plastic ones may also be used—were placed over the protruding implant shafts (Fig. 9-14).

A wax bite and plaster index were taken (Fig. 9-15), with the castings and copings included in the index (Fig. 9-16). (Sometimes copings are not necessary over the implants. Instead, the plaster index picks up the castings covering the natural tooth abutments and only the impression of the protruding implant shafts.) Duplicate size bronze or copper shafts were immediately placed in the index and the master

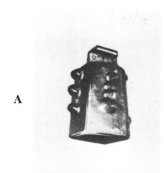

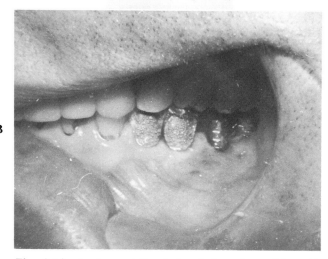

A

B

Fig. 9-14. A, A specially designed interchangeable gold coping fits over the vent-plant shafts. B, The copings are fitted over the protruding implants. (B, From Linkow, L. I.: The radiographic role in endosseous implant interventions, Chron. Omaha Dent. Soc. 29[10]:304-311, 1966.)

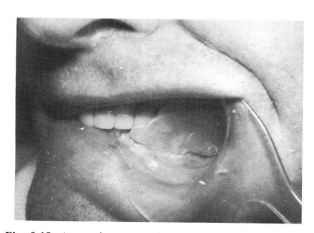

Fig. 9-15. A wax interocclusal record of centric relation is taken.

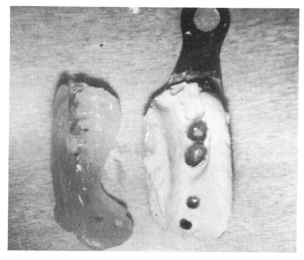

Fig. 9-16. A plaster index is seen in the metal tray. (From Linkow, L. I.: The radiographic role in endosseous implant interventions, Chron. Omaha Dent. Soc. 29[10]:304-311, 1966.)

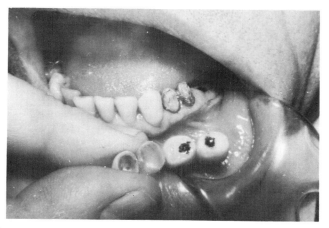

Fig. 9-17. Holes are made through the acrylic splint guided by the indelible pencil markings that were made over the occlusal surfaces of the implants. (From Linkow, L. I.: The radiographic role in endosseous implant interventions, Chron. Omaha Dent. Soc. 29[10]:304-311, 1966.)

stone model poured into the index. This eliminated a double casting technique.

To fit the temporary prefabricated acrylic splint into position over the natural tooth abutments and implant shafts, the occlusal surfaces of the shafts were marked with indelible pencil. The markings were transferred to the tissue-bearing surfaces of the acrylic splint (Fig. 9-17). With a vulcanite bur, two holes were made to accommodate the protruding implant shafts. These holes were very generous and larger than the shafts to ensure an easy fit. Once

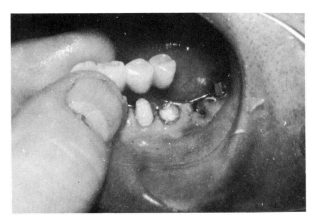

Fig. 9-18. The temporary acrylic splint is fitted into proper position. (From Linkow, L. I.: The radiographic role in endosseous implant interventions, Chron. Omaha Dent. Soc. 29[10]:304-311, 1966.)

proper occlusion had been established, fast-setting acrylic was placed into the holes and the splint was placed over the teeth and implants (Fig. 9-18). It was quickly removed and replaced every 20 seconds or so. This guaranteed that the holes exactly accommodated the implant shafts, yet prevented the acrylic from locking to the implants themselves.

After the acrylic set, all excess on the tissue-bearing surface was removed and the surface was polished with the splint outside the mouth. (When a patient has extremely soft tissue, the splint may be lined with a soft material, such as a rubber base, or with a soft tissue conditioner.) The temporary splint was then cemented into place with a temporary cement (Fig. 9-19). This cement should be used only inside those areas of the splint intended to cover the natural tooth abutments. Otherwise, because the implant

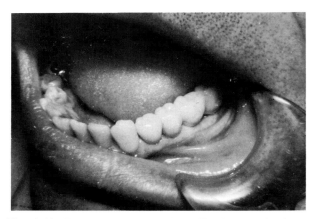

Fig. 9-19. The temporary acrylic splint is affixed with a temporary cement.

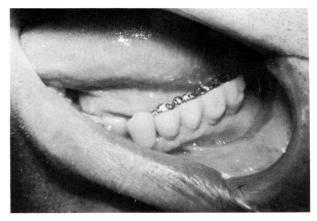

Fig. 9-21. The acrylic-and-gold fixed partial denture is cemented with hard cement. (From Linkow, L. I.: The radiographic role in endosseous implant interventions, Chron. Omaha Dent Soc. 29[10]:304-311, 1966.)

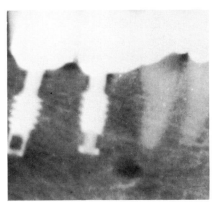

Fig. 9-20. The final prosthesis is in place before cementation.

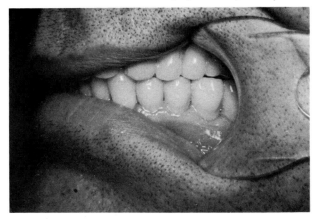

Fig. 9-22. The bridge as seen from the buccal surface.

shafts are not tapered and have parallel walls with sharp line angles that add to their retentive qualities, the splint will be difficult to remove and could dislodge the implants.

The final fixed partial denture was tried in position, ground into proper occlusion, and a final intraoral periapical x-ray taken (Fig. 9-20). The bridge was then cemented into place with one of the permanent type cements (Fig. 9-21), thus completing the implant intervention procedure (Fig. 9-22).

Case 2
Unilateral posterior free-end saddle restoration using spiral-posts and a temporary splint

The spiral-shaft implant of Raphael Cherchève is a post type implant (Fig. 9-23). This means that it can be used only where there is a fairly substantial amount of alveolar bone. Only 4 to 5 mm. of the shaft should extend from the fibromucosal tissue. The length of this implant, however, can be varied by cutting off several spirals. Thus the spiraled portion can be set deeply enough in bone to allow a bony shelf to grow over it, making exfoliation extremely difficult.

The insertion technique for the spiral-shaft implant is similar to that used for inserting the vent-plant, except that special taps must be used to trephine a hole exactly the size of the implant. This step is eliminated when using the vent-plant, which is self-tapping.

In the following case, two Cherchève spiral-post implants and one natural tooth are used to support a five-unit fixed partial denture.

First, intraoral periapical radiographs were taken

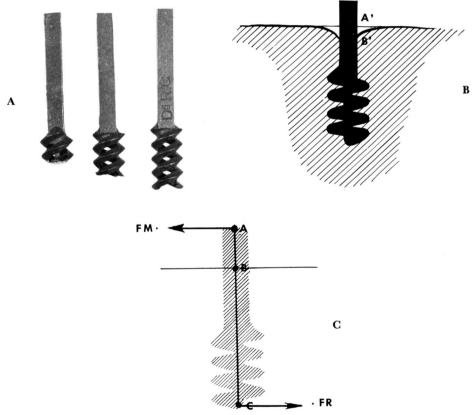

Fig. 9-23. **A,** The spiral-shaft double-helical implants. **B,** A good portion of the shaft should extend into the bone below the alveolar crest *(A')* so that the eventual invagination of the epithelial tissue *(B')* would not extend to the open spirals. **C,** Only about 4 to 5 mm. of the shaft *(A-B)* should extend out of the fibromucosal tissue. The rest of the implant *(B-C)* should be buried in bone. The masticatory forces *(FM)* are applied to the extraosseous portion of the implant while resistance to this force *(FR)* is opposed by the intraosseous portion *(BC)*. Therefore: $FM \times AB = FR \times BC$.

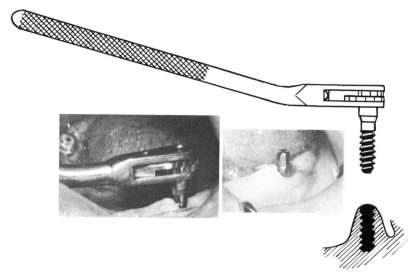

Fig. 9-24. The taps are carefully screwed into the bone using a hand ratchet. (From Cher-chève, R.: Les implants endo-osseoux, Paris, 1962, Librairie Maloine.)

in the area of the intended implant interventions. Then the anterior tooth abutment was prepared for a full coverage restoration. A modeling compound copper tube impression of the prepared tooth and a wax interocclusal record of centric relation were made. An alginate impression of the opposing jaw and an elastic impression of the prepared tooth plus the edentulous space were also made. The technician used these impressions to fabricate a veneer casting and a temporary acrylic splint to cover the natural tooth abutment and implant abutments immediately after insertion.

At the beginning of the second visit, just prior to insertion of the implants, the coping was fitted over the natural tooth abutment and its gingival, marginal, and occlusal relationships adjusted. The acrylic splint was tried in position and ground into proper occlusion. Its tissue-bearing surface was hollowed out in the area of the implants.

To insert the first implant, a No. 6 round bur was placed in a slow-running contra-angle with a water spray attachment. This tool was centered over the alveolar crest and used to drill directly through the mucoperiosteum into the underlying bone until the bur was stopped by the built-in "stop guard" on its shaft. This first bur was left in position, disengaged, and radiographed for parallelism with the prepared coronal portion of the tooth abutment and for its proximity to the mandibular canal.

With the first bur in the alveolus as a parallel guide, a second round bur was drilled into the bone

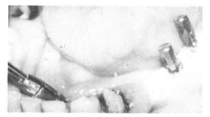

Fig. 9-25. Both taps are parallel to one another and to the bicuspid preparation.

about 4 mm. behind it. Great care was taken not to perforate the buccal or lingual plates of bone. An x-ray was used to ensure this.

Leaving one of the round burs in position, the other was removed. A helical bone bur was drilled deeper through the same hole, making sure that it was parallel both mesiodistally and buccolingually with the prepared tooth and with the extended shaft of the round bur. Another x-ray was taken to reveal the depth of the helical bur, its proximity to the mandibular canal, and its degree of parallelism with the prepared tooth and round bur shaft.

The remaining round bur was removed, and the second helical bur was driven into the alveolus parallel to the shaft of the first helical bur and deeper than the hole created by the preceding round bur. An x-ray was taken to evaluate this.

One of the helical burs was then removed; in its place a tap, set in a hand ratchet, was screwed deep into the bone parallel to the remaining helical

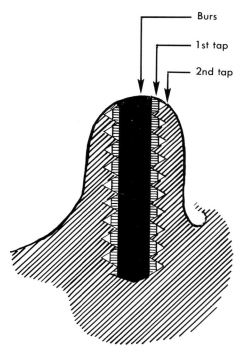

Burs

1st tap

2nd tap

Fig. 9-26. The difference in diameter between the narrower tap as compared to the wider tap is seen in this diagram. (From Cherchève, R.: Les implants endo-osseoux, Paris, 1962, Librairie Maloine.)

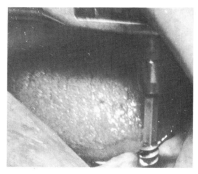

Fig. 9-27. The first implant is screwed into either one of the tap holes.

bur and to the prepared crown (Fig. 9-24). Another x-ray was used to check the accuracy of insertion. The second helical bur was substituted by another tap of the same diameter (Fig. 9-25) and x-rayed.

The first set of taps was exchanged for taps of the same diameter as the spiral portion of the implant. Each tap was carefully screwed into the bone with the hand ratchet to maintain sharp and unbroken threads of bone that fit snugly against the implants (Fig. 9-26). Their positions were checked by x-ray. One of the taps was then removed and the depth of the artificial socket checked with a special bone probe. When measurements for both sockets were approved, the implants were ready for insertion.

A hexagonal prolongator was used to unite the shaft portion of the implant with the head of the ratchet, and the spiral-shaft implant was then screwed into the hole made by one of the previously removed taps (Fig. 9-27). Its depth and direction were checked with an x-ray. The remaining tap was then removed, and the second spiral-shaft implant was carefully screwed into the threaded hole (Fig. 9-28). Another x-ray was taken to check the parallelism and depth of both implants.

The gold casting was then fitted over the prepared bicuspid tooth, and gold copings were placed over the protruding implant shafts (Fig. 9-29). A wax interocclusal record of centric relation was made and a plaster index taken (the index included the castings and copings).

The temporary, prefabricated acrylic splint was then hollowed out sufficiently to generously accept the implant shafts. It was tried over the abutments, both natural and implant, and checked for passive fit. Once proper occlusion had been established, fast-setting acrylic was placed into the hollowed portions that encapsulated the implant shafts, and the splint was placed over the tooth and implants. It was repeatedly removed and replaced to prevent the acrylic from fusing to the implants. After the acrylic set,

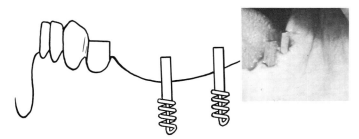

Fig. 9-28. Both implants are seen in position parallel to one another and to the anterior abutment preparation.

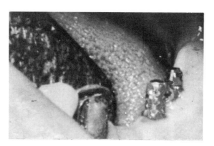

Fig. 9-29. The copings and casting are placed over the implants and bicuspid preparation respectively.

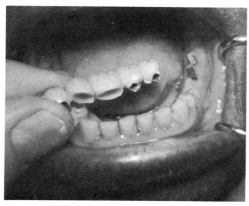

Fig. 9-30. The processed veneer type bridge is fitted. (From Linkow, L. I.: Intra-osseous implants utilized as fixed bridge abutments, J. Oral Implant Transplant Surg. **10**[2]:17-23, 1964.)

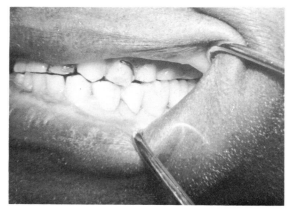

Fig. 9-31. The prosthesis is cemented with hard cement. (From Linkow, L. I.: Intra-osseous implants utilized as fixed bridge abutments, J. Oral Implant Transplant Surg. **10**[2]:17-23, 1964.)

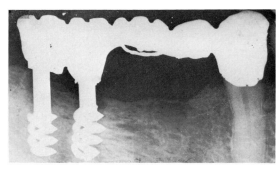

Fig. 9-32. A periapical x-ray showing completed case. (From Linkow, L. I.: Intra-osseous implants utilized as fixed bridge abutments, J. Oral Implant Transplant Surg. **10**[2]:17-23, 1964.)

all excess on the tissue-bearing surface was removed and the splint polished. (The splint may or may not be relined with a soft material.) The splint was inserted, with temporary cement only inside the area to cover the natural tooth abutment.

On the third visit, the final fixed partial denture was tried in position (Fig. 9-30). It was ground into proper occlusion (Fig. 9-31), and a final intraoral periapical x-ray was taken (Fig. 9-32). Cementation of the bridge with one of the permanent type cements was then accomplished.

Case 3
Unilateral posterior free-end saddle restoration using a vent-plant and a triplant

Although there was enough bone height in the patient described in this case to use two post type implants, a tripodial unit was used in symbiosis with one post implant. The triplant was used in the second molar area, and in order to avoid penetrating the mandibular canal the pins diverged 45 degrees from one another.

Before the implant intervention, the two anterior teeth were prepared for full crown restorations and first impressions made. Then the vent-plant was inserted in the region of the first molar, checking the depth and direction of the burs and the implant with x-rays (Fig. 9-33).

With each step carefully analyzed by x-ray, the triplant pins were inserted one by one so as to straddle the canal. The protruding heads were bent together and fused with cold cure acrylic. When the acrylic core hardened, it was prepared for a full crown restoration (Fig. 9-34).

Elastic impressions, with a wax interocclusal record of centric relation, were made for the fabrication of the fixed partial denture (Fig. 9-35). This was

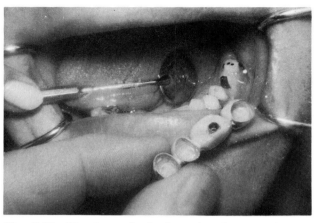

Fig. 9-35. The four-unit fixed partial denture prior to insertion.

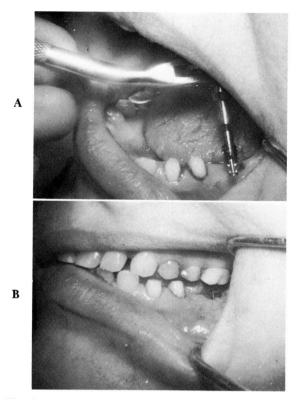

A

B

Fig. 9-33. A, A self-tapping vent-plant is seen prior to its insertion. B, The vent-plant must be set deep enough so that there will be no occlusal interference.

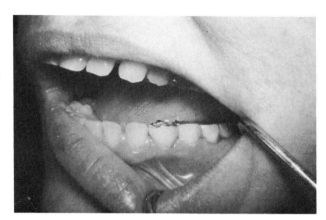

Fig. 9-36. The four-unit fixed partial denture is then cemented with hard cement.

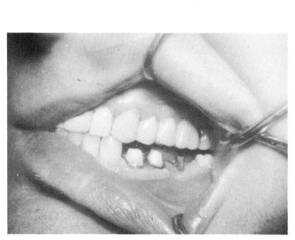

Fig. 9-34. Pin implants are drilled into the bone distal to the vent-plant and fused with an acrylic core that is prepared for a full crown restoration.

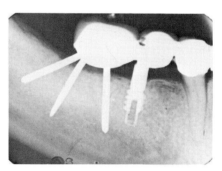

Fig. 9-37. An x-ray reveals the vent-plant and triplant.

cemented with hard cement (Fig. 9-36) and the implants and prosthesis x-rayed (Fig. 9-37).

Case 4
Unilateral posterior free-end saddle restoration using a prefabricated prosthesis and vent-plants

If the operator so chooses, the final fixed partial denture may be fabricated prior to implant insertion. This approach has several advantages.

1. The entire time needed to complete the prosthesis, insert the implants, and cement the bridge takes either two or three visits, depending upon whether elastic impression material or modeling compound tube impressions are used, respectively.

2. Because the finished prosthesis is fitted over the implants immediately after their insertion, fewer postoperative complications occur. Using the temporary splint technique generally involves removing and replacing the acrylic temporary splint several times. Also, the lapse of time between setting the implants and the final processing and cementing of the bridge invites complications. The ideal situation is to place the final prosthesis into position immediately after the implants are screwed into the bone.

With the prefabricated fixed partial denture technique, it is imperative that the patient wear the prefabricated denture for a day or two before the implants are inserted. Also, and even more important, the prosthesis should not be permanently cemented into position immediately after implant insertion. The bridge should be placed in the mouth temporarily, using cement only inside the crowns that cover the natural tooth abutments. The reason for the prosthesis' pretrial is to check for impingement of the pontics on the soft tissues. Severe pain can occur when the tissue-bearing surface of any pontic, usually its buccogingival line angle, presses into the underlying tissues. If there is a severe impingement, the constant pain suffered by the patient can often mislead the inexperienced dentist into believing that the pain results from the implants. A well-placed endosseous implant will cause no pain from the very onset. After a few trial days, the bridge is removed and all necessary adjustments are made prior to cementation with hard cement.

In this case, a three-unit fixed partial denture utilized the second bicuspid as the natural tooth abutment and two vent-plants.

On the first visit, the bicuspid was prepared for a full crown restoration. A full mouth wax interocclusal record of centric relation and an elastic impression, including the bicuspid and posterior

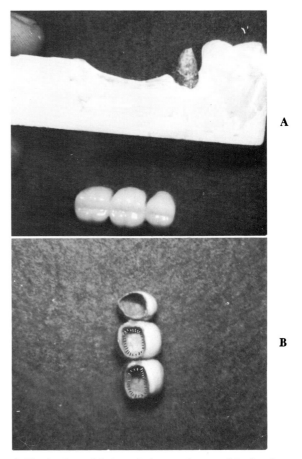

Fig. 9-38. A, A prefabricated three-unit porcelain-fused-to-metal bridge. B, The undersurface of the bridge, showing lumens that accept the abutments. Note the retention pins inside the crowns, which facilitate the procedure.

edentulous area, were obtained. A full mouth upper alginate impression was also taken. The models were carefully articulated and a three-unit fixed partial denture fabricated (Fig. 9-38).

On the second visit, the three-unit fixed partial denture was positioned in the mouth, held only by the bicuspid preparation (Fig. 9-39). All necessary occlusal and gingival adjustments were then made and an x-ray taken to reevaluate the implant site (Fig. 9-40). At this point the operation may vary. If the cantilevered pontics were not made with openings for the implants, their undersurfaces should be marked with small indelible pencil marks. The bridge is replaced in the mouth and the pencil marks transferred to the fibromucosa over the alveolar crest. Generous holes are then drilled in the pontics to accept the implant posts. If the holes were predrilled, their rims should be marked and the marks transferred to the mucosa.

Using the transferred pencil marks as guides, the

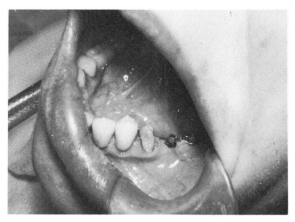

Fig. 9-41. The vent-plants are set into their proper locations in the bone.

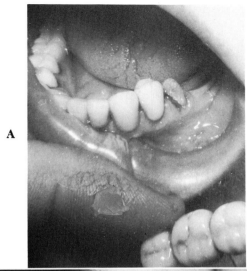

A

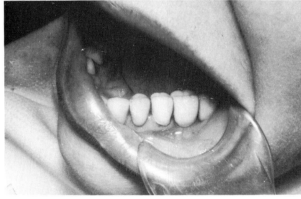

B

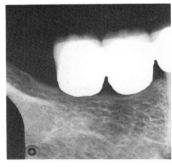

Fig. 9-39. A, The fixed partial denture is tried in the mouth prior to implant insertions. B, The prosthesis in place prior to implant insertions.

Fig. 9-40. The prefabricated bridge is radiographed for the final determination of the implant sites.

implants were set in position (Fig. 9-41). The bridge was tried over the protruding implant shafts and checked for interference with its fit. If a bridge sits too high or cannot be easily slipped over the shafts, the holes should be enlarged. Then fine adjustments of the diameter and depth of the holes should be accomplished so that the implant shafts fit snugly within them. To do this, either of two methods may be followed:

1. The holes may be filled with cold cure acrylic. The bridge is taken on and off at 20-second intervals, and the final hardening is allowed to take place outside the mouth. The excess acrylic along the under-surface of the bridge is then trimmed away and the area polished. Or, if the implant shafts are not parallel with each other, before the acrylic finally hardens, the excess is quickly removed and oxyphosphate of zinc cement is placed inside the bicuspid casting. The bridge is placed back into the mouth for its final setting, with the acrylic bound to the implant shafts.

2. Prefabricated gold copings whose outer surfaces have numerous deep undercuts are placed over the protruding implant shafts (Fig. 9-42). The bridge is then placed in position. If there is any impingement, larger holes are made inside the pontics. After the bridge slips on and off easily, the holes are filled with cold cure acrylic and the bridge is seated over the undercut copings and the bicuspid tooth preparation. When the acrylic hardens, the bridge is removed and the gold cores have now become an integral part of the bridge. The excess acrylic around the margins of the gold copings is removed, and the entire tissue-bearing surface of the crown is trimmed and polished (Fig. 9-43).

As the final operative step, the bridge was ce-

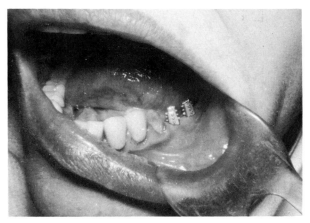

Fig. 9-42. The copings are placed over the implants. (From Linkow, L. I.: Prefabricated endosseous implant prostheses, Dent. Concepts **10:**3-11, 1967.)

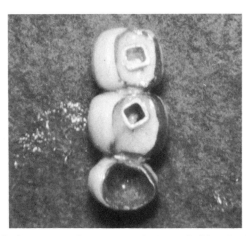

Fig. 9-43. The copings are picked up inside the bridge with quick cure acrylic. (From Linkow, L. I.: Prefabricated endosseous implant prostheses, Dent. Concepts **10:**3-11, 1967.)

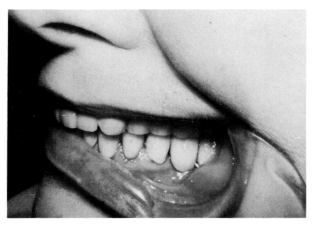

Fig. 9-44. The prosthesis is cemented. (From Linkow, L. I.: Prefabricated endosseous implant prostheses, Dent. Concepts **10:**3-11, 1967.)

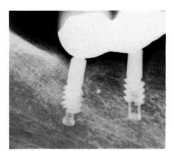

Fig. 9-45. The postoperative x-ray.

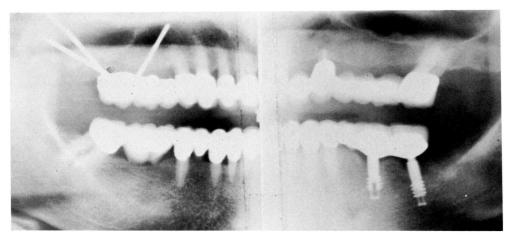

Fig. 9-46. A Panorex roentgenogram shows the implants in position. (From Linkow, L. I.: Prefabricated endosseous implant prostheses, Dent. Concepts **10:**3-11, 1967.)

mented with oxyphosphate of zinc cement (Fig. 9-44). Postoperative x-rays illustrate the bridge (Fig. 9-45). In this case, the remainder of the arch was also splinted, as seen in the Panorex (Fig. 9-46).

Case 5
Unilateral posterior free-end saddle restoration using a prefabricated prosthesis and mixed implants

Sometimes it is difficult or too risky to use two post type implants to stabilize a prosthesis in a posterior free-end saddle area. As it was in this case, this may be caused by the presence of widely spaced trabeculae. Such alveolar bone sometimes occurs in the second lower molar region, and post type implants are inadvisable because fairly dense bone is needed to stabilize them. In this case it was necessary to immediately replace a vent-plant with a triplant. From the moment of the vent-plant's insertion it was loose, even though the intervention proceeded cautiously and without mistake.

The triplant pins were driven across the socket vacated by the vent-plant and into the surrounding bone (Fig. 9-47). (Again, it is necessary to note that only a type of implant that can extend into the bone around an open socket should be used.) As each pin was inserted, its depth and direction were radiographed. When the three pins were in place, angled as obliquely as possible without perforating the buccal or lingual plates of bone, the excess portion protruding into the mouth was trimmed.

Normally, the pins are then fused together with acrylic, using the paintbrush technique to avoid air bubbles, and final impressions taken for completing the bridge. In this case, however, a prefabricated bridge was processed prior to the interventions (Fig.

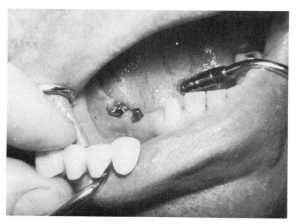

Fig. 9-48. The ends of the pin implants are shortened and the bridge is tried in position.

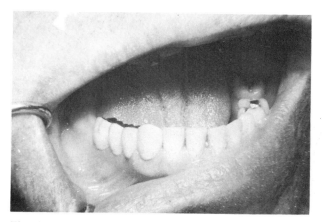

Fig. 9-49. After the pins are fused together with acrylic, the bridge is cemented into position.

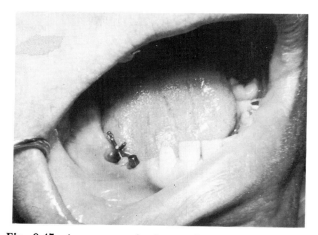

Fig. 9-47. A post type implant and a triplant are seen.

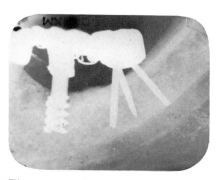

Fig. 9-50. The postoperative x-ray.

9-48). After fusing the pins together, the prosthesis was then cemented with hard cement (Fig. 9-49). An x-ray shows the bridge set over the two types of implants, which seem to complement one another (Fig. 9-50).

Case 6
Unilateral posterior free-end saddle restoration using a prefabricated prosthesis and the hollow-mill technique

The construction of a four-unit prefabricated fixed partial denture replacing two missing mandibular molars and secured by two bicuspids and two posterior vent-plants will be described. Here a bone plug will be placed inside the vent-plants as an autogenous transplant. The plug acts as a matrix for the speedier deposition of new bone. Eventually the plug is replaced by new bone or collagenous tissue.

As a preliminary procedure, an intraoral roentgenogram was made of the implant region and the anterior abutment teeth. At the first operative visit, the two bicuspid teeth were prepared for full crowns and compound tube impressions were made of them. A wax interocclusal record of centric relation was taken. Because the tube impressions were used, an alginate (irreversible hydrocolloid) impression of the teeth in the opposing dental arch and a plaster index of the prepared teeth were included.

At the second visit, the two veneer castings, or metal copings for porcelain, were tried on their respective prepared teeth, and all necessary occlusal and gingival adjustments were made. The shade of the teeth was selected, and a wax interocclusal record of centric relation and a plaster index including the edentulous region were taken.

At the third visit, the four-unit veneer fixed partial denture had been completed (Fig. 9-51). It was tried in the mouth to check for occlusal and gingival fit. All necessary adjustments of the interproximal contacts and gingival contour were made prior to inserting the implants.

The restoration was removed from the mouth, and the mucosa over the alveolar crest was marked with an indelible pencil in the exact area where, according to the roentgenograms, the implants were to be inserted (Fig. 9-52). The fixed partial denture was once more seated firmly and removed, with the indelible pencil markings transferred to the basal surface of the molar pontics (Fig. 9-53). Holes deeper and larger in diameter than the implant shafts were drilled inside the pontics with large burs.

A No. 6 round bur was positioned over the first

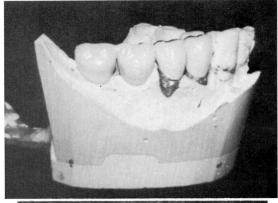

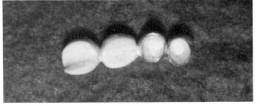

Fig. 9-51. A, A four-unit gold occlusal, acrylic veneer type bridge is prefabricated prior to implant insertions. **B,** The undersurface of the bridge. (From Linkow, L. I.: Prefabricated mandibular prostheses for intra-osseous implants, J. Prosth. Dent. **20**[4]:365-375, 1968.)

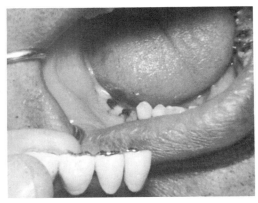

Fig. 9-52. Indelible pencil markings indicate the location for the implants. (From Linkow, L. I.: Prefabricated mandibular prostheses for intraosseous implants, J. Prosth. Dent. **20**[4]:365-375, 1968.)

marked spot on the mucoperiosteum and drilled about 5 mm. into the bone, parallel with the preparations on the two anterior abutment teeth. The round bur was left in the mouth as a guide for drilling the second hole parallel to the first one. Another No. 6 round bur was then employed to drill the second hole at the other point marked with indelible pencil (Fig. 9-54). Roentgenograms were made after each bur was drilled into position.

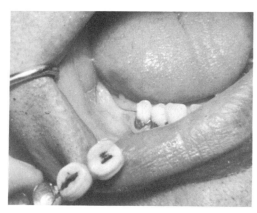

Fig. 9-53. The markings are transferred to the tissue-bearing surfaces of the pontics and then the properly sized holes are made. (From Linkow, L. I.: Prefabricated mandibular prostheses for intraosseous implants, J. Prosth. Dent. **20**[4]: 365-375, 1968.)

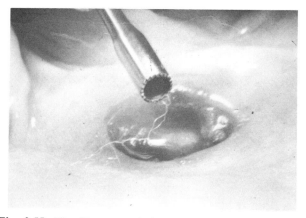

Fig. 9-55. The fibromucosal tissue in the area of the mandibular symphysis is incised and the tissue reflected, exposing the underlying bone. A "hollow-mill" trephine is attached to the contra-angle. (From Linkow, L. I.: Prefabricated mandibular prostheses for intraosseous implants, J. Prosth. Dent. **20**[4]:365-375, 1968.)

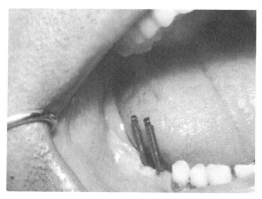

Fig. 9-54. The starting holes are made with spear-point burs followed with helical type burs. (From Linkow, L. I.: Prefabricated mandibular prostheses for intraosseous implants, J. Prosth. Dent. **20**[4]:365-375, 1968.)

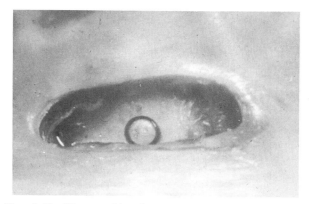

Fig. 9-56. The trephine is rotated through the cortical plate and into the deeper alveolar bone. (From Linkow, L. I.: Prefabricated mandibular prostheses for intraosseous implants, J. Prosth. Dent. **20**[4]:365-375, 1968.)

Since vent-plants were to serve as the implant abutments, helical burs of a corresponding size were employed. One of the round burs was removed and the other one was left in position as a parallel guide for the helical bur.

If the "hollow-mill" technique is to be used, as it was in this case, the operator has two choices. He can try to get a good bone plug from the implant site itself or from the symphysis area, just behind the cortical plate of bone on the labial aspect of the mandible. In obtaining a plug from the site itself, the hole made by the helical bur is restricted to the same depth reached by the round bur. A "hollow-mill" trephine the same diameter as the implant is inserted with a slow-running contra-angle to

the depth where the vent-plant will rest. When this depth is reached, the hollow mill is carefully taken out of the bone. The core of the patient's bone is then set inside the vent-plant, which is then screwed into the artificial socket to its predetermined depth.

If the bone in the region where the vent-plant is to be placed is too cancellous, an autogenous plug of bone can be obtained from the mandibular symphysis. To do this, the tissue in the mouth over the symphysis is incised to expose the underlying bone (Fig. 9-55). A "hollow-mill" trephine is placed in a contra-angle handpiece and is slowly drilled into the exposed bone, cooled continuously with water, to a depth of ⅛ to ¼ inch to create a bone plug (Fig. 9-56). The bone plug is removed from the trephine

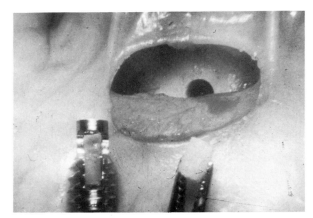

Fig. 9-57. The plug of bone is removed and then placed inside the vent-plant. (From Linkow, L. I.: Prefabricated mandibular prostheses for intraosseous implants, J. Prosth. Dent. **20**[4]:365-375, 1968.)

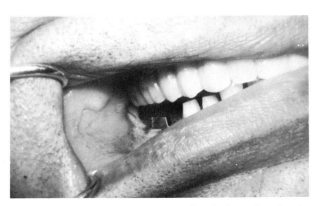

Fig. 9-58. The vent-plants are set deeply into the alveolar bone. (From Linkow, L. I.: Prefabricated mandibular prostheses for intraosseous implants, J. Prosth. Dent. **20**[4]: 365-375, 1968.)

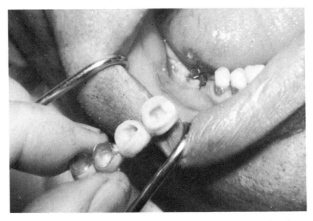

Fig. 9-59. The bridge is fitted into position over the implants and then removed. (From Linkow, L. I.: Prefabricated mandibular prostheses for intraosseous implants, J. Prosth. Dent. **20**[4]:365-375, 1968.)

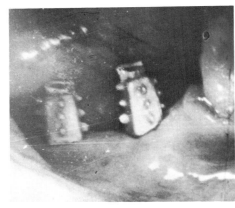

Fig. 9-60. Gold copings are placed over the implants and picked up inside the bridge.

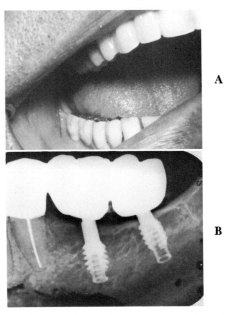

Fig. 9-61. A, The fixed prosthesis is cemented with hard cement. **B,** The postoperative radiograph. (From Linkow, L. I.: Prefabricated mandibular prostheses for intraosseous implants, J. Prosth. Dent. **20**[4]:365-375, 1968.)

and placed into the vent (Fig. 9-57). Then the implant is screwed into its socket, which was prepared to its full depth by helical burs.

With the vent-plants seated (Fig. 9-58), the operation proceeded in the normal manner. The bridge was tried over the implants and any necessary adjustments in the size of the holes made (Fig. 9-59). Gold copings were placed over the implants (Fig. 9-60), acrylic was placed inside the holes to pick up the copings, and the prosthesis was trimmed, polished, and permanently seated with oxyphosphate of zinc cement (Fig. 9-61).

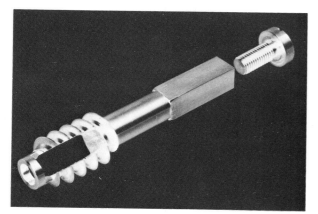

Fig. 9-62. The internally threaded vent-plant.

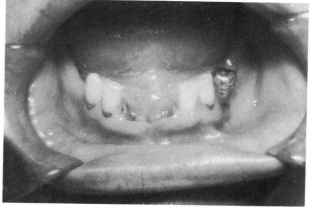

Fig. 9-63. The preoperative picture shows only five teeth remaining.

Case 7
Two unilateral bridges fixed to a template using internally threaded vent-plants

In this case, two separate bridges were screwed to a template incorporating full crown restorations. The implants used to secure the prosthesis were internally threaded vent-plants (Fig. 9-62).

The patient had five teeth remaining (Fig. 9-63). On the first visit, these were prepared for full crown restorations. On the next visit, the castings were tried and balanced. The internally threaded vent-plants were then screwed into the bone posteriorly (Fig. 9-64).

A wax bite, an alginate impression of the opposing jaw, and a full lower plaster index were made. Internally threaded duplicate shafts were placed in the plaster index, and the master stone model was poured and articulated. The small set screws protruded from the duplicate shafts just enough to be slightly short of the opposing jaw master model when the articulator was closed in centric occlusion (Fig. 9-65). The threads of these screws were ground away so that the screws were able to be lifted out of the duplicate shafts with the wax pattern.

The castings were soldered to one another and a wax template built around the protruding set screws. The template was cast and soldered to the anterior castings. The acrylic veneer facings were then processed (Fig. 9-66). (Sometimes the two posterior templates are constructed so that their anterior sections are not rigidly soldered to the nearest crown restorations but slip over them. In this manner the entire template can be removed to expose the implants.)

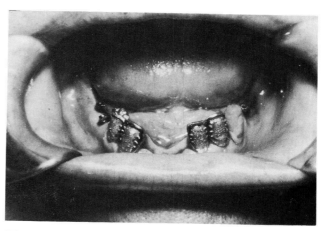

Fig. 9-64. Veneer type castings were made for the prepared teeth and internally threaded vent-plants were set into the bone ending close to the fibromucosal tissue.

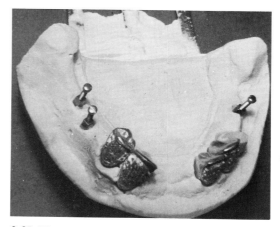

Fig. 9-65. The master stone model with the five castings and three duplicate implant shafts with their set screws attached.

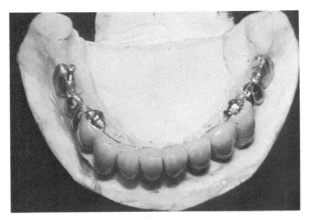

Fig. 9-66. The anterior portion of the prosthesis was processed with acrylic facings. Extending from it and soldered to it are both the scalloped templates.

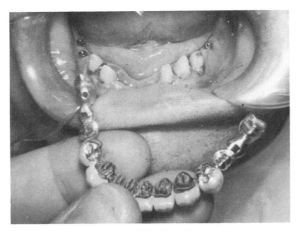

Fig. 9-67. The prosthesis is fitted into position and then cemented.

At the next visit the prosthesis was tried in the mouth and seated with soft cement (Fig. 9-67), and the set screws were screwed through the template and into the internally threaded vent-plants (Fig. 9-68). The bite was checked anteriorly, and all adjustments were made.

A final bite and a full mouth impression of the lower jaw with the prosthesis in place were taken (Fig. 9-69). From this the two unilateral fixed partial dentures were fabricated (Fig. 9-70).

Both of the unilateral bridges were set into position over the template with temporary cement (Fig. 9-71). In this manner, if any future trouble were to arise, the two bridges could easily be removed.

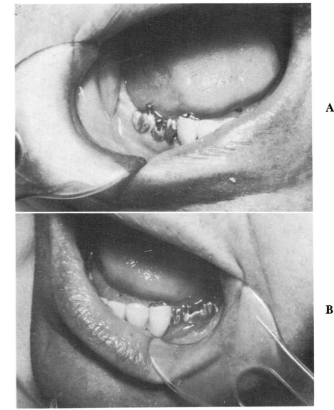

A

B

Fig. 9-68. A, The set screws are screwed through the template and into the internally threaded underlying vent-plants on the right side. **B,** The set screws are then inserted on the left side.

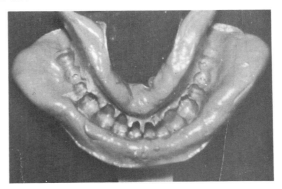

Fig. 9-69. A rubber base impression is taken for the fabrication of both posterior superstructures.

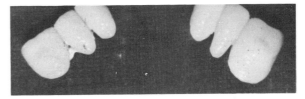

Fig. 9-70. The processed superstructures.

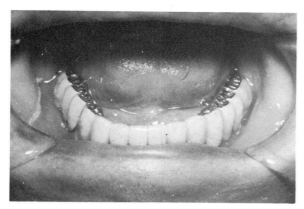

Fig. 9-71. The superstructures are cemented over the templates with a soft cement.

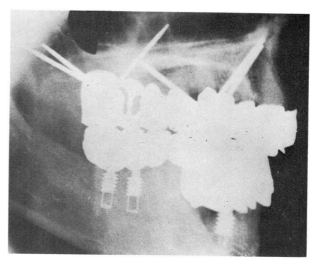

Fig. 9-73. Lateral plate roentgenogram showing superstructures in position

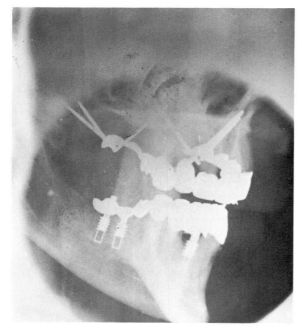

Fig. 9-72. Lateral plate x-ray revealing screws going through template.

Fig. 9-72 shows the three vent-plants and the template with its set screws connecting the template to the implants. Fig. 9-73 illustrates the bridges over the template.

BILATERAL RESTORATIONS

When inserting implants in a mandible where both posterior quadrants of teeth are missing, the same basic steps are taken as for a unilateral free-end saddle bridge. However, it must first be determined whether both bridges are to be fabricated

independently or whether they will be incorporated into one complete full arch splint.

A number of factors can influence the operator's decision:

1. Whether or not both bicuspids on each side of the arch are present can aid in the determination. If no bicuspids, or only one on each side, are available, then a full arch splint should be used.
2. If both bicuspids are present in each quadrant, the density of the bone surrounding them and the condition of their periodontal attachments should be evaluated. If the bone has resorbed a good deal and the teeth are mobile, then a full arch splint should again be chosen.
3. The condition of the anterior teeth should be considered. The absence of decay and the lack of fillings should certainly influence the operator, as well as the patient, as to the diagnosis of two independent fixed partial dentures instead of a full arch prosthesis.
4. If the maxillary arch contains a full complement of teeth, a full arch fixed lower prosthesis might be considered. However, the presence of a full or a partial maxillary denture may indicate unilateral splints for the mandible.
5. The absence or presence of bruxism and other adverse habits such as pipe smoking should be taken into consideration.
6. The height, thickness, and density of the osseous structures in the edentulous areas affect the choice. The less ideal the site, the more effective a full mouth splint.

The restorative procedures required for the preparation of the teeth and the fabrication of the fixed partial dentures are relatively the same for almost all types of implants. The bridge should always be permanently affixed as rapidly as possible after implant insertion.

Case 8
Bilateral posterior restorations using a full arch splint and mixed implants

In this case a full arch splint was secured by mixed implants and natural tooth abutments. First, all remaining teeth in the arch were prepared for full crown restorations (Fig. 9-74). The necessary compound tube impressions, as well as the bite registrations and opposing jaw impressions, were taken (Fig. 9-75). From these impressions, the full crown restorations and the full arch temporary acrylic splint were made.

At the beginning of the next visit, the temporary acrylic splint was inserted, balanced, and equilibrated with the teeth of the opposing jaw. The castings were then placed over the prepared abutment teeth and checked for proper marginal adaptations, gingival contours, contact points, and articulation with the opposing teeth (Fig. 9-76). Another full mouth plaster index was taken, with the castings seated over the teeth, in order to solder them together. At this time, the implants could either be set into their predetermined locations or, preferably, implantation delayed until the bridge was completely prefabricated.

At the next visit, the soldered castings were tried in the mouth and again checked for any discrepancies. When everything was satisfactory, a wax bite and plaster index of the entire lower arch were taken and the prosthesis was fabricated in the laboratory (Fig. 9-77).

The implants were inserted into the right lower quadrant according to the methods already described. The burs were placed parallel to each other and to the prepared teeth (Fig. 9-78). They were replaced by three spiral-post type implants: a Cherchève implant (Fig. 9-79), a Muratori implant (Fig. 9-80), and a Sandhaus crystalline bone screw (CBS) (Fig. 9-81). As each implant was inserted, the bridge was replaced by drilling a hole into the tissue-bearing surface of its corresponding pontic. The holes were made larger than the implant shafts to accommodate any lack of parallelism and to facilitate insertion (Fig. 9-82).

After the lower right implants were inserted and

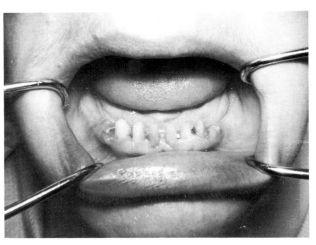

Fig. 9-74. The remaining six anterior teeth are prepared.

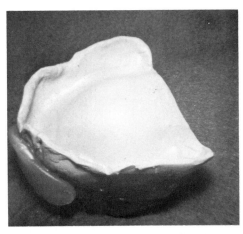

Fig. 9-75. An impression of the upper edentulous maxilla is taken as well as a wax interocculusal record of centric relation.

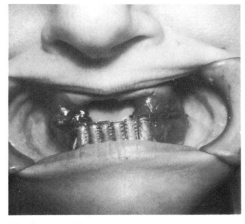

Fig. 9-76. The castings are fitted and once again an interocclusal record of centric relation is taken.

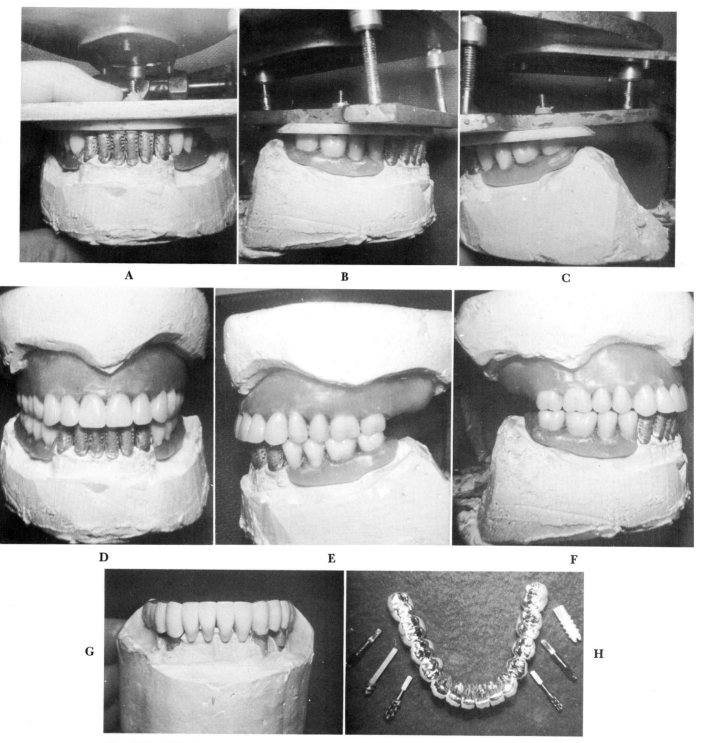

Fig. 9-77. With the use of a specially designed occlusal template, denture teeth were temporarily used posteriorly on both sides to establish geometrically parallel occlusal planes. **A to F,** The upper denture teeth were waxed up to meet with the established lower plane. These were then tried in the mouth again for accuracy and esthetics. **G,** The lower full arch fixed denture was then fabricated from the original six anterior castings after the upper denture was processed. **H,** The completed prosthesis with the different implants that are to be used.

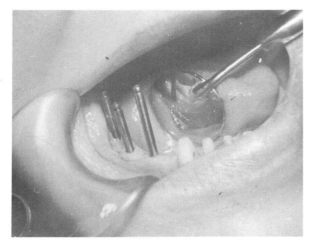

Fig. 9-78. Holes are prepared with various types of burs.

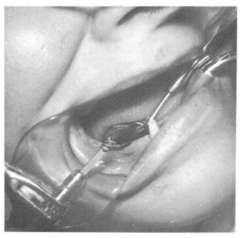

Fig. 9-79. A Vitallium spiral-shaft implant (Cherchève) is placed in the right bicuspid region.

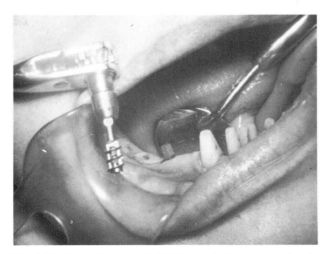

Fig. 9-80. A titanium spiraled (Muratori) implant is placed in the first molar region.

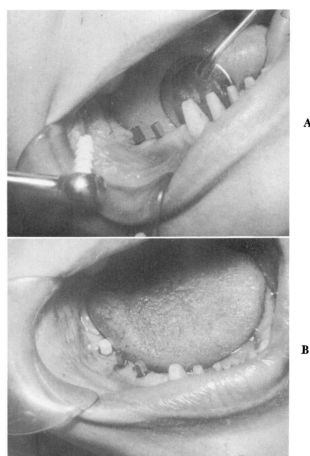

A

B

Fig. 9-81. A, An aluminum oxide (synthetic sapphire method of Sandhaus) implant (also called CBS bone screw) is placed in the second molar area. **B,** All three implants (Figs. 9-79 to 9-81, *A*) are seen in their proper positions.

the bridge fitted over them with no interference, the implants on the left side were inserted one by one. Here a Michel Cherchève narrow ridge implant (Fig. 9-83) and two Linkow vent-plants (Fig. 9-84) were used. Once again, and in the same manner as on the right side, holes were made inside the tissue-bearing surfaces of the pontics to house the protruding implant shafts (Fig. 9-85). The jaw now had three implants in each side (Fig. 9-86). The bridge was again tried over all the implants (Fig. 9-87).

At this point, if the implant shafts on both sides of the jaw are parallel, interchangeable gold copings are placed over them. The bridge is tried over them and then removed. Cold cure acrylic is placed inside

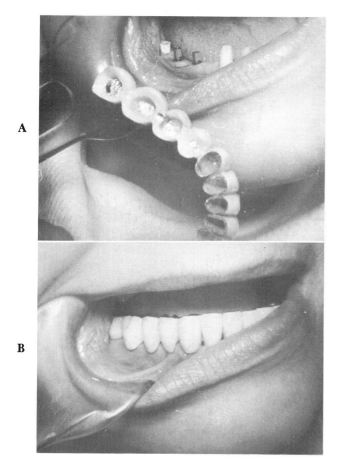

A

B

Fig. 9-82. A, Holes are made inside the pontics corresponding to the implant locations. B, The bridge must fit with
no interferences from the implants.

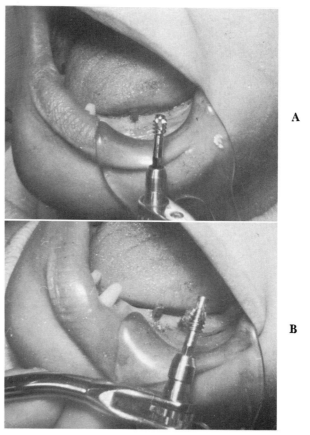

A

B

Fig. 9-84. A, A titanium vent-plant (Linkow) is placed in
the first molar region. B, A wider vent-plant is set into the
second molar region.

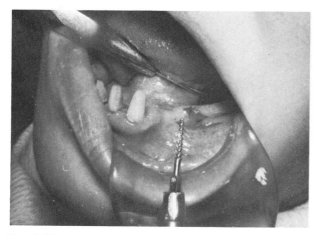

Fig. 9-83. A narrow ridge (Michel Cherchève) titanium
implant is placed in the lower left bicuspid area.

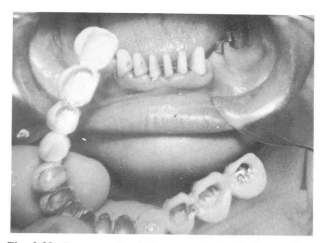

Fig. 9-85. Corresponding holes are made inside the pontics.

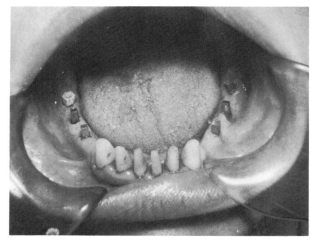

Fig. 9-86. The six different implants as well as the six tooth abutments are easily seen to be parallel to one another.

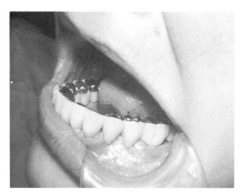

Fig. 9-87. The bridge is tried over the implants.

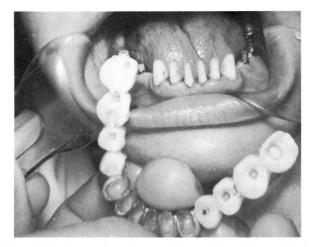

Fig. 9-88. The undersurface of the bridge with modified lumens.

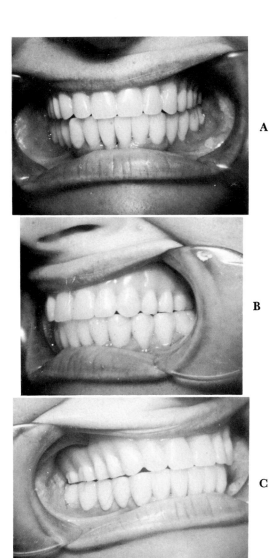

Fig. 9-89. A, The prefabricated full arch fixed denture is cemented with hard cement. **B,** The occlusion from the left side. **C,** The occlusion from the right side.

the holes in the pontics, and the bridge is placed back into the mouth while the patient bites into centric occlusion. When the acrylic hardens, the bridge is removed with the gold copings fixed to the pontics and the excess acrylic is highly polished. Finally, the entire prosthesis is cemented into position with hard cement.

If the implants are not parallel and telescopic copings are undesirable, cold cure acrylic may be placed inside the holes made in the pontics and the bridge seated directly over the implant shafts without the gold copings. However, when doing this, it is imperative to remove the bridge in an up-and-

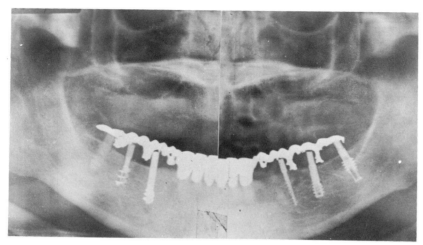

Fig. 9-90. A Panorex reveals all six implants. Since the prefabricated prosthesis had all acrylic pontics (which cannot be seen on radiographs) the retention bars and loops of the gold work make the prosthesis appear to have uneven margins.

down fashion while the acrylic is hardening. The bridge should never be left in the mouth to harden. Not only will it be almost impossible to remove, but the rough knife-like edges of the hardened acrylic can injure the soft tissues. Therefore the bridge must be hardened outside of the mouth and all excess acrylic trimmed and polished. Also, the holes must be made wider to compensate for the implant's lack of parallelism (Fig. 9-88). The bridge is permanently seated with a hard cement (Fig. 9-89). A final x-ray is then taken (Fig. 9-90).

Case 9
A full arch splint for a partially edentulous mandible using bilateral posterior implants

In this case only two lower cuspid teeth were present. From impressions and bites, two gold copings were cast to cover the cuspids, and two veneer crown castings were made to fit over the copings. A temporary acrylic splint was fabricated with a trench along the tissue-bearing surface of the free-end pontics to accommodate and support the implants (Fig. 9-91).

The gold copings were cemented over the cuspid teeth, and the cuspid veneer castings were placed over the copings. An accurate wax bite and plaster index of the lower jaw were taken and articulated with the opposing model. From this the anterior quadrant was cast and soldered together and a wax-up of their facings was accomplished.

The six-unit anterior splint with the wax facings was placed over the two cuspid copings and checked for accuracy and esthetics. The implants were set

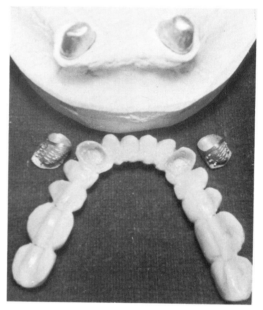

Fig. 9-91. Two gold copings and two veneers are cast to fit over the only remaining cuspid teeth. A temporary full arch acrylic splint is also made.

into their positions and interchangeable gold copings placed over them. The interocclusal space was checked while the patient bit in centric occlusion to make sure that there was no interference from the copings (Fig. 9-92). An accurate wax interocclusal record of centric relation was then taken with the castings and copings in position.

A full lower plaster index was also made, pick-

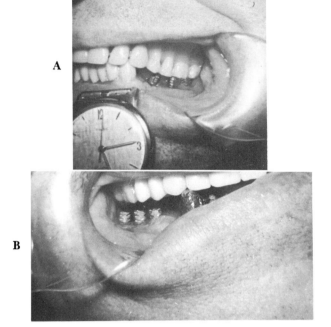

Fig. 9-92. A, Three vent-plants are set into the bone on the right side. B, Three vent-plants are set into the bone on the left posterior quadrant.

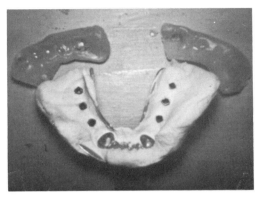

Fig. 9-93. The gold copings are picked up in the plaster index.

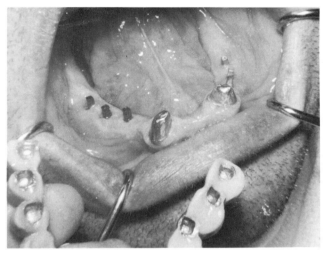

Fig. 9-94. The full arch fixed denture was processed and ready to be cemented. Note the darker type of screw shafts on the right side (tantalum) as compared to the lighter colored ones (titanium) on the left side. (From Linkow, L. I.: The era of endosseous implants, J. D. C. Dent. Soc. 42[2]:14-19, 1967.)

ing up all the castings and copings (Fig. 9-93). (If copings are not used over the implant shafts, the plaster will pick up the impressions of the shafts themselves. Duplicate shafts are placed inside the copings or in the impressions of the shafts, and the duplicate tooth dies are placed inside the castings.) The master stone model was poured, allowed to harden, and then articulated with the model of the opposing jaw.

The full arch fixed denture was made. Wax-ups can be accomplished directly over the implant copings for the final contoured crown restorations and fabricated with the double casting technique, or the wax-ups can be accomplished directly over the duplicate implant shafts after first removing the copings from them. Prior to waxing directly over these shafts, however, at least two coats of nailpolish or lacquer should be painted over that portion of the shafts that will support the castings. In this manner, the final castings will not fit too snugly. This allows room for cement and compensates for any errors in parallelism of the implant shafts.

The finished prosthesis was inserted (Fig. 9-94). The marginal fits of the castings and occlusion and articulation with the opposing jaw were thoroughly checked (Fig. 9-95). It was quite important at this time to check the tissue-bearing surfaces of all the castings that fit over the implants. These surfaces are much wider than the implant shafts themselves and, unless relieved considerably, often impinge on the soft tissues directly under them.

Prior to final cementation, radiographs were taken of the finished prosthesis in place (Fig. 9-96).

THE PARTIALLY EDENTULOUS MANDIBLE

As long as there is sufficient alveolar bone, implants may be used in any part of the mandible to act as abutments for fixed bridgework. The following cases illustrate some of these situations.

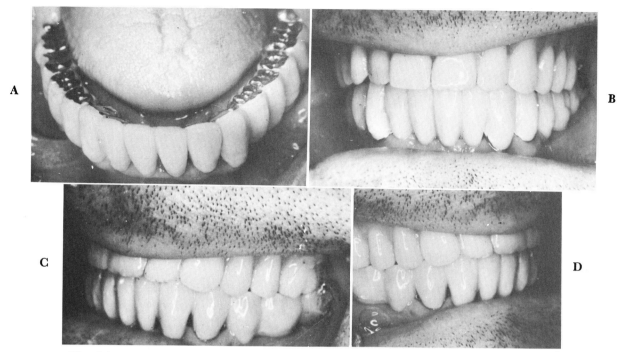

Fig. 9-95. A, The cemented prosthesis. The occlusion as seen from the B, front, C, left side, and D, right side.

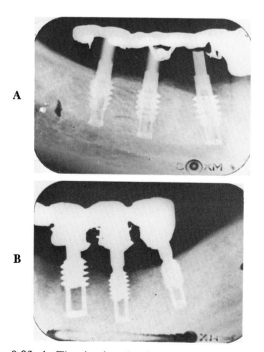

Fig. 9-96. A, The titanium implants on the left side. B, The tantalum implants on the right side. Note again, the acrylic saddle areas are not seen.

Case 10
Posterior restorations for a mandible with anterior teeth previously restored with fixed bridgework

Occasionally implants are desired for the posterior quadrants of a mandible in which the remaining anterior teeth have been previously restored with fixed, splinted restorations. Especially in those situations where the restorative work was done exceptionally well, it would be unwise to destroy it, considering the extra financial burden on the patient and the impracticality of unnecessary steps for the dentist.

There are basically two methods of utilizing the preexisting splint for support of the implants. The first method is used for bilateral cases having cantilevered pontics posterior to the last abutment tooth on each side or for a unilateral case having a single cantilevered pontic. The second method is used in a jaw in which no cantilevered pontics exist in the fixed splint. The first method, involving preexisting cantilevered pontics, will be illustrated by a mandibular restoration case. A maxillary case involving no cantilevered pontics will be included in the following chapter.

On the first visit, the pontic was prepared for a full crown preparation, making sure not to reduce the mesial interproximal surface too much so as not to weaken the solder joint (Fig. 9-97). A rubber base impression of the preparation and edentulous area, a bite, and an opposing jaw alginate impression were taken.

On the second visit, the veneer casting was tried over the pontic preparation and adjusted. The implants were set into sites determined by radiographs taken at the previous visit. In this case, a single triplant was used (Fig. 9-98). Its pins were built up with acrylic, and then the acrylic core was prepared for a full crown restoration. (When post implants are used, interchangeable gold copings are fitted over the implant posts and a wax bite and plaster index are taken. These should cover the natural abutment tooth as well as the copings over the implant shafts.)

An impression was taken with a soft impression material. (Plaster should be avoided because it might leak underneath the acrylic core, wedging between it and the soft tissue and causing dislodgment when the hardened plaster is removed.)

The temporary acrylic splint was fitted over the abutments and adjusted. It was affixed with temporary cement, and care was taken not to place any inside that portion of the splint that covered the implants. The splint was fabricated from the same master stone model that was used for fabricating the veneer casting.

On the third and final visit, the completed prosthesis was tried in the mouth and radiographed (Fig. 9-99). Any further adjustments were made, and then the bridge was cemented with hard cement (Fig. 9-100).

This method is not only useful where cantilevered

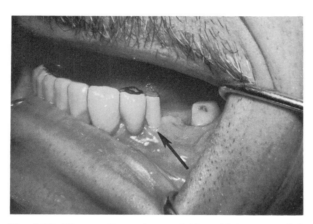

Fig. 9-97. The cantilevered second bicuspid is prepared for a full crown preparation, making sure not to sever its mesio-proximal solder joint. An acrylic core supporting a triplant is seen posteriorly. (From Linkow, L. I.: The versatility of implant interventions, Dent. Concepts 2:5-17, 1966.)

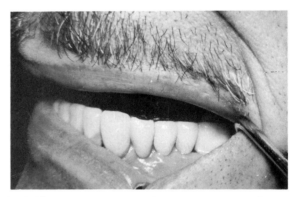

Fig. 9-99. The completed partial bridge is cemented. (From Linkow, L. I.: The versatility of implant interventions, Dent. Concepts 2:5-17, 1966.)

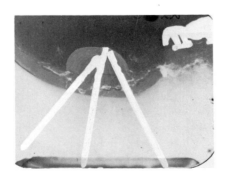

Fig. 9-98. The three pins are driven deep into the bone and diverge from each other at almost 45-degree angles. (From Linkow, L. I.: The versatility of implant interventions, Dent. Concepts 2:5-17, 1966.)

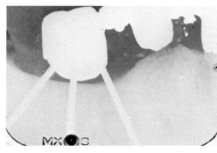

Fig. 9-100. The postoperative radiograph. (From Linkow, L. I.: The versatility of implant interventions, Dent. Concepts 2:5-17, 1966.)

pontics exist, but it also applies to those situations in which the posterior abutment of an existing bridge must be extracted. After complete healing of the extraction site, an implant bridge may be diagnosed. The old bridge is cut distal to the cantilevered pontic.

Case 11
Full arch restoration for a partially edentulous mandible using mixed anterior and posterior implants

When few teeth remain, it is often desirable to place endosseous implants in both the anterior and posterior regions, providing there is enough alveolar

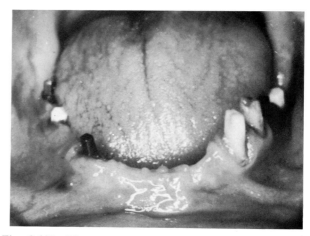

Fig. 9-103. Three vent-plants and two synthetic sapphire implants are seen, as well as the only two remaining tooth abutments.

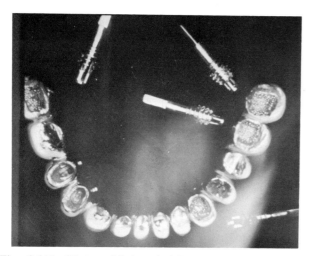

Fig. 9-101. The prefabricated full arch denture reveals hundreds of tiny bubbles inside the crowns that are to fit over the vent-plants.

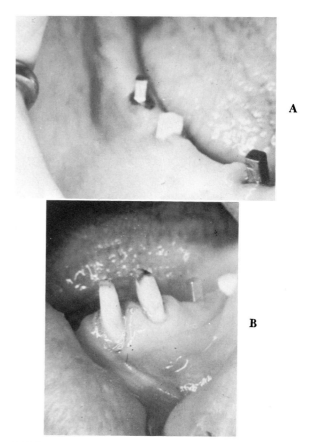

A

B

Fig. 9-104. A, A close-up of the right side reveals the synthetic sapphire implant between both titanium vent-plants. B, The left side includes the two teeth, the vent-plant, and synthetic sapphire implant.

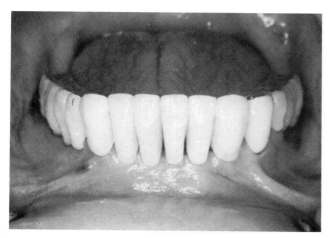

Fig. 9-102. The bridge is tried in the mouth prior to implant insertions.

bone. Such a case will now be presented. Only two teeth, the left first and second bicuspids, remained. A prefabricated full arch denture was processed in acrylic and gold (Fig. 9-101), and the patient wore it temporarily for 24 hours to test for comfort and pontic interferences on the soft tissue (Fig. 9-102). Areas where the pontics infringed on the soft tissues were trimmed accordingly.

The implants were placed in one by one (Fig. 9-103). In this case titanium vent-plants were combined with synthetic sapphire implants (Fig. 9-104). As each implant was inserted, the bridge was fitted over it and the corresponding pontic hollowed out. After all the implants were in the bone and the prosthesis properly fit, cold cure acrylic was added inside the pontics to get a closer adaptation of pontics to implants. The patient wore the bridge

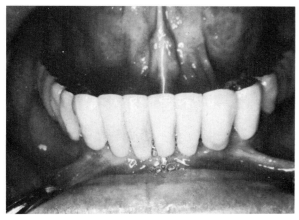

Fig. 9-105. The bridge is cemented with oxyphosphate of zinc.

temporarily for a few more days to ensure that none of the pontics impinged on the underlying tissues. The prosthesis was then cemented with hard cement (Fig. 9-105). A Panorex clearly illustrates the implants and fixed full arch denture (Fig. 9-106).

Case 12
Full arch restoration for a partially edentulous mandible using internally-threaded vent-plants

Certain post type implants, including those of Jeanneret, Cherchève, Muratori, Benaim, and Linkow, have internally threaded hollow posts that accept small bolts. This is a good feature for several reasons:

1. The superstructure needs not be cemented; instead, it can be screwed into position.
2. The implants need not be parallel to each other, as they must be with solid shaft implants. This facilitates the operation.
3. Because the fixed prosthesis is screwed into, rather than cemented over, the shafts, the hollow-shafted implants need not extend more than 0.5 to 1 mm. out of the mucosa. Thus temporary splints need not necessarily be fabricated to help stabilize the implants and protect the tongue, cheeks, and lips from protruding shafts.
4. If an implant should have to be removed, the procedure is less complicated.

The patient used to illustrate the technique had only three remaining teeth in the mandible. These supported a removable partial denture (Fig. 9-107). The three remaining teeth were prepared for smooth-surfaced gold copings with interproximal extensions

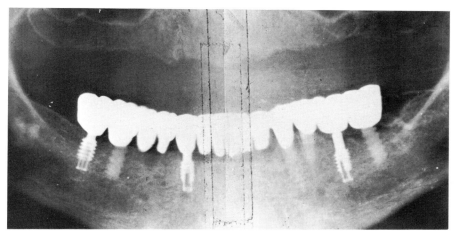

Fig. 9-106. A postoperative Panorex reveals all five implants and the two teeth.

(Fig. 9-108). The extensions were fabricated distoproximally on the lower right lateral and lower left cuspid copings, while the extension on the molar coping was fabricated on the mesioproximal surface.

The copings were tried over the three prepared abutments for proper fit. They were left in position

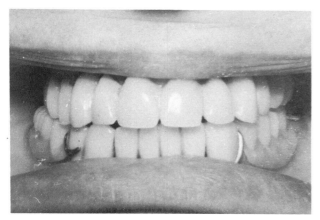

Fig. 9-107. A preoperative photograph shows a lower removable appliance with a six-unit anterior splint with a posterior removable partial denture.

A

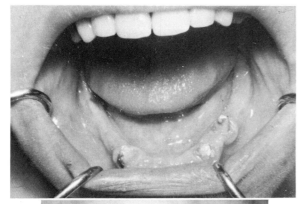

B

Fig. 9-108. A, Only three teeth remained. **B,** Copings with atypical extensions were made for the three remaining teeth.

while the implants were being inserted. To insert the implants, No. 6 round burs were drilled through the fibromucosa (Fig. 9-109). Helical burs were then used until the sites were wide enough to accommodate the taps (Fig. 9-110). Implants with hollow-threaded shafts were set deep enough so that the shafts were almost flush with the fibromucosa (Fig. 9-111).

An accurate wax or stone bite, including both arches, was taken. Round copper rods were placed inside the hollow shafts. These extended about 5 mm. above the shafts and were used merely to emphasize the implant sites, thus facilitating the laboratory technique.

A full upper alginate impression was taken. With the proper size tray, a full lower plaster index was allowed to set in the mouth and then removed. Duplicate, hollow-threaded shafts were then placed in their proper positions in the plaster index. (The

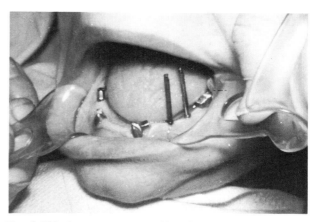

Fig. 9-109. Burs were then drilled into the bone to create the sockets for the implants.

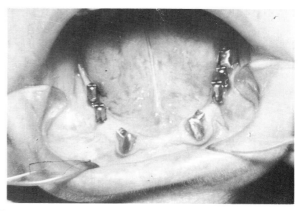

Fig. 9-110. Taps were then used to widen the holes.

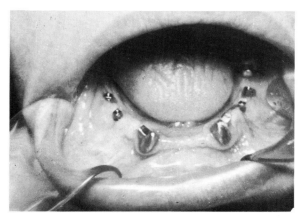

Fig. 9-111. Internally threaded implants were then "hand-ratcheted" into the bone. (From Linkow, L. I.: Internally threaded endosseous implants, Dent. Concepts 10:16-20, 1967.)

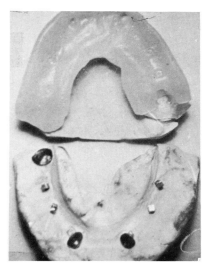

Fig. 9-112. The plaster index with the gold copings and duplicate implant shafts is seen, as well as the wax interocclusal record of centric relation.

index should include the three gold copings, the copper rods, and the duplicate shafts [Fig. 9-112].) A master stone model was poured into the plaster index. After it hardened, it was articulated with the model of the opposing jaw (Fig. 9-113). Two integral units—the mesostructure and the superstructure—were fabricated from the master stone model.

The mesostructure was constructed as two separate units, one for each side of the jaw. Thus, if an implant in the left quadrant, for example, became troublesome, the operator needed to remove only the mesostructure on the involved side. Each mesostruc-

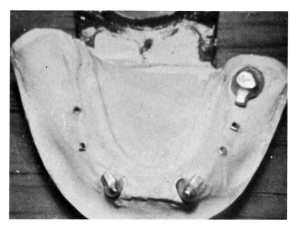

Fig. 9-113. The master stone model. (From Linkow, L. I.: Internally threaded endosseous implants, Dent. Concepts 10:16-20, 1967.)

ture contained two set screws for insertion into the implant shafts and two units to accept the screws of the superstructure (Fig. 9-114).

To fabricate the mesostructure, the set screws were partially inserted in the duplicate hollow-threaded implant shafts, leaving a good portion of the screw sticking out of the shaft. The amount of protrusion desired was determined by occlusal clearance—there should be at least 2 mm. between the heads of the screws and the occlusal surfaces of the opposing teeth. When the height of the screws had been adjusted, a wax-up of the mesostructure was accomplished. The wax was built up to a proper bulk, with no undercuts around the set screws. The wax-up also contained at least four sets of internal threading to accept the set screws of the superstructure and thus stabilize it. These threaded units were made separately. Hollow-threaded shafts that were duplicates of the implant shafts were fabricated with the line angles of their shafts undercut with a carborundum disk. The separate shafts were then placed strategically in the wax mesostructure, and wax was built up around them. The wax-up was then sprued, invested, and cast. The duplicated shafts were locked permanently into position in the gold casting.

The cast mesostructure was then tried on the master model (Fig. 9-115). It included the four set screws for insertion into the implant shafts and four threaded shafts to accept the superstructure's screws.

The superstructure was fabricated as a full arch splint, a restoration that reduced the buccolingual movements of the teeth and implants more than any other type of prosthesis.

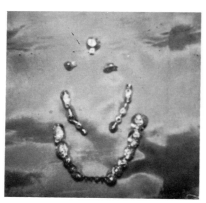

Fig. 9-114. The copings (with hollow recesses made in their extensions), the mesostructures, and a superstructure are fabricated.

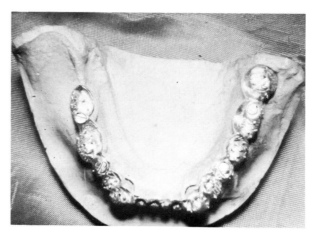

Fig. 9-116. The superstructure fits exactly over the mesostructures and secures itself to them with its four set screws. (From Linkow, L. I.: Internally threaded endosseous implants, Dent. Concepts 10:16-20, 1967.)

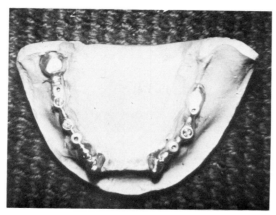

Fig. 9-115. The mesostructures have two sets of screws that fasten it to the internally threaded portions of the duplicate implant shafts. They also contain two sets each of internal threadings that allow the superstructure to be screwed into them. (From Linkow, L. I.: Internally threaded endosseous implants, Dent. Concepts 10:16-20, 1967.)

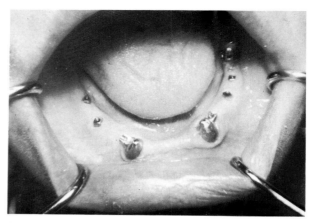

Fig. 9-117. The copings over the prepared teeth and the healed implant sites. (From Linkow, L. I.: Internally threaded endosseous implants, Dent. Concepts 10:16-20, 1967.)

The superstructure could also have been fabricated from the master model by first waxing over the mesostructure, removing the completed wax-ups, spruing, and then casting it (Fig. 9-116). Alternately, the mesostructure could first have been tried in the mouth and returned to the master model before fabricating the superstructure.

At the next visit, after inserting the three copings (Fig. 9-117), the mesostructure was screwed into its proper position (Fig. 9-118) and radiographed. The superstructure was then screwed into the threading of the mesostructure (Fig. 9-119) and radiographed. An accurate wax interocclusal record of centric re-

lation was taken, then the superstructure, mesostructure, and gold copings were all removed from the mouth and reset on the master model. The superstructure was then processed. In this case it was fabricated in acrylic (Fig. 9-120).

On the final visit the copings, the mesostructure, and the processed superstructure were tried in the mouth and equilibrated. After necessary adjustments, everything was removed. The three remaining teeth were dried, and the three gold copings were cemented over them with a hard cement. Using a soft, temporary cement mixed with some Vaseline, the mesostructure was cemented over the copings and

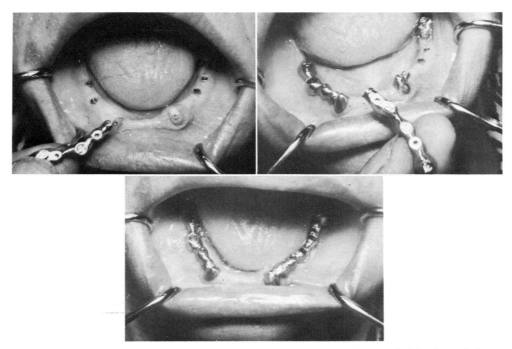

Fig. 9-118. The mesostructure is fitted over and into the internally threaded implant shafts. (From Linkow, L. I.: Internally threaded endosseous implants, Dent. Concepts **10**:16-20, 1967.)

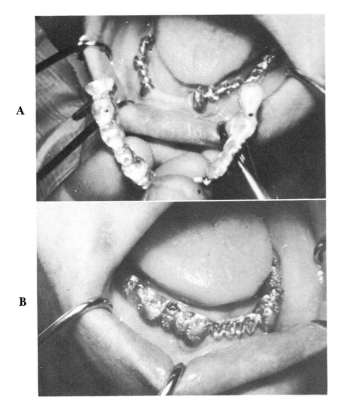

Fig. 9-119. The superstructure is then fitted over both mesostructures.

then screwed into the implants. With the same mix, the superstructure was seated. After the mixture hardened, the excess was removed (Fig. 9-121). The patient's mouth was once more checked for any prematurities or interferences in occlusion, then the four set screws secured the superstructure to the mesostructure (Fig. 9-122).

Patients usually do not mind the silver color of the four set screws. For those that do, the screws may be set below the occlusal surfaces of the crowns and covered with acrylic. To remove the bridge, the shallow acrylic coverings should be drilled out. Proper occlusion is most important, as always (Fig. 9-123).

The entire case may be summarized with radiographs. Fig. 9-124 shows the four implants in the mandible. Fig. 9-125 shows the mesostructure over the implants and Fig. 9-126, the superstructure screwed to the mesostructure.

Case 13
Precision fitted denture for a partially edentulous mandible using anterior vent-plants

Sometimes, in order to more perfectly balance the occlusal forces and to prevent tipping of a full denture, implants are placed on one side of the midline to complement the natural teeth on the other side. In this case, two vent-plants were planned to

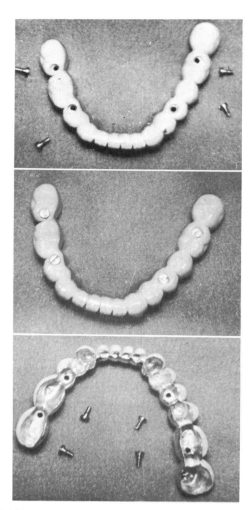

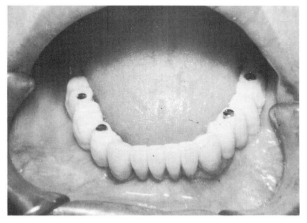

Fig. 9-122. The screws are screwed through internal threadings that are part of the superstructure framework.

Fig. 9-120. The prosthesis is processed with acrylic. (From Linkow, L. I.: Internally threaded endosseous implants, Dent. Concepts 10:16-20, 1967.)

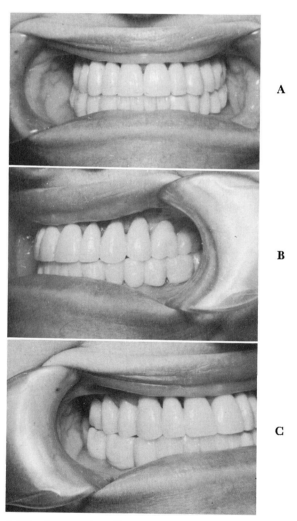

A

B

C

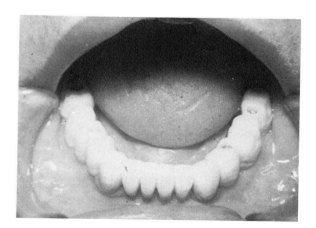

Fig. 9-121. The processed superstructure is seated.

Fig. 9-123. A, Anterior, B, left posterior, and C, right posterior sections of the completed case. (From Linkow, L. I.: Internally threaded endosseous implants, Dent. Concepts 10:16-20, 1967.)

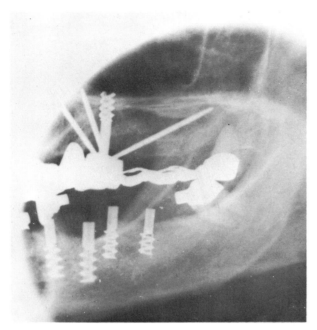

Fig. 9-124. An immediate postoperative roentgenogram reveals the four internally threaded implants, the three atypically shaped copings, and a triplant and spiral-shaft implant in the maxilla.

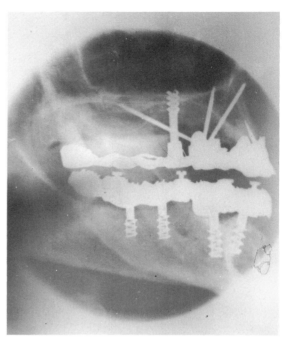

Fig. 9-126. The lateral plate x-ray shows the superstructure screwed into both mesostructures. (From Linkow, L. I.: Internally threaded endosseous implants, Dent. Concepts 10: 16-20, 1967.)

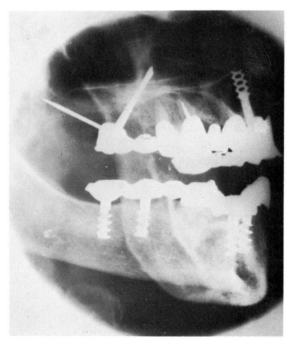

Fig. 9-125. Same patient as in Fig. 9-124 as viewed from the other side, showing the mesostructures in position over the implants.

balance the four remaining teeth: the right central, lateral, cuspid, and first bicuspid. All were prepared for full crown restorations (Fig. 9-127).

To insert the vent-plants, round burs were drilled through the fibromucosal tissue and into the bone (Fig. 9-128). These were followed with the varying sizes of helical burs (Fig. 9-129). The vent-plants were then self-tapped into the deep bone structures (Fig. 9-130).

Impressions were taken of the prepared teeth and implant shafts, and a soldered gold coping splint was cast. A one-piece gold superstructure casting to fit over the copings was processed with it in the denture (Fig. 9-131).

The structure was then cemented over the prepared teeth and implant shafts (Fig. 9-132) and the denture fitted and balanced (Fig. 9-133). The radiograph of the superstructure over the copings reveals the extremely long vent-plants used in this case (Fig. 9-134). Because very few nerve endings exist in the anterior region of the mandible, long post type implants were possible.

THE EDENTULOUS MANDIBLE

There are several considerations and alternatives in planning a full arch fixed denture for a

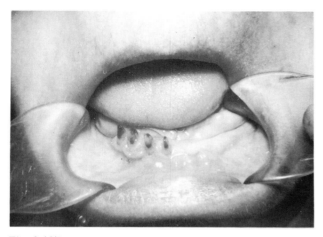

Fig. 9-127. Four remaining anterior teeth are prepared.

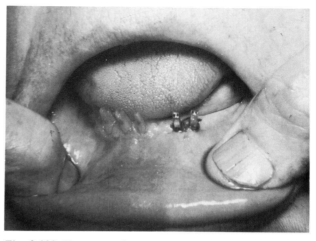

Fig. 9-130. Two vent-plants are screwed into the holes.

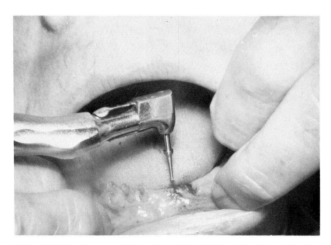

Fig. 9-128. A round bur is drilled directly through the fibromucosal tissue and into the bone.

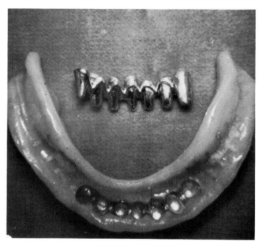

Fig. 9-131. A seven-unit gold splint was fabricated, as well as a denture with an internal framework of gold, to create an accurate and frictional grip over the splint.

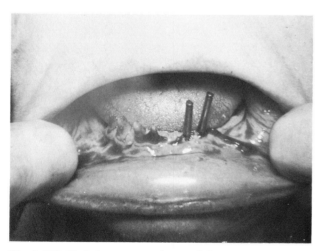

Fig. 9-129. Both burs are made parallel to each other.

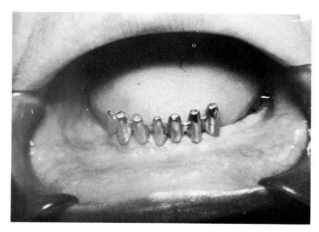

Fig. 9-132. The gold splint is cemented with oxyphosphate of zinc.

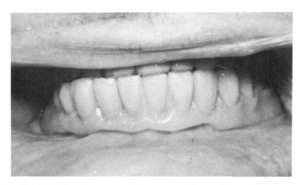

Fig. 9-133. The denture with processed acrylic teeth is seen in position.

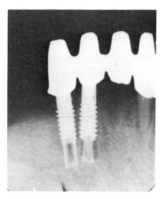

Fig. 9-134. An intraoral postoperative x-ray.

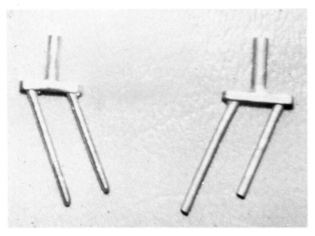

Fig. 9-135. The bifid implants of Bordon and Azoulay. (From Linkow, L. I.: Clinical evaluation of the various designed endosseous implants, J. Oral Implant Transplant Surg. **12:**35-46, 1966.)

completely edentulous mandible. If there is not enough bone above the mandibular canal, a sub-periosteal implant with a removable snap-on denture can be very successful. When there is enough bone, the patient can usually tolerate a conventional denture and implants are not needed. In those cases, however, where the patient has a full or partial complement of natural teeth in the maxilla, a conventional lower denture is usually not satisfactory. It is in such situations that endosseous implants benefit the patient. Vertical post type implants, blades, triplants, bifid implants, or a combination can be utilized. The use of a template in completely edentulous mandibles is not compulsory, as it is when using triplants in the maxilla.

Case 14
Full arch splint for an edentulous mandible using bifid implants

The architectural design of some implants limits their use to certain areas in the maxilla or mandible. One example of a good, although limited, design is the bifid implant of Bordon and Azoulay (Fig. 9-135). Because of its design, the bifid must be set into the jaw in pairs, rather than as a single implant, to obtain maximum retention. A single one can be pulled out without too much resistance. However, when two are set into bone so that their endosseous pin portions are going in opposite directions and are splinted in the oral cavity with a fixed partial denture or connecting bar attachment, they become extremely retentive.

The location of bifid implants is limited mostly to the anterior portions of the maxillae and mandible, from cuspid to cuspid. They work well in resorbed edentulous mandibles where, for a number of reasons, a subperiosteal implant is contraindicated. Bifids have also been successful in the anterior regions of both jaws when the ridges are extremely narrow.

In this case, bifid implants were used as the abutments in an edentulous mandible. Because the bar between the two legs of each bifid must sit directly on bone, rather like a subperiosteal implant, the crest of the anterior portion of the alveolar ridge was exposed by incising and retracting the mucosal tissue with a scalpel (Fig. 9-136).

Using an acrylic template guide against the crest of the ridge in the cuspid areas, a spiraled bur the same diameter as an implant leg was drilled deep into the bone. The bur was then removed and a duplicate pin, the same diameter and length as the implant leg, was placed through the template and

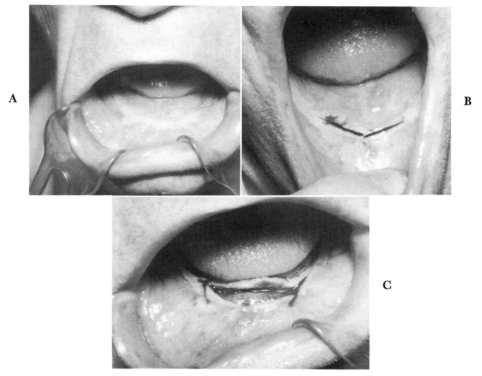

Fig. 9-136. A, The operative site. B, A clean cut is made down to the bone. C, The fibro-mucosal tissue is reflected with a periosteal elevator to expose the underlying bone.

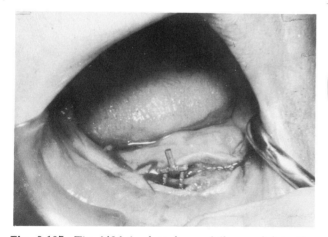

Fig. 9-137. The bifid implant is carefully eased into the holes made by the twist drills.

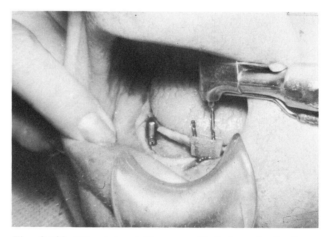

Fig. 9-138. The twist drills are guided through the bone for the second implant using a plastic template.

into the bone and left there. Still holding the template, the second hole was made in the bone with the helical bur. Both the helical bur and duplicate implant pin were then removed from the bone and the template, and the template was taken out of the mouth.

The bifid implant was then inserted for a trial

fit (Fig. 9-137). The two parallel, but angulated, pins of the implant should slide through the two artificially-made holes in the bone. All adjustments were made until it fit properly.

When the implant was finally seated to its proper depth in the bone, the horizontal bar touched the alveolar crest. The implant was then removed. A small rectangular seat for the horizontal bar the same size and depth as, or slightly larger than, the bar was then created in the crest of the ridge with a fissure bur.

The implant was once again tried in the mouth. (If the horizontal bar is not seated deeply enough and if its superior surface is protruding from the crest of the ridge, the site needs more attention. The implant must be removed and the template once

again introduced to guide the spiraled bur to make deeper holes until the implant fits flush.)

Twist drills for the second bifid implant were then used in the cuspid area on the other side of the arch (Fig. 9-138), making sure that the pins went in the opposite direction from those of the first implant. The horizontal bar spanning the legs of this implant must also fit flush with the alveolar crest (Fig. 9-139).

To give added retention and to help prevent dislodgment by buccolingual movements of the tongue, a vent-plant was inserted midway between the bifid implants, ending deep into the cortical bone along the inferior border of the mandible (Fig. 9-140).

Before the soft tissues were sutured over the horizontal portions of both implants, a full lower plaster

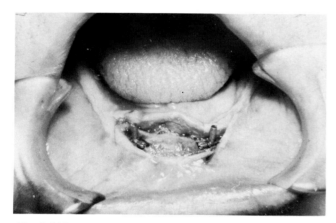

Fig. 9-139. Both bifid implants in place.

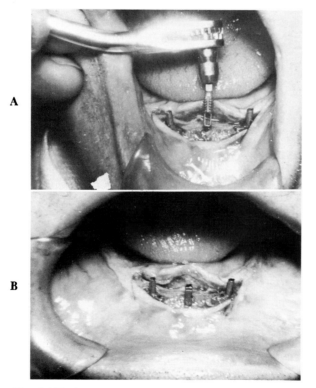

Fig. 9-140. A, A vent-plant is also used to help support the two bifid implants. **B,** The three implants in position.

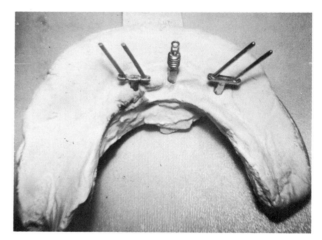

Fig. 9-141. A plaster index is taken of the three implants as well as the rest of the lower arch. Duplicate implants were used in the index to facilitate laboratory procedures.

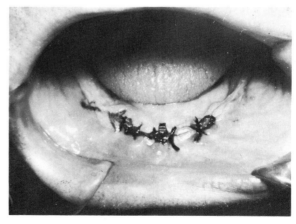

Fig. 9-142. The tissue was then sutured around the protruding shafts.

index was taken, as well as the necessary bites and opposing jaw impressions. Duplicate implant posts were placed inside the plaster index (Fig. 9-141). The tissue was then sutured (Fig. 9-142), with the sutures being removed about 4 or 5 days later.

The master model was poured and articulated. A specially designed gold superstructure containing two Gerber stress-breaker type attachments was then fabricated (Fig. 9-143). These resilient attachments de-

flected some of the load brought to bear upon the implants. The superstructure was cemented over the three protruding posts with hard cement (Fig. 9-144). A full upper denture and a full lower denture with built-in internal female attachments were made. To obtain geometric parallelism of the occlusal planes on both sides of the arch, various types of occlusal templates, with and without a curve of Spee, are sometimes used. These templates are de-

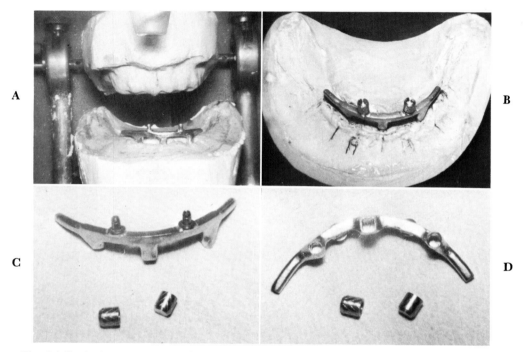

Fig. 9-143. A, A superstructure framework with a center-poise attachment is fabricated using the Hanau articulator. B to D, Two resilient type Gerber attachments were used. The female attachments will be processed inside the lower denture. The undersurface of the superstructure has copings that fit over the implant shafts.

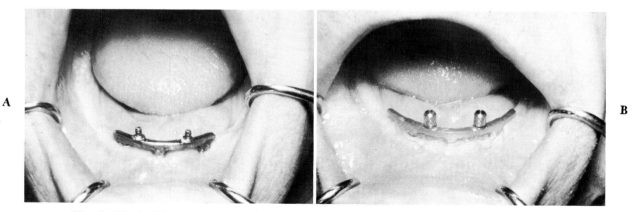

Fig. 9-144. A, The superstructure is cemented with hard cement over the implants. B, The female attachments are placed over the male attachments.

signed to attach to most of the three-dimensional articulators (Fig. 9-145). After the wax-up had been tried and the occlusion carefully checked in the mouth, both dentures were processed. Final adjustments were made on the articulator, with minute adjustments made in the mouth (Fig. 9-146).

Cross-sectional occlusal films (Fig. 9-147), lateral plate roentgenograms (Fig. 9-148), and a postero-anterior film show these implants in position (Fig. 9-149).

Case 15
A permanent prosthesis for the completely edentulous mandible using post type implants

After careful examination to determine the feasibility of using all post type implants, impressions were taken. These included a lower alginate impression of the entire edentulous mandible (Fig. 9-150),

an opposing full upper alginate impression (irreversible hydrocolloid) of the maxillary teeth, and the proper wax interocclusal record of centric relation. The models were articulated, and a full lower temporary acrylic splint was fabricated (Fig. 9-151). The entire tissue-bearing surface of the splint was hollowed out. For splints that are not hollowed out, the following procedure is recommended.

The vertical post implants were set into the jaw one at a time (Fig. 9-152). After each implant was inserted, the occlusal surface of each post was marked with an indelible pencil (Fig. 9-153). The mark was transferred to the acrylic splint and a generous hole drilled to accept the implant. The acrylic splint was then replaced and adjusted so that no impingement prevented proper seating. Following this procedure, by the time the last implant was placed into the mandibular bone, only one adjust-

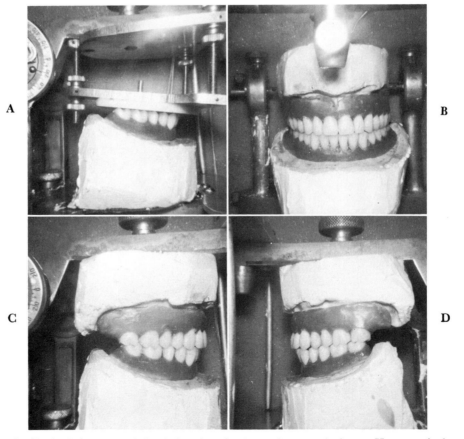

Fig. 9-145. A, Using a specially designed occlusal template attached to a Hanau articulator the lower teeth are waxed so that both occlusal planes are geometrically parallel. (Courtesy E. Glueck.) **B to D,** The upper teeth are then waxed up to the lower teeth.

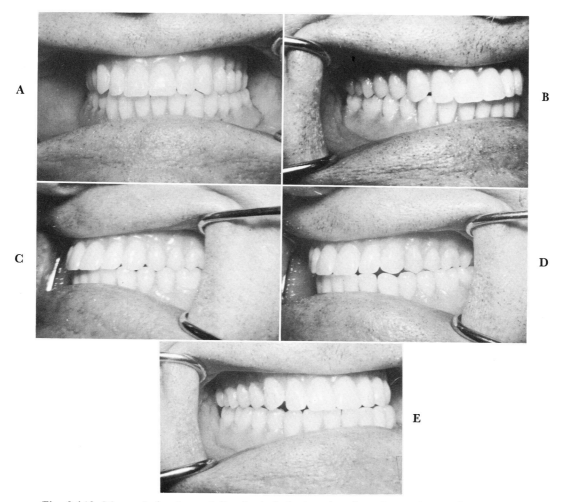

Fig. 9-146. The occlusion is carefully checked. **A,** Anterior view of teeth in centric occlusion. **B,** Right posterior view of centric occlusion. **C,** Left posterior view of teeth in centric occlusion. **D and E,** Left and right working sides, respectively.

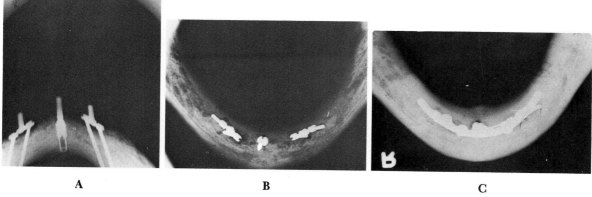

Fig. 9-147. A, A cross-sectional x-ray reveals the three implants. **B,** The three implants are also seen from an occlusal view. **C,** An occlusal view as seen after the superstructure was cemented over the implants.

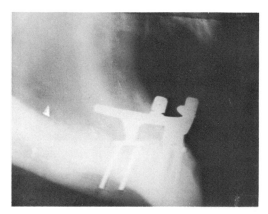

Fig. 9-148. A lateral oblique radiograph showing the position of the implants.

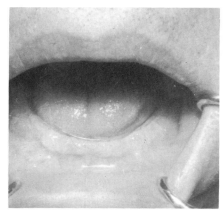

Fig. 9-150. The edentulous mandible.

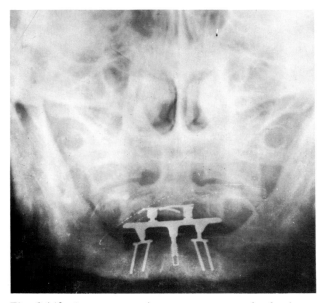

Fig. 9-149. A posteroanterior roentgenogram clearly shows the two bifid implants, the vent-plant, and the superstructure attachment.

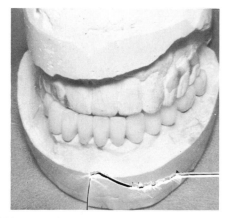

Fig. 9-151. A prefabricated temporary acrylic splint.

ment inside the hollow splint was necessary. If the splint was not adjusted until all of the implants were set, the splint probably would never have fit properly and might have broken during the crude adjustments.

Cold cure acrylic was added inside the holes, and the splint was then placed over all of the implants. It was quickly removed and replaced about every 20 seconds or so and finally allowed to harden outside the mouth. It was then carefully trimmed and polished. Vaseline (or any antibiotic salve) was placed inside the holes—no cement of any kind should be used—and the temporary splint was set

over the implants (Fig. 9-154). At this point the splint was not secured in the mouth and could easily be removed.

During the same visit, impressions for the final prosthesis were taken. This can be done by either of two methods. By one method interchangeable gold copings are slipped over the protruding shafts (Fig. 9-155) and a wax interocclusal record of centric relation is made and a plaster index taken (Fig. 9-156). The full arch fixed denture is then processed from the master model using the double casting technique, thereby utilizing the gold copings. The copings may also be used merely as transfer copings. In this latter procedure, duplicate implant shafts are placed inside the gold copings while they are still in the plaster index (Fig. 9-157). When the master stone model is poured, allowed to harden, and then separated from the plaster index, the copings are removed from the duplicate shafts. The shafts are then coated with three layers of lacquer, and then the full arch

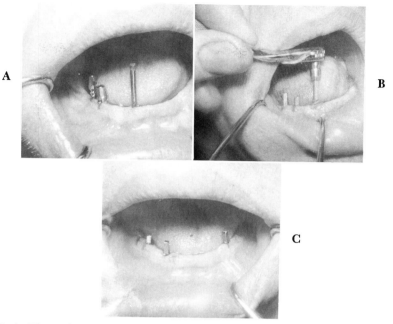

Fig. 9-152. A, The various burs and taps are seen making the necessary holes for insertion of the implants. B, The implants are inserted. C, The implants should be as nearly parallel as possible to one another.

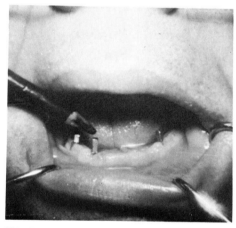

Fig. 9-153. The occlusal surface of the implant shafts are marked with an indelible pencil.

wax-up is fabricated directly over the shafts. The case is finally processed and cemented into place after final occlusal adjustments are made (Fig. 9-158).

The other method involves eliminating the copings entirely. A full lower plaster index is taken of the protruding shafts, and duplicate shafts are placed inside the plaster. The master model is then poured and articulated, and the prosthesis is fabricated di-

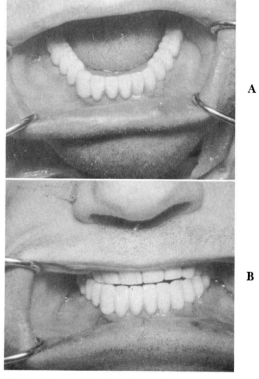

Fig. 9-154. A, The prefabricated acrylic splint is fitted into position. B, It is carefully articulated.

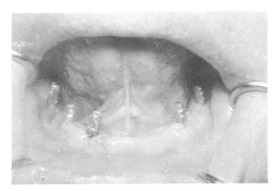

Fig. 9-155. Copings are placed over the implant shafts.

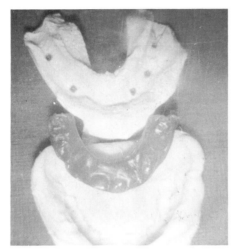

Fig. 9-156. The copings are picked up with a plaster index.

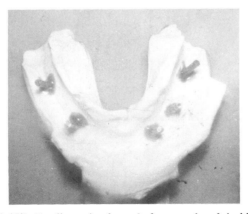

Fig. 9-157. Duplicate implant shafts are placed inside the plaster index.

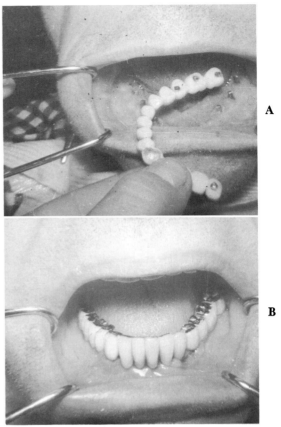

Fig. 9-158. A, The processed full arch fixed denture. B, The finished prosthesis affixed with hard cement.

rectly over the duplicated shafts. The final impression can also be accomplished with elastic impression materials, if desired.

Case 16
A removable prosthesis for an edentulous mandible using vertical post implants with a connecting bar

When a fixed full arch denture that is easily removable is desired, the following technique can be used. In the patient in this case, the implants were first set into the bone (Fig. 9-159). Interchangeable copings were then placed over them.

A plaster index was immediately taken and the master model poured. A round or oval gold bar can be soldered to the copings in an around-the-arch fashion (Fig. 9-160), or a vertical connecting bar may be cast and soldered to the copings (Fig. 9-161). The prosthesis, with a groove made on its undersurface, will fit over the bar (Fig. 9-162). The completed superstructure, consisting of copings connected by a gold bar, was cemented over the implants with hard cement (Fig. 9-163).

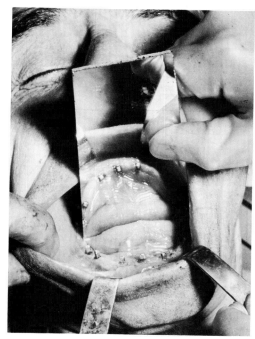

Fig. 9-159. Spiral-post implants in an edentulous mandible. (From Cherchève, R.: Les implants endo-osseoux, Paris, 1962, Librairie Maloine.)

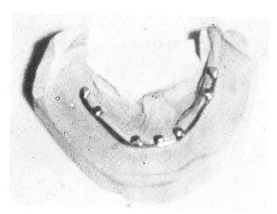

Fig. 9-160. Sometimes the protruding implant shafts are splinted together with gold copings connected to each other by a dolder connecting bar.

Bites and a rubber base impression were taken, making sure to prevent the impression material from seeping into the space between the bar and the fibromucosa at the crest of the ridge.

A removable denture may be fabricated with either an all-acrylic frictional grip, internal clip bar attachment (Fig. 9-164), or a Gerber or Ceka type attachment. After processing and adjustment, the denture was slipped over the bar. Radiographs show

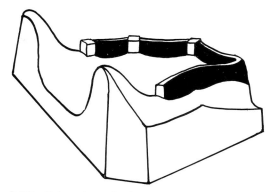

Fig. 9-161. Other times the implants are connected to each other with a vertical connecting bar.

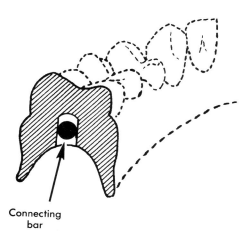

Connecting bar

Fig. 9-162. The removable denture is attached to the dolder bar with just a closely adapted acrylic frictional grip. (From Cherchève, R.: Les implants endo-osseoux, Paris, 1962, Librairie Maloine.)

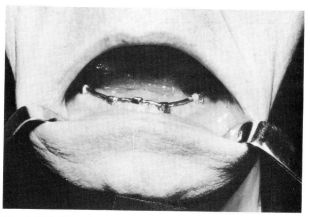

Fig. 9-163. The linked copings cemented over the implants. (From Cherchève, R.: Les implants endo-osseoux, Paris, 1962, Librairie Maloine.)

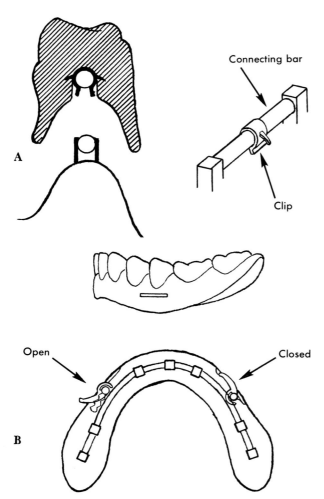

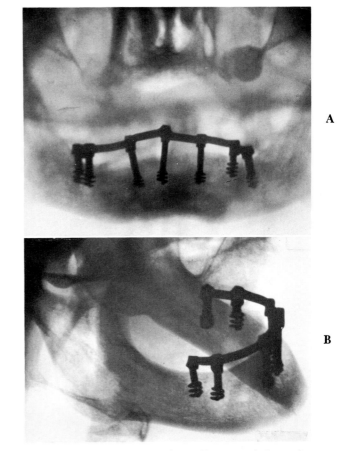

Fig. 9-164. A, The bridge may contain clips that snap onto the connecting bar. B, Another variation of clips that snap onto the connecting bar. (From Cherchève, R.: Les implants endo-osseoux, Paris, 1962, Librairie Maloine.)

Fig. 9-165. A, A posteroanterior radiograph of the patient. B, A lateral oblique radiograph of the same patient. (From Cherchève, R.: Les implants endo-osseoux, Paris, 1962, Librairie Maloine.)

the implants and connecting bar soldered to the copings (Fig. 9-165).

Case 17
A permanent full arch restoration for an edentulous mandible using vertical post implants with a mesostructure

Sometimes it is necessary to fabricate a mesostructure over post type implants to more equitably distribute stress and to provide balance. The implants are placed into the bone so that their shafts protrude 4 mm. into the oral cavity. Interchangeable gold copings are placed over the protruding shafts.

A full mouth plaster index of the lower jaw and a wax interocclusal record of centric relation were made, and an alginate (irreversible hydrocolloid)

impression of the opposing jaw was taken. A scalloped template, which was to be tissue-bearing, was constructed and soldered to the copings. Protruding from the template between the copings were vertical posts that would help stabilize the final prosthesis. After this mesostructure template was tried in place over the implants, another bite was taken and the final prosthesis was fabricated, using the mesostructure as the framework. At the final visit, everything was cemented into position.

Case 18
A full arch restoration for the completely edentulous mandible using triplants

It is generally inadvisable to support a full arch with triplants. This type of implant must be set in extremely wide alveolar bone so that its legs can be angled far apart. Such sites are rare in a full arch, and other implants should be used in combination with triplants. In some rare cases, however, an arch completely supported by triplants may be attempted.

First, an elastic impression of the entire mandible was taken. A metal template was then processed. The template was placed over the mucosal tissue and held firmly with a denture adhesive, and radiographs of the jaw were taken, using the template as a guide for making the pin holes. The template was removed and the pin holes drilled through it. The perforated template was replaced, and the pins were driven through the holes one by one. The ends were built up with acrylic cores, using the brush-on technique, and then prepared for full crown restorations.

A full lower elastic impression, a wax interocclusal record of centric relation, and an alginate (irreversible hydrocolloid) impression of the opposing jaw were made. The master model was fabricated and articulated.

From the master model, either a full arch fixed denture can be fabricated or a connecting superstructure bar can be constructed to be cemented permanently over the acrylic cores, with the additional fabrication of a removable denture with internal attachments.

Case 19
A full arch restoration for an edentulous mandible using internally threaded implants

In this case the implants were set so that their shafts did not protrude more than 1 mm. from the fibromucosa. In this way no temporary splint was needed. A plaster index of the entire mandible was taken, and duplicate shafts were placed inside the index. From the master model, three types of restorations could have been fabricated: a mesostructure with a set of screws for insertion into the implants (the mesostructure must contain internally threaded shafts to accept the screws of the superstructure); only a superstructure (this is actually the full arch splint, but it contains strategically situated internal thread systems across its length for screws that will fasten the bridge directly to the internally threaded implants); and a template with at least four protruding vertical posts to support the fixed denture. The template itself could have been ce-

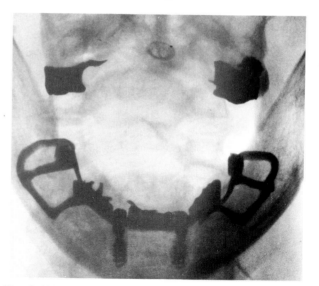

Fig. 9-166. An endentulous mandible restored with endosseous and subperiosteal implants. The implants are connected by a solid type vertical bar. (From Cherchève, R.: Les implants endo-osseoux, Paris, 1962, Librairie Maloine.)

mented onto or screwed into the implants. The prosthesis, fabricated to conform to the peripheral scalloping of the template, was cemented over the protruding posts of the template.

Case 20
Full arch resorations for the edentulous mandible using combined endosseous and subperiosteal implants

Occasionally x-rays will reveal that the alveolar crest has unevenly resorbed. Although there may still be enough alveolar bone in the anterior region to support endosseous implants, the posterior regions have completely resorbed unilaterally or bilaterally and require subperiosteal implants.

In the case illustrated in Fig. 9-166, a subperiosteal implant was inserted posteriorly on each side, following routine subperiosteal insertion techniques. Two post type implants were inserted anteriorly, again using routine procedures. The anterior posts of the subperiosteal implants were joined to the endosseous implants by a connective bar with built-in snap attachments. Impressions were taken, and a prosthesis was constructed to be supported by the implant posts and the connecting bar spanning them.

CHAPTER 10

Maxillary endosseous
implant interventions

Maxillary restorations have caused more prob-lems than mandibular ones. The character of the bone and its height can vary a great deal more than in the mandible. In addition to problems arising from the bone's patterns of resorption and porosity, gravity and occlusal forces complicate the picture. Whereas a mandibular restoration sits on the jaw, a maxillary restoration is suspended. This means that the restora-tion must be firmly anchored not only against move-ments of the cheeks, tongue, and lips but also against gravity. Because bone resorption may leave little definition of the arch, there may be difficulties in balancing the prosthesis. Also, resorption leaves little bone between the floors of the various sinuses and the crest of the ridge. This means that implant place-ment may have to be diverted elsewhere, such as to the nasal septum or the tuberosities.

The first implant restorations for the maxillae were unsuccessful for several reasons. A major cause of implant failure was unequal balance and lack of sup-port as a result of an insufficient number of im-plants. This insufficiency resulted not from poor judgment but from the limited suitability of early implant designs. The redistribution of stress and the better balance provided by the use of a template helped alleviate some problems.

There was also a weight problem. Eliminating excess bulk by carefully designed prostheses, some-times in more than one part, helped. These and other factors contributing to the prognoses of max-illary implants will be discussed in the following cases. In each case reasons for the choice of pros-thesis and implant are presented. Some failures will be included so that the reader may understand the rationale underlying the development of the more successful implantation procedures. All the implants discussed here were either post or pin type implants. Maxillary interventions using the blade-vent will be discussed in the chapter devoted exclusively to that type of implant.

UNILATERAL RESTORATIONS

The problems encountered when dealing with maxillary posterior free-end saddle areas are very different from those arising in the mandible. The main concerns are anatomic: the porosity of the alveolar bone, the location of the antral floor, and the amount of bone between alveolar crest and the floor of the sinus, as well as the buccopalatal thickness of the residual crest. In some cases there is enough bone for two post type implants; other cases require either the use of triplants or a combination of the two types of implants.

When contemplating a fixed posterior bridge for the maxillae, an intraoral radiograph is taken to de-termine the types of implants to be used as well as their locations. At least two teeth anterior to the edentulous area are prepared, and impressions for full crown coverage—either porcelain, gold, or acrylic—are taken. If two vertical spiral-post implants are to be used, an alginate or elastic impression of the entire side of the arch, including the prepared abutment teeth and the edentulous area, should be taken. This is needed to fabricate a temporary acrylic splint for immobilizing the posts. If triplants only are to be utilized, the temporary acrylic splint is not necessary. However, if a triplant and post type implant are combined, a temporary splint is necessary to stabilize the post type implant.

Case 1
A unilateral posterior free-end saddle restoration using a triplant and a template

A highly significant factor in the success of a maxillary posterior fixed partial denture is the Linkow scalloped template, which acts as a stress-distributing

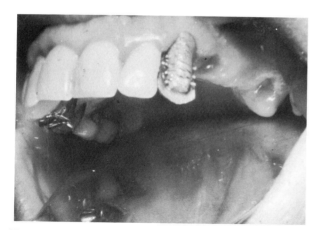

Fig. 10-1. A veneer crown casting is fitted over the cuspid preparation, which will be the anterior abutment for the contemplated four-unit fixed partial denture.

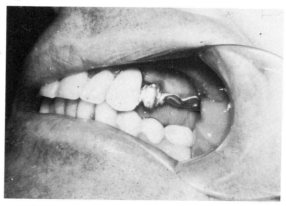

Fig. 10-2. The scalloped template is soldered to the cuspid casting and the acrylic facing is processed to it. It is then fitted in the mouth.

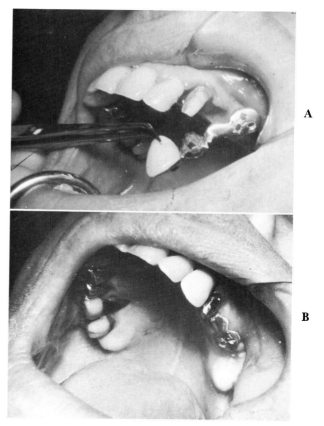

A

B

Fig. 10-3. A, From an intraoral radiograph the locations of the holes in the template are determined. B, Hard cement is placed inside the cuspid crown and it is cemented into place.

bar. In this case, a four-unit fixed partial denture with scalloped template was the restoration. The abutments were the left cuspid and a single triplant.

On the first visit, the cuspid tooth—the most anterior abutment tooth—was prepared. A modeling compound tube impression of it was taken, as well as a wax bite and an opposing jaw impression. From this impression a gold veneer casting was fabricated.

On the second visit, the cuspid veneer casting was fitted and adjusted (Fig. 10-1). A wax interocclusal record of centric relation and a plaster index, including the cuspid casting and entire edentulous area, were taken. The cuspid on the master stone model acted as the anterior abutment for the fabrication of the scalloped template. Immediately distal to the cuspid casting, a wax vertical post was fashioned with a shoulder all around its gingival border, which continued interproximally as a shoulder and buccally or labially as either a shoulder, chamfer, or feather edge.

The template, which was attached to the disto-proximal surface of the wax vertical post, was waxed in such a fashion that its buccolingual and inter-proximal contour took on a scalloped shape in order to follow the predetermined ridge lap of the teeth. The shape was predetermined by placing various sized acrylic denture teeth against the gingival surface of the master stone model until the proper sizes were determined.

The template was no thicker than a very thin sheet of green wax, and its buccal and lingual peripheral borders were rolled slightly so the template would not interfere with the soft tissues. The wax template was carefully removed from the master

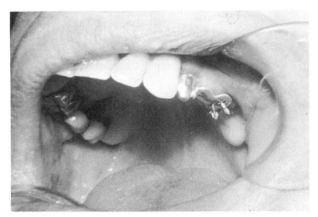

Fig. 10-4. The pin implants are slowly driven through the template in their predetermined directions in order to circumvent the maxillary sinus in an anteroposterior direction.

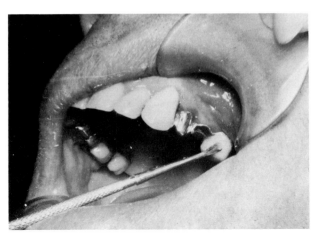

Fig. 10-5. The ends of the pins are fused to each other with cold cure acrylic resin.

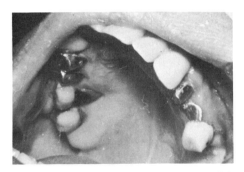

Fig. 10-6. The hardened acrylic core is prepared for a full crown restoration, making sure it follows the peripheral outline of the gold template.

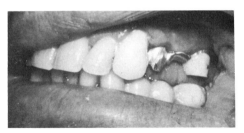

Fig. 10-7. The interocclusal clearance between the prepared acrylic core and the opposing lower tooth is determined by having the patient bite in centric relation.

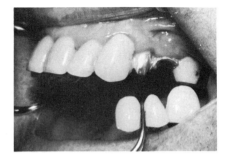

Fig. 10-8. From an elastic impression and wax interocclusal record of centric relation, the completed (one-piece casting) superstructure is fitted into position over the acrylic core and gold post extending from the template.

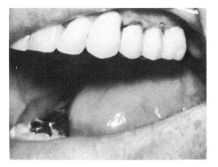

Fig. 10-9. The superstructure is cemented.

stone model and cast in gold. It was soldered to the veneer crown cuspid casting, which was then waxed for a veneer facing and processed.

On the third visit, the processed acrylic veneer cuspid crown with the attached template was tried in the mouth and adjusted (Fig. 10-2). An intraoral periapical radiograph, made using the long cone technique, was taken to show the relationship of the template to the maxillary sinus. From this x-ray guide, three holes were made in the template (Fig. 10-3). The holes were slightly wider than the pins to allow them to enter at oblique angles. The holes also helped guide the pins in their circumvention of the sinus.

The framework, which included the processed acrylic-and-gold veneer crown with the vertical post and template attached to it, was then permanently set into position by filling the cuspid crown with oxyphosphate of zinc cement. It was held firmly in place until the cement hardened, at which time the excess was removed.

The implant pins were driven through the three predetermined holes of the template and deep into the osseous structures, passing mesially and distally to the maxillary sinus (Fig. 10-4). The ends of the pins were built up with an acrylic core (Fig. 10-5), which was prepared for a full crown restoration (Fig. 10-6).

A wax interocclusal record of centric relation was made. An elastic impression of the left side, from the cuspid crown to the posterior acrylic core, was taken, making sure that there was no interference occlusally from the acrylic core when the patient bit into centric occlusion (Fig. 10-7).

On the fourth, and final, visit, the posterior unilateral veneer type fixed partial denture, or superstructure, was fitted over the gold abutment post and the acrylic core abutment (Fig. 10-8). It was checked for marginal adaptation and proper articulation (Fig. 10-9) and radiographed (Fig. 10-10).

The fixed partial denture was cemented permanently over both abutments. When the cement hardened, it was trimmed and the patient dismissed.

Case 2
Unilateral posterior free-end saddle restoration using the simplified template technique

To save the dentist and the patient an additional visit, the template and fixed partial denture can be completed together. To illustrate the technique, a case will be given in which a four-unit bridge using the two maxillary right bicuspids as the anterior abutments and replacing the two missing molars with a triplant was used.

On the first visit, the two anterior teeth were prepared for full crown coverage restorations (Fig. 10-11). At the next visit, the veneer crowns were tried in the mouth and properly balanced (Fig. 10-12). A wax interocclusal record of centric relation was made and a plaster index was taken, making sure to include the edentulous area distal to the bicuspid as well as the castings themselves. From this impression and bite the entire prosthesis was fabricated.

The two castings were soldered together, and the

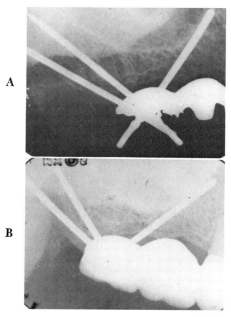

Fig. 10-10. A, The pins are driven through the scalloped template. **B,** The cemented superstructure.

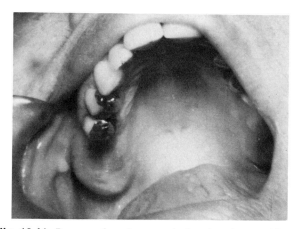

Fig. 10-11. Preoperative photograph showing the two bicuspid teeth and the edentulous area posterior to it.

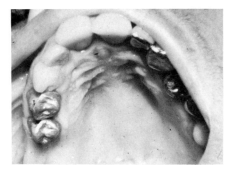

Fig. 10-12. Two veneer crown castings are fitted over the prepared teeth.

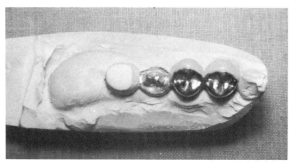

Fig. 10-14. The quick-setting stone previously poured over the mushroom pin heads is prepared for a full crown restoration.

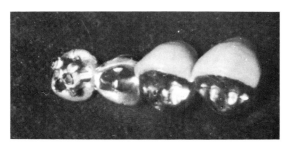

Fig. 10-13. The veneer crown castings are soldered together and processed with acrylic facings after the posterior scalloped template, including the vertical mushroom pin heads, is soldered to the second bicuspid restoration.

template was soldered to the castings. The first portion of the template was the vertical post, which supported the anterior crown of the two-unit, one-piece superstructure casting that fitted over it. The second portion of the template included vertical mushroom posts. These mushroom posts, which could either have been cast with the template or later soldered to it, helped increase the bond between the acrylic core and the gold template. They could be bent in any direction if they interfered with the pin implant insertions, or all but one could have been removed. Instead of the mushroom posts, gold wires could also have been soldered to the area to serve the same purpose. Only one end of a wire is soldered; the other is bent into a loop.

Acrylic was processed onto the two anterior crowns (Fig. 10-13). At this point, because the mushroom heads would interfere with taking an impression of the template for making the superstructure, a fast-setting stone mix was poured over and in between the mushroom projections. When this hardened, it was prepared for a full crown restoration (Fig. 10-14). This stone core simulated the eventual acrylic core that would act as the posterior abutment.

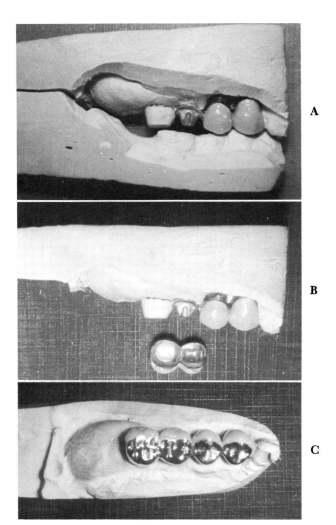

Fig. 10-15. A, The stone core is prepared so that when the models are articulated there is enough room occlusally for a restoration. B, The one-piece superstructure is fabricated from an elastic impression. C, The superstructure is seen accurately fitted over the template.

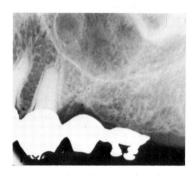

Fig. 10-16. An intraoral radiograph is taken with the template in the mouth to determine where to place the holes to accommodate the pins in circumventing the antral floor.

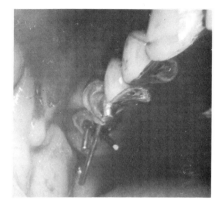

Fig. 10-18. The pin implants are driven through the template.

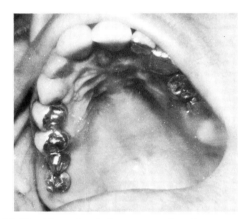

Fig. 10-17. After the holes are made, the two anterior crowns are cemented over the prepared teeth.

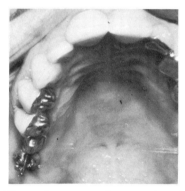

Fig. 10-19. The ends are cut short so that they will not interfere with the insertion of the superstructure.

It was then possible to take an elastic impression of both vertical extensions of the template for fabricating the one-piece casting of the two-unit superstructure (Fig. 10-15).

The stone core was then tapped off the template, and the bridge was placed in the mouth with the superstructure and equilibrated. The superstructure was then removed, leaving the template attached to the two bicuspid crowns still in the mouth. It was imperative at this time to check that the scalloped template did not impinge on the fibromucosal tissue; it must fit passively. An x-ray was then taken in the sinus area to determine where the holes were to be made through the template in relation to the sinus (Fig. 10-16). The template was removed from the mouth and the holes drilled through it.

Hard cement was then placed inside the two bicuspid crowns and the prosthesis cemented into position over the two dried bicuspid teeth (Fig. 10-17).

The individual pin implants were slowly driven through the template in the various directions predetermined by the radiographic interpretations (Fig. 10-18). The excess length of the pins was removed (Fig. 10-19). The pins were then locked together with acrylic and the two-unit superstructure was cemented over the template (Fig. 10-20). (A good method of cementation is to use oxyphosphate of zinc cement inside the anterior crown, which fits over the gold post in the template. The posterior crown should be filled with acrylic after roughening the inside of the crown and notching the acrylic core. In this manner, an acrylic-to-acrylic bond is achieved posteriorly.)

Once again, the bridge was checked for occlusion, and any excess cement was removed (Fig. 10-21).

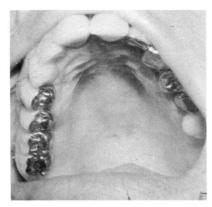

Fig. 10-20. After the pins are fused together and to the template with acrylic, the superstructure is cemented.

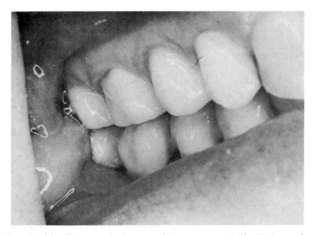

Fig. 10-21. The occlusion, which was carefully balanced prior to the implant insertion, is again checked after the superstructure is cemented.

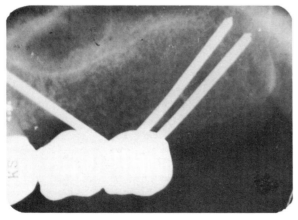

Fig. 10-22. The completed case.

The postoperative x-ray shows the three pins circumventing the sinus floor (Fig. 10-22).

Case 3
Full arch splint for a posterior unilaterally edentulous area using a triplant

This is an early case, done before the advent of the scalloped template. Here the pin implants were driven directly through the fibromucosal tissue and into the bone. Today, when triplants are used, some type of template is added for extra stabilization. This case details the procedures involved in inserting a simple triplant. Except for the addition of a template, the procedures are similar to current techniques.

A 40-year-old woman, who was wearing a maxillary unilateral partial removable denture to replace the posterior left quadrant of teeth distal to the first bicuspid, desired a fixed denture.

Because a large anterior diastema existed between her two central incisors and because there was decay under an old fixed partial denture in her right posterior quadrant, a full arch splint was desirable. A triplant was planned to circumvent the sinus as the posterior abutment in the left edentulous side.

The teeth were prepared for veneer crown restorations. The crowns were carefully fitted over the prepared abutments and all necessary occlusal, gingival, and interproximal adjustments were made (Fig. 10-23). With a slow-running contra-angle attached with a water attachment and special chuck, the first pin implant was slowly drilled through the fibromucosal tissue in a mesial direction through the center of the alveolar crest (Fig. 10-24). The angulation and depth of the pin relative to the anterior extent of the antral floor were radiographed as the pin was inserted.

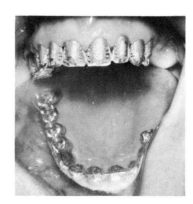

Fig. 10-23. The soldered castings are fitted and the occlusion carefully balanced.

The second pin was driven through the soft tissue and into the bone in a distopalatal direction, and the third pin driven in a distobuccal direction (Fig. 10-25). It is imperative to circumvent the maxillary sinus along its mesial and distal extensions. If an attempt is made to circumvent the sinus buccopalatally, the pins inevitably terminate in the sinus.

The three pins were carefully locked to each other with acrylic monomer and polymer, using the brush-on technique, until a dense core was built (Fig. 10-26). When the core hardened, it was prepared for a crown preparation with a tapered diamond stone (Fig. 10-27).

Impressions were then taken. Elastic impression material, either in a tray or copper tube, should be used for this purpose. When the casting was made, it was fitted over the acrylic core and a wax interocclusal record of centric relation made. A full mouth plaster index was then taken of all the castings. (A

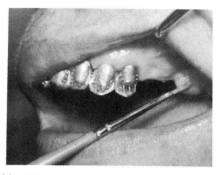

Fig. 10-26. Using the brush-on technique, the pins are fastened to one another with the polymer and monomer.

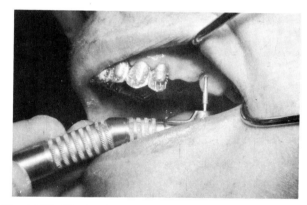

Fig. 10-27. The hardened acrylic core is prepared for a full crown restoration with a tapered diamond stone.

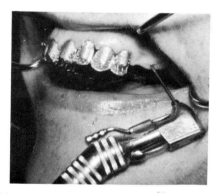

Fig. 10-24. With a slow-running contra-angle and a water spray, the first pin is driven through the mucoperiosteal tissue and into the bone.

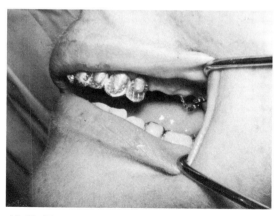

Fig. 10-25. Two other pins are driven in different directions into the bone.

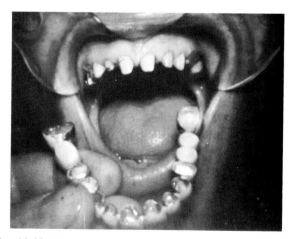

Fig. 10-28. The completed full arch fixed denture prior to cementation.

compound tube impression should never be used for duplicating an acrylic core, because some compound might lodge under the tissue-bearing surface of the core, thereby loosening the triplant.)

A full arch acrylic-and-gold veneer fixed denture was then fabricated and tried in the mouth (Fig. 10-28). After balancing for fine adjustments, the prosthesis was affixed with hard cement (Fig. 10-29). A final periapical intraoral radiograph reveals the posterior abutment (Fig. 10-30).

Case 4
Full arch splint for a long unilateral span using mixed implants

The patient, a woman in her middle sixties, was edentulous from the left maxillary cuspid and had been wearing an all-acrylic removable denture for the past 12 years (Fig. 10-31).

A full arch splint was planned, with three implants as posterior abutments: a titanium vent-plant, a cobalt-chrome spiral-shaft implant, and a tantalum triplant. The teeth were prepared (Fig. 10-32). A vent-plant was placed in the first bicuspid area, and a spiral-shaft implant was set in the second bicuspid area (Fig. 10-33). Pins were driven in the molar area and fused with acrylic. The core was prepared for a crown restoration (Fig. 10-34).

All necessary impressions and bite registrations

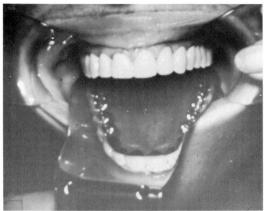

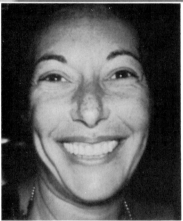

Fig. 10-29. The cemented prosthesis.

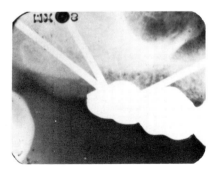

Fig. 10-30. The intraoral radiograph showing the tripodial implant acting as the most posterior abutment.

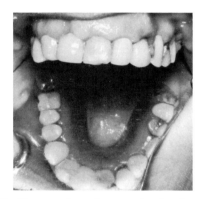

Fig. 10-31. Preoperative photograph showing remaining teeth and an all-acrylic removable partial denture.

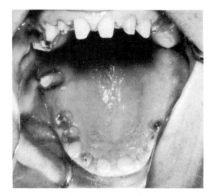

Fig. 10-32. All the teeth are prepared.

were taken to make a gold occlusal acrylic veneer full arch fixed denture (Fig. 10-35). The prosthesis was then fitted (Fig. 10-36) and cemented with hard cement (Fig. 10-37). A lateral plate roentgenogram shows the vent-plant, spiral-shaft implant, and triplant (Fig. 10-38).

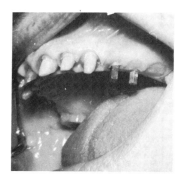

Fig. 10-33. A vent-plant and a spiral-post implant are seen in position.

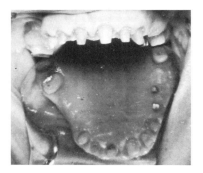

Fig. 10-34. A prepared acrylic core affixing the posterior triplant is seen behind the spiral-post implant.

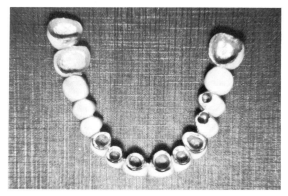

Fig. 10-35. A one-piece full arch fixed denture is fabricated.

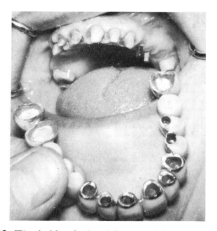

Fig. 10-36. The bridge is fitted into position and last-minute adjustments in occlusion and gingival adaptation are done prior to its cementation. All three dissimilar metals plus the gold showed no evidence of galvanic action. The case is still functioning after 6 years.

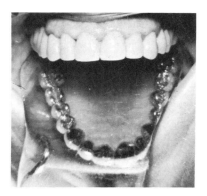

Fig. 10-37. The cemented restoration.

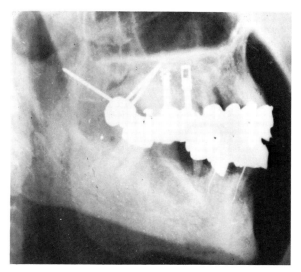

Fig. 10-38. A lateral plate roentgenogram clearly reveals the vent-plant, spiral-shaft implant, and triplant.

Case 5
A full arch acrylic veneer bridge for a unilaterally edentulous posterior area using a template and a triplant

This patient's remaining teeth were in poor condition and very unattractive (Fig. 10-39). After all periodontal conditions had been alleviated, the teeth were prepared for full crown restorations (Fig. 10-40).

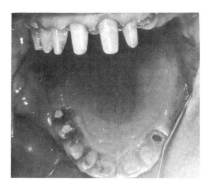

Fig. 10-39. Preoperative photograph reveals caries, separation of teeth, and lack of proper occlusion.

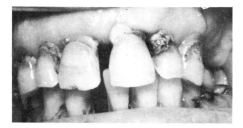

Fig. 10-40. The remaining teeth are prepared after proper periodontal therapy.

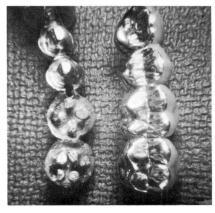

Fig. 10-41. A prefabricated full arch fixed denture is completed. Here the tiny projections that help fuse the pin implants to the template are seen extending vertically from the scalloped template.

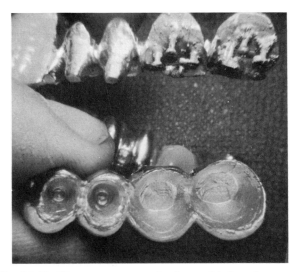

Fig. 10-42. The superstructure is also prefabricated.

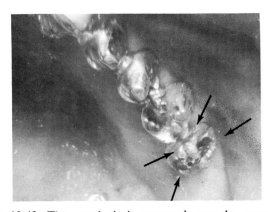

Fig. 10-43. The prosthesis is cemented over the prepared abutment teeth with hard cement and then the pin implants (arrows) are driven through the template.

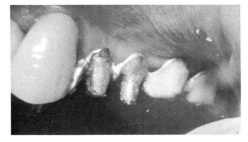

Fig. 10-44. The pins are affixed together with cold cure resin material.

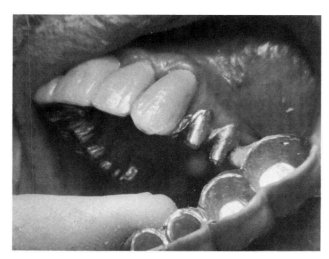

Fig. 10-45. The superstructure is fitted into position.

All necessary impressions were taken, including a wax interocclusal record of centric relation, with various try-ins until the final full arch fixed denture with its posterior scalloped template was processed. The template, which was rigidly attached to the upper left cuspid, had a vertical post and vertical mushroom-shaped pin heads (Fig. 10-41). The peripheral borders of the template were scalloped to allow the mucosal tissue, over which the template fitted passively, to blend itself into the interproximal embrasures.

The impression for the one-piece four-unit bridge, or superstructure, was accomplished by first pouring quick-setting stone over the pin heads. When the stone hardened, it was prepared for full crown restorations. An elastic impression was taken over the stone cores and gold posts from which the superstructure was to be waxed, cast, and processed (Fig. 10-42).

The full arch splint was then tried in the mouth and adjusted. A radiograph was taken of the area

A

B

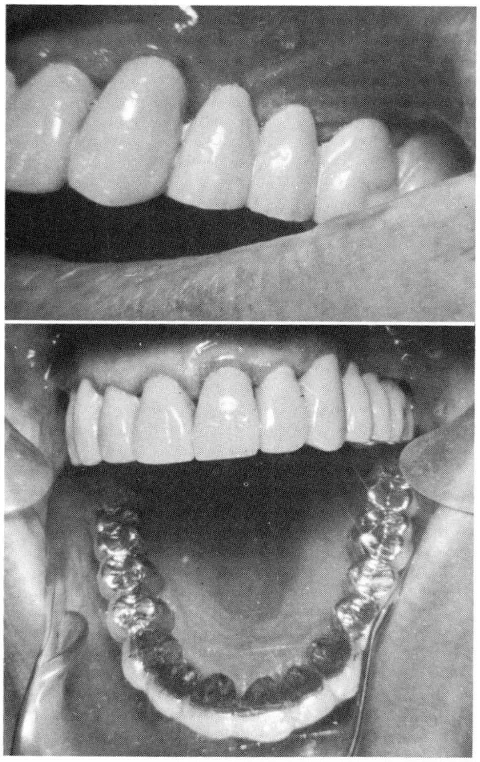

Fig. 10-46. **A,** The superstructure is finally fixed to the template with hard cement. **B,** The entire full arch fixed denture.

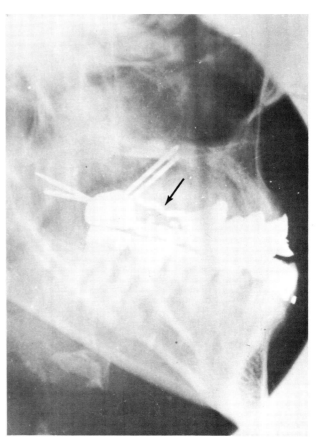

Fig. 10-47. An extraoral lateral plate roentgenogram of the case. Arrow points to the scalloped template.

where the triplant was contemplated, and the bridge removed for drilling holes to accommodate the pins. The bridge was then cemented in position with hard cement, which was chipped away when set.

One by one the pins were carefully driven through the template and fibromucosa and into the bone (Fig. 10-43). The pins were x-rayed for proper angulation in circumventing the maxillary sinus. They were fused together and to the vertical mushroom heads of the template with acrylic. The hardened acrylic cores were prepared for full crown restorations (Fig. 10-44).

The superstructure was tried in position (Fig. 10-45) and, after all necessary adjustments, cemented over the template (Fig. 10-46). A final lateral plate radiograph shows the triplant and template (Fig. 10-47).

Case 6
A full arch porcelain-baked-to-metal bridge for a unilaterally edentulous posterior arch using a template and triplant

The patient's remaining teeth were prepared for full coverage (Fig. 10-48). The restoration included the full arch porcelain-baked-to-metal bridge with a posterior scalloped template and a two-unit superstructure (Fig. 10-49).

The prosthesis was tried in the mouth (Fig. 10-50) and removed for the drilling of holes in the template for the pins. The prosthesis was returned to the mouth and cemented with oxyphosphate of zinc cement over the prepared abutment teeth. The pin implants were then carefully drilled through the holes in the template and into the bone. All excess length of the pins protruding into the oral cavity was removed (Fig. 10-51). The pins were fastened with acrylic to form a core, which was then prepared. A soft mix of acrylic was placed inside the posterior

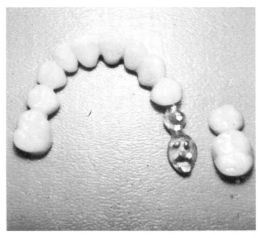

Fig. 10-49. The completed porcelain-baked-to-metal full arch denture with its scalloped template and superstructure is prefabricated prior to insertion of the implants.

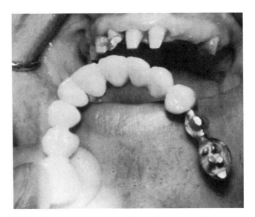

Fig. 10-50. The prosthesis is fitted into position.

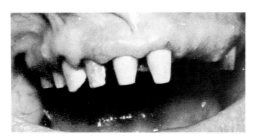

Fig. 10-48. All of the remaining teeth are prepared for full coverage restorations.

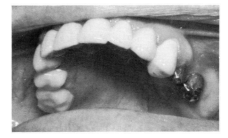

Fig. 10-51. After the holes are made through the template, the prosthesis is cemented over the prepared teeth. The pin implants are then properly angulated through the template and into the bone.

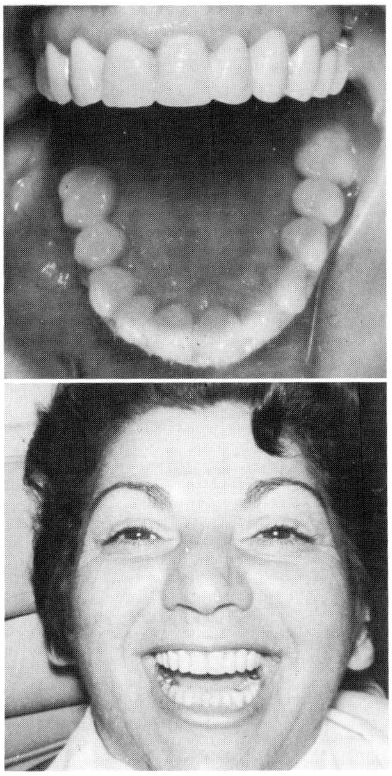

crown, and oxyphosphate of zinc cement was placed inside the anterior crown to seat the superstructure. The excess acrylic was removed while still soft, but the excess zinc cement was not removed until it hardened (Fig. 10-52). An intraoral radiograph clearly shows the triplant pins avoiding the maxillary sinus (Fig. 10-53).

BILATERAL RESTORATIONS

Many patients lack posterior teeth on both sides of the arch yet retain a number of anterior teeth. For these patients, a fixed denture can be useful and successful. When enough bone exists posteriorly below the sinus floor, post type implants can be used. As long as there is enough bone flanking the sinus, it can be circumvented with a triplant. In those cases where the floor of the sinus has dropped to the resorbed alveolar crest, a blade implant can be inserted in the maxillary tuberosity distal to the most distal extent of the maxillary sinus.

In addition to the type of implant, other considerations apply. These will be explored in detail under the sample case presentations.

Case 7
Bilateral posterior restorations using triplants and templates

This patient was bilaterally edentulous (Fig. 10-54). An alginate, or irreversible hydrocolloid, impression of the remaining unprepared anterior teeth and both edentulous areas of the maxillae was taken, as well as an opposing jaw alginate impression.

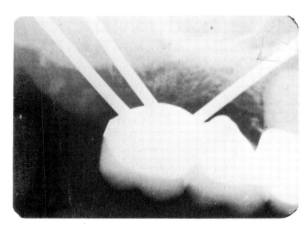

Fig. 10-52. The completed prosthesis.

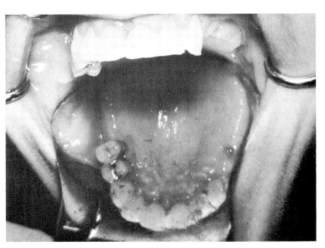

Fig. 10-53. A final intraoral periapical radiograph clearly reveals the circumvention of the sinus floor using the pin implants.

Fig. 10-54. The patient was bilaterally edentulous in the posterior region.

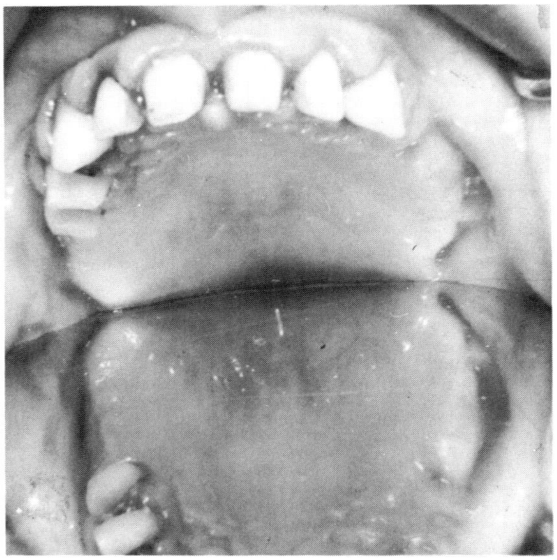

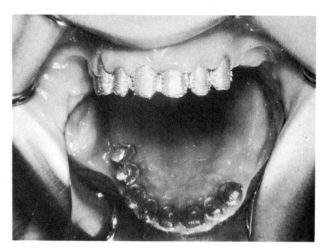

Fig. 10-55. The teeth were all prepared.

Fig. 10-56. Gold castings to support acrylic teeth were fitted over the preparations.

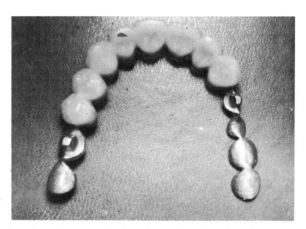

Fig. 10-57. The prefabricated prosthesis included the processed acrylic teeth and the scalloped templates. (From Linkow, L. I.: Maxillary endosseous implants, Dent. Concepts 10[1]:14-24, 1966.)

All of the remaining teeth were prepared (Fig. 10-55) and compound tube impressions and a wax interocclusal record of centric relation were taken.

Cold cure acrylic of the desired shade was then squeezed into the teeth impressions inside the alginate impression. The alginate impression was carefully positioned over the prepared teeth, which had been lubricated with Vaseline, using the posterior edentulous areas as guides for proper seating. The impression was held motionless in the patient's mouth for approximately 5 minutes, until the acrylic hardened, and then it was removed. The resulting acrylic splint was carefully trimmed, fitted, and adjusted along its gingival and occlusal margins and cemented in with one of the soft temporary cements.

At the next visit, gold copings were fitted over the abutment teeth (Fig. 10-56). A wax interocclusal record of centric relation was made and a full mouth plaster index taken.

A full arch fixed denture was fabricated; in this case it was made of acrylic over gold. All the copings were soldered and processed with acrylic teeth. The scalloped template, which extended over the edentulous areas, began distal to the last abutment on each side of the arch (Fig. 10-57). Just behind the last natural abutment on each side was a vertical post. This bore the first crown in each bridge. The scalloped template continued distal to each post, ending where the last tooth in the bridge sat. The outline, design, and contour of the scalloped areas were determined by the contour of denture teeth, which were placed on the master stone model before the template was made. The teeth should esthetically complement the anterior teeth of the arch. Because the template should always fit passively over the soft tissue, no "ditching" should be made on the master cast prior to the waxing of the template.

The prosthesis was then fitted in position over the prepared abutment teeth (Fig. 10-58), and all necessary gingival and occlusal adjustments were done. The adaptation of the template to the underlying soft tissue was also carefully evaluated for passive fit.

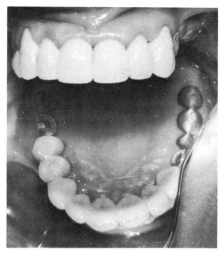

Fig. 10-58. The prosthesis was tried in the mouth for accuracy of its fit and passivity of template to the tissues.

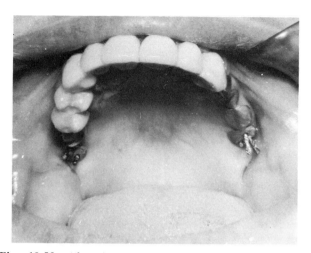

Fig. 10-59. After it was cemented, pin implants were driven through the previously prepared holes in the template. (From Linkow, L. I.: Maxillary endosseous implants, Dent. Concepts 10[1]:14-24, 1966.)

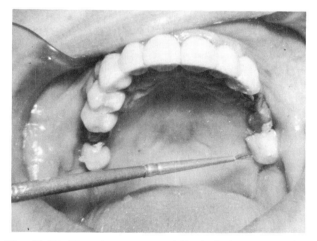

Fig. 10-60. The pins were carefully locked to each other with acrylic liquid and powder, using the brush-on technique. (From Linkow, L. I.: Maxillary endosseous implants, Dent. Concepts 10[1]:14-24, 1966.)

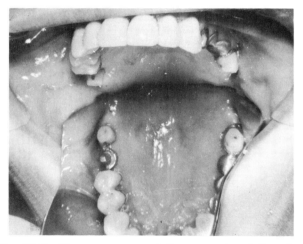

Fig. 10-61. The cores are carefully prepared to follow the peripheral outline of the gold template.

Intraoral radiographs of both posterior edentulous areas were taken with the prosthesis still in the mouth to evaluate the relationship of the maxillary sinus to the scalloped template.

The prosthesis was then removed from the mouth, and holes were drilled with a No. 557 fissure bur through the template for the pins. These holes should be angulated in the direction in which the pin implants must go in order to avoid the sinus. They must also be slightly larger than the pins; otherwise, the inserted pins can distort the template, thereby tending to dislodge the prosthesis or to create a great deal of pressure and tension, which could lead to failure.

Hard cement (oxyphosphate of zinc) was then placed inside the crowns, the teeth were thoroughly dried, and the prosthesis was placed into proper position and held firmly until the cement hardened. The excess cement was then removed.

The pin implants were then slowly drilled through the holes in the template, angulated in their proper positions (Fig. 10-59). Each step was carefully

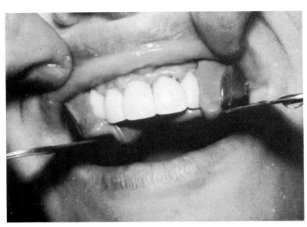

Fig. 10-62. Rubber impressions are taken of the templates, which must include the acrylic cores and the gold posts for the fabrication of the two bilateral fixed superstructures.

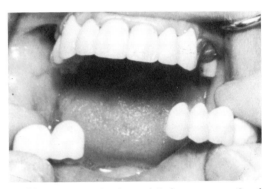

Fig. 10-63. The two fixed partial dentures are fitted and carefully checked for any occlusal interferences. (From Linkow, L. I.: Maxillary endosseous implants, Dent. Concepts **10**[1]:14-24, 1966.)

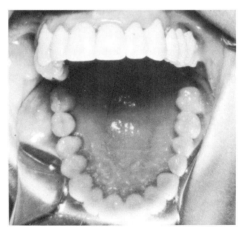

Fig. 10-64. The bridges are cemented over the templates. (From Linkow, L. I.: Maxillary endosseous implants, Dent. Concepts **10**[1]:14-24, 1966.)

x-rayed. The pins were fused together with acrylic using the brush-on technique (Fig. 10-60). (Note that in this case, one of the first scalloped template cases, no vertical mushroom pin heads were included to fuse the pins to the template.) With a tapered diamond bur, the hardened acrylic cores were prepared for full crown restorations. Their outlines followed the underlying contour of the gold template (Fig. 10-61).

At this point either a full arch elastic impression or—as in this case—two unilateral rubber impressions may be taken (Fig. 10-62). The impressions included the gold vertical posts, the prepared acrylic cores, and the scalloped template existing between them. A wax interocclusal record of centric relation was also taken. From the impressions two unilateral fixed partial dentures were waxed, cast (usually in one piece), and processed.

At the next visit, the tissue around the implants and crowns covering the teeth was checked carefully for any impingement from remaining cement or acrylic. The two fixed partial dentures were tried in the mouth (Fig. 10-63) and balanced, and then the

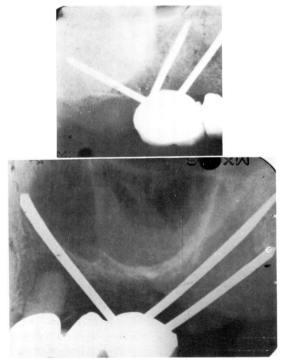

Fig. 10-65. Postoperative periapical radiographs of both triplants.

prostheses were cemented with hard cement (Fig. 10-64). Postoperative radiographs were taken of each area (Fig. 10-65).

Case 8
Bilateral restorations using a scalloped template with precision attachments and triplants

When the long-term fate of a triplant in a posterior edentulous area is dubious for any reason, a template with precision attachments may be used. To facilitate removal, the template bears on its most anterior portion a male attachment that fits into a female attachment on the most distal portion of the restoration spanning the prepared abutment teeth. This type of template may be used for bilateral restorations, in which case a template is made for each side of the jaw, or for a unilateral restoration. The following case illustrates one of the reasons why such a template procedure may prove handy.

The patient, a 58-year-old woman, was very suspicious about the longevity of implants and wanted assurance that there would not be much future work

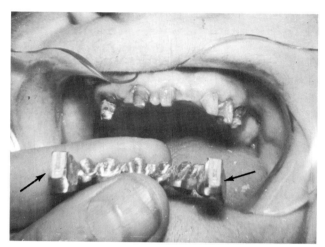

Fig. 10-66. Female precision attachments *(arrows)* are soldered to the distoproximal surfaces of the last abutment castings on each side of the arch.

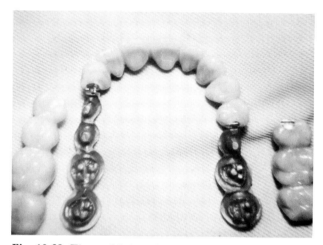

Fig. 10-68. The prefabricated porcelain-baked-to-metal prosthesis includes the splinted porcelain-to-metal anterior portion, two posterior scalloped templates with male precision attachments that attach them to the anterior quadrant, and two porcelain-baked-to-metal superstructures.

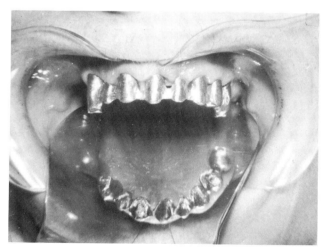

Fig. 10-67. The soldered copings are fitted over the prepared teeth.

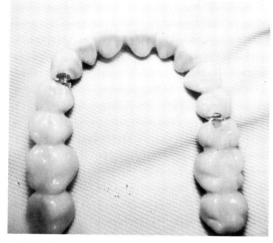

Fig. 10-69. The posterior superstructures are fitted over the templates.

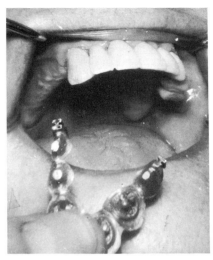

Fig. 10-70. The anterior quadrant is cemented and the two templates are tried for accuracy.

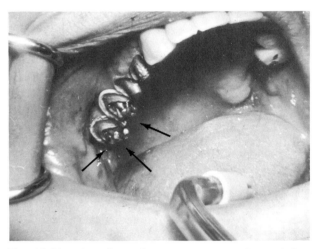

Fig. 10-71. After the male attachments are inserted into the female attachments, the pin implants are driven through the template.

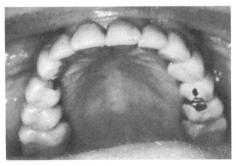

Fig. 10-72. The two superstructures are then cemented over both templates.

necessary in case the implants had to be removed. The procedure was explained, with no promises as to longevity, and she agreed to it.

Her remaining six teeth—the maxillary right central and cuspid, left central and cuspid, and bicuspids—were prepared for full crown restorations. Metal castings were fabricated, fitted, and then soldered together. Included in the metal splint at the distoproximal ends of the right cuspid and left second bicuspid castings were two female precision attachments (Fig. 10-66). The soldered castings with the attachments were fitted in position over the prepared teeth (Fig. 10-67). A wax interocclusal record of centric relation and a full arch maxillary plaster index were taken. The completed prosthesis included the completely processed six teeth (porcelain over gold), the scalloped templates with male precision attachments, and the two superstructures, processed in porcelain over metal (Fig. 10-68). The bilateral templates were attached to the anterior quadrant of teeth by the male attachments fitting into the female attachments, while the superstructures were easily fitted into position over the templates (Fig. 10-69).

The anterior restoration was cemented over the prepared abutment teeth with hard cement, and the two templates with holes for the triplant pins were placed into their correct positions (Fig. 10-70).

Pin implants were driven through the template and then locked with acrylic (Fig. 10-71). The superstructures were then cemented into position over the templates with soft cement (Fig. 10-72). By using soft cement, the superstructure need be removed only by tapping with a crown and bridge remover. A Panorex of the completed case appears in Fig. 10-73.

The precision attachments can be attached in a different manner, if desired. Instead of designing the prosthesis so that the template, or templates, is separate from the anterior quadrant of teeth, the template can be made a rigid part of the anterior quadrant by soldering it directly to the last abutment crown. However, the female precision attachment is also soldered on the distoproximal surface of the last crown so that it rests on the most anterior portion of the template (Fig. 10-74).

Case 9
Bilateral restorations when anterior teeth have been previously restored with fixed bridgework

To utilize a preexisting splint for the support of implants, the following procedures may be used. In this case, the patient had a seven-unit anterior porce-

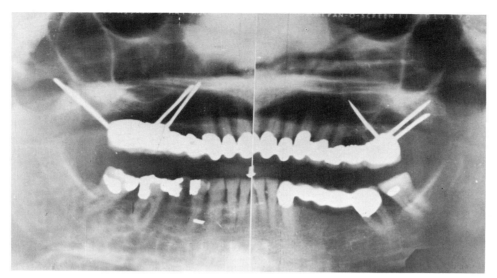

Fig. 10-73. A Panorex of the completed case.

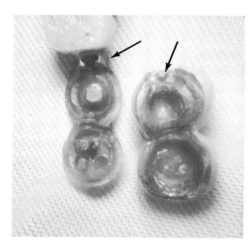

Fig. 10-74. Another case shows the female precision attachment soldered distally to the last abutment porcelain crown. The template extends distally to attachment. The superstructure with its male attachment is also seen. Arrows point to male and female precision attachments.

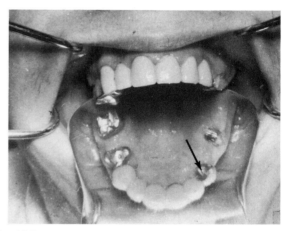

Fig. 10-75. An anterior porcelain-baked-to-metal fixed partial denture existed prior to implant insertions. In order not to have to destroy the bridge, an atypical inlay preparation (arrow) was accomplished on the upper left cuspid crown.

lain-baked-to-metal bridge (Fig. 10-75). The right side was restored conventionally, but implants were needed in the left as posterior abutments.

To prepare for the implant-supported restoration, the left cuspid casting was prepared for an atypical Class II inlay preparation with a fairly deep lingual shoulder, the location of which was determined by the contour of the gold crown in the area. (It was not necessary in this case to make this in the gingival third of the crown. Also, if possible, a few parallel vertical pits may be drilled through the occlusal

pulpal floor of the Class II preparation.) Caution was necessary while preparing the previously made crown to prevent exposing the pulp chamber of the tooth.

An accurate impression of the inlay preparation was taken and the inlay fabricated. The impression also included the entire edentulous area for the fabrication of a temporary acrylic splint.

On the second visit, the inlay was tried in the prepared cuspid crown restoration. After checking for accurate fit, it was removed and the implants

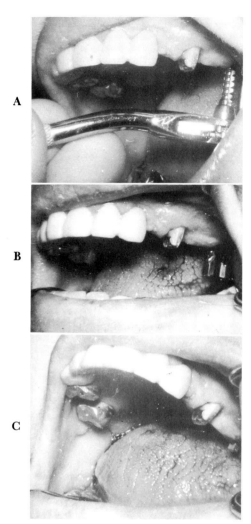

Fig. 10-76. A, Since the earlier spiral type implants were used at that time, the bone was prepared with taps. **B,** Both taps should be parallel to each other and to the anterior abutment tooth. **C,** The implants were then screwed into position.

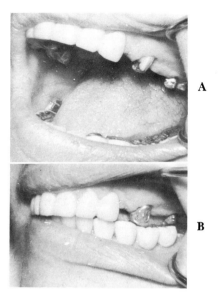

Fig. 10-77. A, Gold copings (prefabricated) were placed over the protruding implant shafts. **B,** The veneer casting was fitted over the bicuspid tooth preparation.

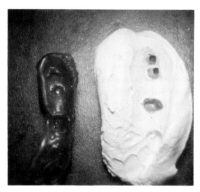

Fig. 10-78. A wax interocclusal record of centric relation and a silicone index were taken.

were inserted into the edentulous area (Fig. 10-76).

The inlay was replaced and prefabricated gold copings were placed over the implant shafts, making sure that neither the inlay nor the gold copings interfered with centric occlusion (Fig. 10-77).

A wax interocclusal record of centric relation and silicone index were taken (Fig. 10-78), and the temporary splint was placed in the mouth. The master stone model was poured from the impressions (Fig. 10-79) and the fixed partial denture com-

pleted. The prefabricated gold copings could have been used only as transfer copings or as the framework for the restorations, using the double casting technique.

On the third visit, the required radiographs of the bridge in place before final cementation were taken. Then the bridge was cemented with hard cement, using the anterior inlay preparation and the posterior implants as the abutments (Fig. 10-80).

Six years later a Panorex shows the spiral posts in the maxillary molar area (Fig. 10-81).

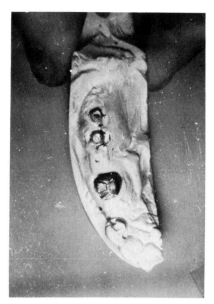

Fig. 10-79. The master model shows the veneer casting, implant copings, and the atypical inlay preparation made on the existing cuspid crown.

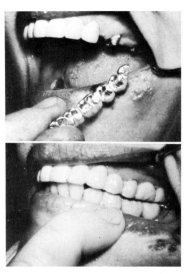

Fig. 10-80. The completed prosthesis with its anterior inlay preparation was cemented into position.

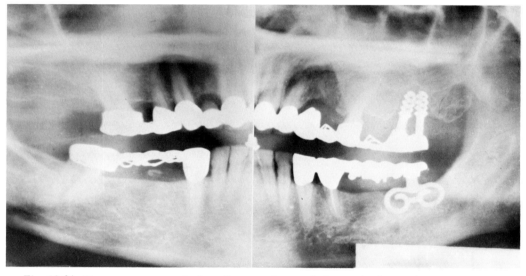

Fig. 10-81. Six years postoperatively, a Panorex shows spiral posts in the maxillary molar area. In spite of the fact that the screws were placed too close to one another and the solid shafts were never buried in bone, the patient is still able to masticate with no discomfort. A blade was placed 1 year prior to x-ray of lower left side.

Case 10
A full arch splint for bilateral free-end saddle areas using spiral-shaft implants and a temporary splint

An important decision in planning restorations for a bilaterally edentulous maxilla is whether to include all the implants in one complete full arch splint or to fabricate two unilateral fixed partial dentures instead.

The choice should be based upon the number of teeth remaining and their condition. Generally, however a full arch splint is preferable when both posterior quadrants are edentulous. The following case illustrates the procedure using spiral-post implants.

Radiographs of the edentulous areas were taken. For more accurate definition of the septal floors of the sinus, good intraoral roentgenograms are pref-

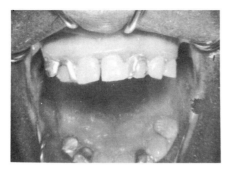

Fig. 10-82. Posteriorly, teeth were absent.

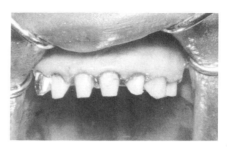

Fig. 10-83. The remaining teeth were prepared for full coverage restorations.

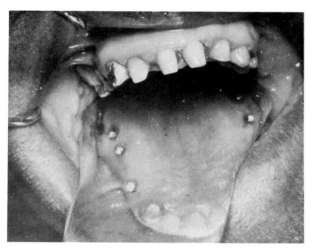

Fig. 10-84. Spiral-post implants were placed in both posterior quadrants, avoiding the maxillary sinus.

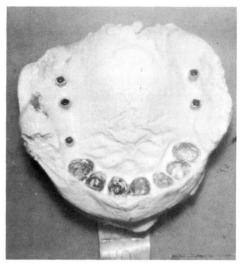

Fig. 10-85. Castings were made for the teeth and copings for the implants. All were picked up with a plaster index.

erable to extraoral ones. Better still is the long cone paralleling technique using super-speed, intraoral films. From radiographic interpretation and the number and spread of the roots of the remaining abutment teeth, the types of implants to be used can be determined.

Because both posterior quadrants were edentulous and the remaining teeth in poor condition (Fig. 10-82), all the teeth were prepared (Fig. 10-83). Impressions for their castings were taken. For the fabrication of a temporary full arch splint, a full mouth elastic impression, a lower full jaw alginate impression, and an accurate wax interocclusal record of centric relation were also made.

At the second visit, the temporary acrylic splint was tried in the mouth. It fit accurately at the gingival marginal areas of the natural tooth abutments, as well as passively against the mucoperiosteal tissue

in the free-end saddles. The occlusion was articulated and balanced. The splint was then removed from the mouth and the gold castings tried for accuracy in fit and occlusion. An accurate full mouth, wax interocclusal record of centric relation with the castings in place was made, followed by a full mouth plaster index. The master stone model with the castings was then articulated and the castings soldered to each other.

At the beginning of the next visit, the soldered gold splint was tried in the mouth. When everything was satisfactory, the patient was ready for implant interventions.

Five spiral-post implants were inserted one by one (Fig. 10-84). The soldered gold castings were placed back on the anterior teeth, and interchangeable gold castings were placed over the implant shafts. A wax interocclusal record of centric relation

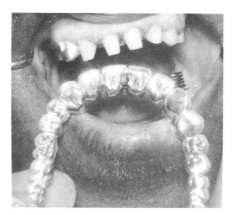

Fig. 10-86. The completed full arch fixed denture is cemented in with hard cement.

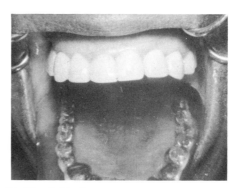

Fig. 10-87. The finished case.

and a plaster index of the entire maxilla were again taken (Fig. 10-85).

The master stone model was poured and both arches articulated on an articulator. The upper full arch splint was fabricated. Because this patient's bite was too strong for porcelain, an acrylic-and-gold veneer type bridge was chosen.

At the next visit, the temporary acrylic splint was carefully removed, and the completed prosthesis was tried (Fig. 10-86). After checking articulation and gingival adaptation, the prosthesis was cemented in position with hard cement (Fig. 10-87).

A lateral plate x-ray reveals the maxillary implants as well as the remaining abutment teeth and bridge (Fig. 10-88). Notice that two unilateral fixed partial dentures with posterior implants also exist in the mandible.

THE PARTIALLY EDENTULOUS MAXILLA

The major problems in planning a restoration for a partially edentulous maxilla are the anatomic configurations and the condition of the remaining teeth. The structure of the bone and the length of the gap between the teeth help determine the type, number, and most advantageous location of the implants. The state of the remaining teeth helps determine whether or not the bridgework will consist of one or more sections. The following cases illustrate some of the ways in which spiral-post implants and triplants have been used as abutments for restorations.

Case 11

A full arch splint for a partially edentulous maxilla using non–self-tapping vent-plants

Here vent-plants of an early design were used. These were too long between the apical ring and the

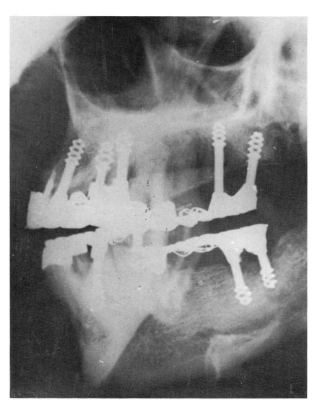

Fig. 10-88. A lateral plate x-ray reveals lower as well as upper implants.

last thread, leaving the broadest part of the implant too close to the alveolar crest. They were non–self-tapping, made of tantalum—which is heavy—and almost entirely hand-fashioned. Because of too many adverse characteristics, these have been discarded in favor of the more successful, modern, self-tapping vent-plants. However, despite the flaws of these early

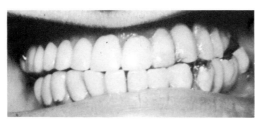

Fig. 10-89. Existing bridges revealed lack of occlusion as a result of extreme mobility of existing abutment teeth.

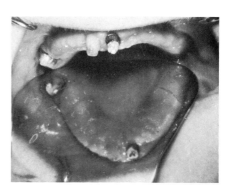

Fig. 10-90. Three upper teeth were saved.

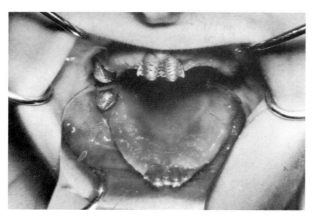

Fig. 10-91. Gold castings were fabricated and fitted.

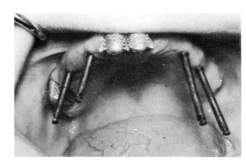

Fig. 10-92. The various sized burs were used to perforate the osseous structures prior to the implant insertions.

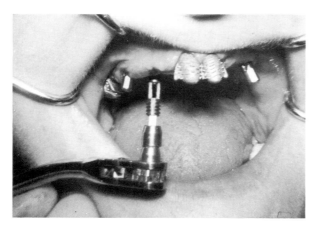

Fig. 10-93. The earliest type of tantalum vent-plants (non-self-tapping) were then screwed into the holes made by the burs and taps.

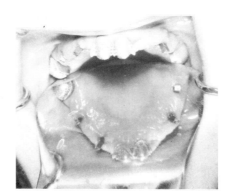

Fig. 10-94. The implants in place.

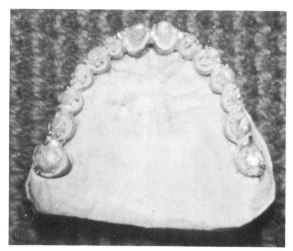

Fig. 10-95. The gold framework was cast and designed for acrylic restorations.

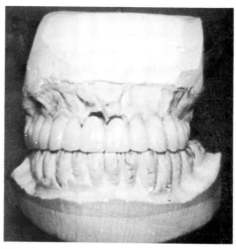

Fig. 10-96. The completed acrylic-over-gold prosthesis.

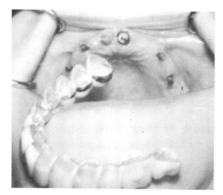

Fig. 10-97. The prosthesis is fitted.

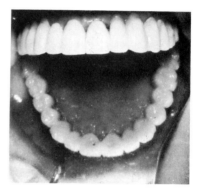

Fig. 10-98. The prosthesis is cemented with hard cement.

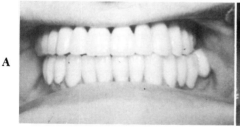
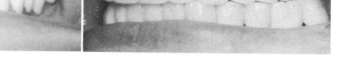

Fig. 10-99. A, The lower jaw was also restored. B, The articulation was carefully balanced.

vent-plants, this case has been functioning for 6 years to date.

The patient, a woman in her early fifties, had completely collapsed upper and lower arches. Her old bridges were made in three sections. Her remaining teeth had loosened to such an extent that every time she would bite, both posterior quadrants

of bridgework would flare out buccally while her upper and lower anterior quadrants would collapse labially (Fig. 10-89).

The three remaining upper teeth that were saved included two central incisors and an upper right second molar. These teeth were prepared for full crown coverage (Fig. 10-90). All necessary impres-

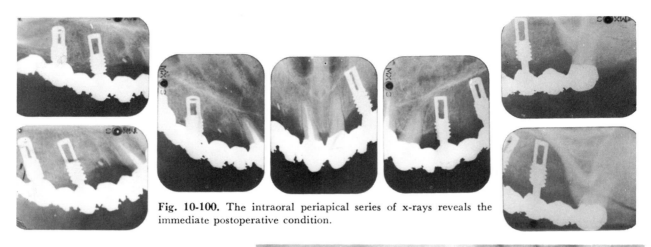

Fig. 10-100. The intraoral periapical series of x-rays reveals the immediate postoperative condition.

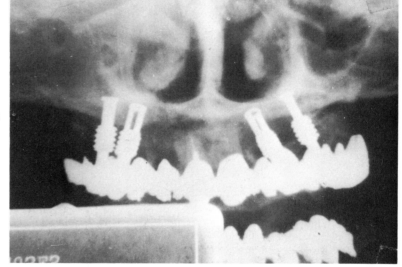

Fig. 10-101. A posteroanterior roentgenogram of the completed case.

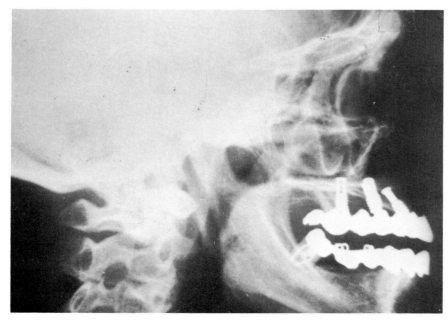

Fig. 10-102. A lateral head roentgenogram.

sions and bite registrations were taken so that three castings could be fabricated to fit over the remaining teeth (Fig. 10-91).

Because the lower teeth could interfere with the proper angulation of a straight handpiece and cause the bur to perforate the palate, a contra-angle was used. Spear-point burs were first used to penetrate the mucosa, submucosa, and superficial alveolar bone. These were followed by various sized helical burs (Fig. 10-92). The tantalum vent-plants, which were non–self-tapping, were then screwed into holes made

in the bone by specially designed and sized taps (Fig. 10-93).

After all the vent-plants had been inserted (Fig. 10-94), a wax interocclusal record of centric relationship and a full maxillary plaster index including the three copings and impressions of the implant shafts were taken. Duplicate shafts were set inside the plaster index, and the master stone model was poured and articulated with the lower cast. The gold framework was then completed in one segment (Fig. 10-95), and the acrylic teeth were processed to the gold (Fig. 10-96).

At the next visit, the upper full arch splint was tried in the mouth (Fig. 10-97) and cemented with oxyphosphate of zinc cement (Fig. 10-98). The lower full arch splint was also processed and cemented (Fig. 10-99).

Immediate postoperative radiographs included intraoral periapical radiographs (Fig. 10-100), a posteroanterior roentgenogram (Fig. 10-101), a lateral head roentgenogram (Fig. 10-102), and a cross-sectional occlusal film (Fig. 10-103).

A 6-year postoperative Panorex film reveals some areas of bone resorption caused specifically by the improper architectural design in these early models. However, no pain or mobility exists and the patient is extremely happy (Fig. 10-104).

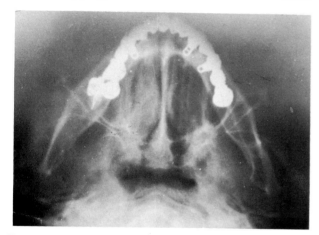

Fig. 10-103. A cross-sectional occlusal film.

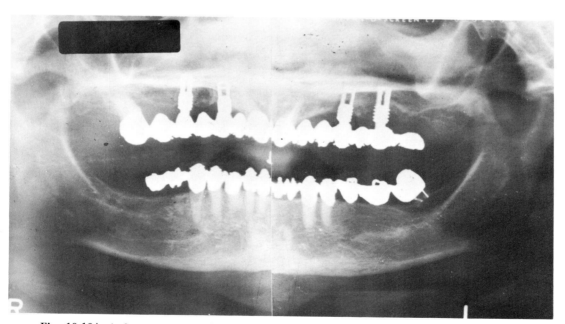

Fig. 10-104. A 6-year postoperative Panorex roentgenogram reveals some bone loss resulting mainly from the earlier improperly designed vent-plants.

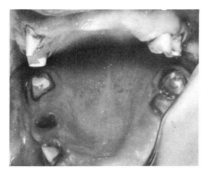

Fig. 10-105. The remaining teeth were prepared.

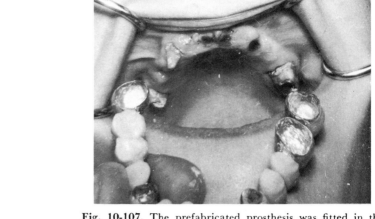

Fig. 10-107. The prefabricated prosthesis was fitted in the mouth and indelible pencil marks were used on the fibro-mucosal tissue in the areas where the implants would be inserted. These markings were transferred to the tissue-bearing surfaces of the pontics, at which time large holes were made through the restorations to accommodate the implant shafts.

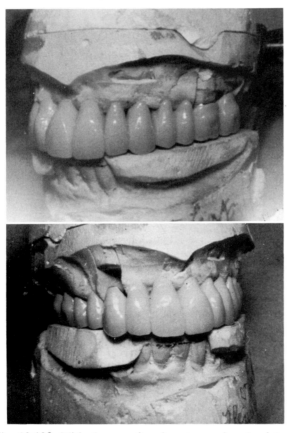

Fig. 10-106. With the use of various types of occlusal templates, the occlusal planes of both posterior quadrants of the full arch fixed denture were fabricated to be geometrically parallel to one another.

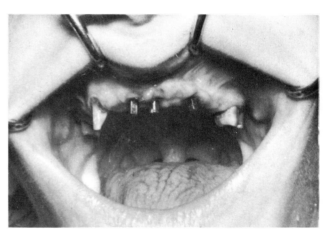

Fig. 10-108. The implants were set properly into the bone.

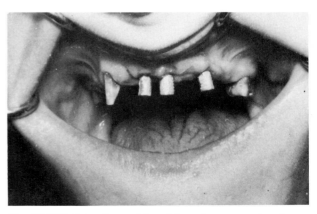

Fig. 10-109. Interchangeable gold copings were placed over the implants.

Case 12
A full arch restoration for long edentulous spans using a prefabricated fixed denture

Not only do implants splinted to remaining natural teeth in a full arch denture help stabilize the prosthesis, they also reduce the vertical and lateral loads on the teeth themselves. In this case, a woman in her late forties was edentulous from the right cuspid to the left second bicuspid. Her remaining teeth were prepared for full crown restorations (Fig. 10-105).

A prefabricated full arch fixed denture was made (Fig. 10-106). With an indelible pencil, the areas determined by x-ray for implant insertion were marked on the fibromucosal tissue (Fig. 10-107). The marks were then transferred to the pontics, which were hollowed out to receive the implant abutments. Post type implants were then inserted (Fig. 10-108).

Interchangeable gold copings were placed over the implants (Fig. 10-109) and picked up with acrylic placed inside the holes of the corresponding pontics (Fig. 10-110). After the acrylic had been

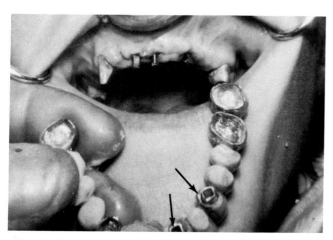

Fig. 10-110. By placing cold cure acrylic inside the openings made in the pontics, seating the bridge, and allowing the acrylic to harden, the copings *(arrows)* become an integral part of the bridge.

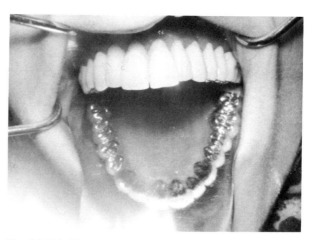

Fig. 10-111. The prosthesis was cemented with oxyphosphate of zinc cement.

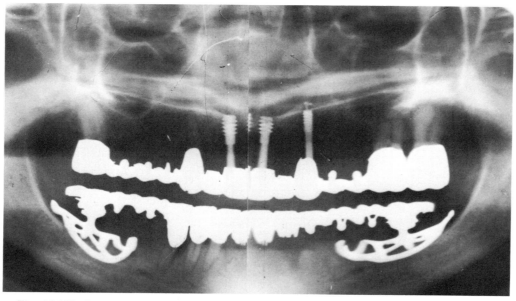

Fig. 10-112. Panorex of completed case. Bilateral subperiosteal implants are seen in the mandible 4 years after their insertion.

trimmed and polished, the final prosthesis was affixed with hard cement (Fig. 10-111). Fig. 10-112 is a Panorex of the completed case.

Case 13
A prefabricated full arch splint for a partially edentulous maxilla using the coping "pick-up" technique

Interchangeable gold copings can act only as transfer copings if desired. Duplicate shafts may be placed into the copings while they are still in the plaster index. The master stone model is poured and

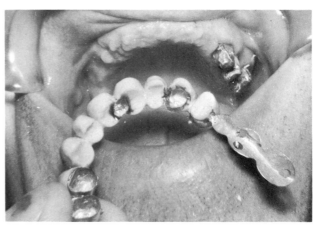

Fig. 10-115. Holes are made through some of the pontics and marked with indelible pencil, and the bridge is seated.

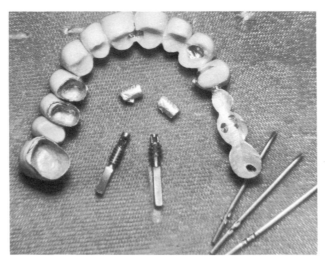

Fig. 10-113. A prefabricated full arch acrylic-veneer-and-gold prosthesis is shown with the vent-plants and triplant pins that are to be used for its support. Also seen are interchangeable gold copings.

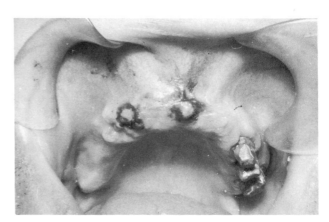

Fig. 10-116. The pencil markings are transferred to the fibromucosal tissue.

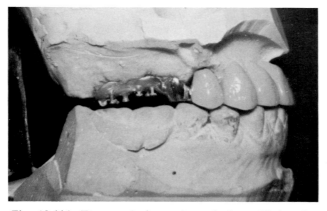

Fig. 10-114. The prosthesis on the articulator. Notice the "vertical mushroom pin heads" extending from the template.

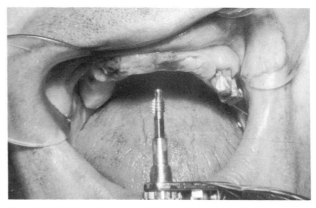

Fig. 10-117. One by one each vent-plant is carefully screwed into its proper location.

the copings are then removed, exposing the duplicate shafts onto which new castings are made. Or the gold copings may be used as a base for the wax-ups of properly contoured crowns that will be double-cast to the copings. A case in point shows a prefabricated maxillary, full arch denture with some of its vent-plants and triplants (Fig. 10-113). The scalloped template is distal to the upper right first bicuspid (Fig. 10-114).

The bridge was seated in the mouth and all necessary adjustments accomplished. To determine the final location of the implants, periapical radiographs of the entire maxilla were taken with the bridge in place. Indelible pencil was used on the tissue-bearing surfaces of the pontics intended to house the implants (Fig. 10-115). The marks were transferred to the fibromucosal tissue by firmly pressing the prosthesis against the gums (Fig. 10-116). At this point holes were also made in the template to accommodate the pin implants.

The implants were then inserted deep into the bone, using the indelible pencil marks as starting guides (Fig. 10-117). As each implant was inserted, the tissue-bearing surfaces of its pontic were hollowed out. For easy fit, each hole was made much larger than its corresponding implant shaft.

Interchangeable prefabricated gold copings were seated over the protruding implant shafts (Fig. 10-118) and the bridge reseated and checked for impingement. Cold cure acrylic was then added to the hollowed-out pontics and the bridge reseated. After the acrylic hardened, the bridge was removed with the gold copings locked inside the pontics. All excess acrylic was trimmed away and polished. The full arch splint was then cemented in with a hard type of cement (Fig. 10-119).

After the bridge was cemented, the triplants were driven through the template (Fig. 10-120). Their heads were fused together with acrylic (Fig. 10-121)

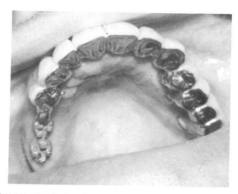

Fig. 10-119. With hard cement the prosthesis is cemented over the teeth and implant abutments.

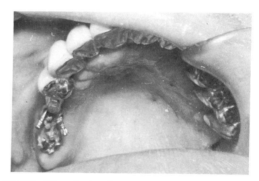

Fig. 10-120. The pin implants are driven through the template.

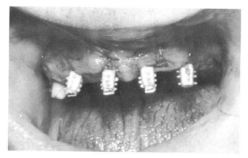

Fig. 10-118. Interchangeable gold copings are placed over the protruding implant shafts.

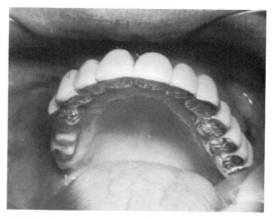

Fig. 10-121. The pins are affixed to each other with acrylic resin and the hardened cores are prepared for crown preparations.

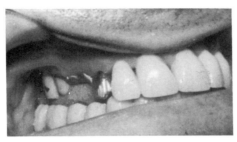

Fig. 10-122. Occlusally, the acrylic cores should be cut short enough to allow room for full crown restorations.

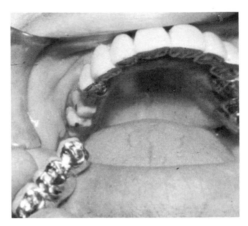

Fig. 10-123. The superstructure is cemented over the template.

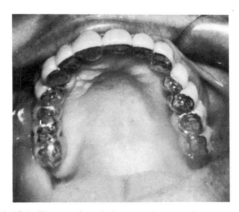

Fig. 10-124. The entire full arch denture is seen.

and the cores prepared and checked to avoid interference with occlusion (Fig. 10-122).

A rubber base impression of the posterior area with the prepared acrylic cores and the vertical gold post extending from the template was then taken with the necessary wax bite. Finally, at the next visit, the small unilateral fixed partial denture was cemented over the vertical gold post and acrylic cores (Fig. 10-123). It thus became an integral part of

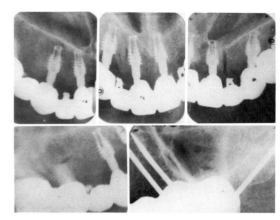

Fig. 10-125. Intraoral radiographs of the vent-plants and triplant case are seen.

the full arch splint (Fig. 10-124). Intraoral radiographs show the implants in place (Fig. 10-125).

Case 14
A full arch restoration for long edentulous spans using the template technique

Whether or not a template is used to span the gaps between natural tooth abutments depends on a number of influencing factors: the firmness of the fibromucosa, the degree of support provided by the bone around the abutment teeth, the periodontal condition, conditions in the opposing arch, and the patient's habits, including bruxism and oral hygiene.

When abutment teeth are weak for any reason and screws or pin implants are to be used, the template should be included as part of the prosthesis. When the fibromucosa is flabby and thick, it must be removed before a template is used. When triplants and, usually, internally threaded implants are used, a template is necessary. This is never necessary when using blade implants. Templates have been frequently criticized by periodontists as well as dentists practicing general dentistry, who claim that they irritate the soft tissues. Linkow has removed many fixed free-end saddles done by other dentists, some of which were in the mouth longer than 10 years. He has never seen any inflammatory reactions of the soft tissues. Isikovitz from Sweden has done hundreds of superplants with the same results.

On the first visit of this patient, the remaining teeth were prepared for full crown restorations and impressions for the castings were taken. Ideally, in maxillary cases, gold copings for the fabrication of full coverage acrylic restorations are preferred be-

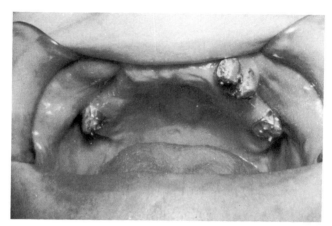

Fig. 10-126. Gold castings are designed to support acrylic teeth.

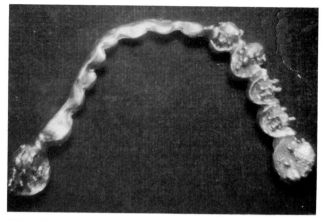

Fig. 10-128. A scalloped template that encompasses the large edentulous area is soldered to the remaining copings.

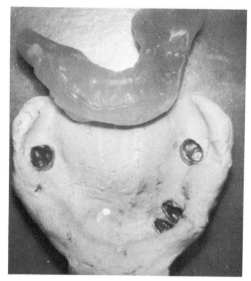

Fig. 10-127. A wax interocclusal record of centric relation and a plaster index are taken.

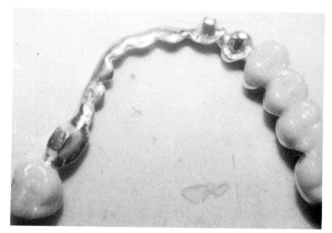

Fig. 10-129. Acrylic teeth are processed to the crown copings.

cause gold is lightweight, a considerable help when few abutment teeth are present. A wax bite and opposing jaw impression were taken, and the master model was poured in stone and articulated.

On the second visit, the castings were fitted over the remaining natural tooth abutments (Fig. 10-126). An accurate wax interocclusal record of centric relation and a plaster index of the entire arch were taken (Fig. 10-127). The template was waxed, cast, and soldered to the copings (Fig. 10-128). Acrylic full crown restorations were processed over the copings (Fig. 10-129).

At the next visit, the substructure was tried in the mouth (Fig. 10-130). Radiographs of the edentulous bone area along the entire region of the tem-

plate were taken. The template acted as a landmark for angulating the pins to avoid the nasal vestibulum and maxillary sinus. From the radiography, the series of holes for the triplants was determined; these holes were then drilled into the template outside the mouth.

The template was fixed in the mouth by cementing the acrylic-over-gold crowns over the tooth abutments with hard cement. The triplant pins were driven through the template (Fig. 10-131) and their ends notched and shortened to the proper intermaxillary occlusal lengths.

The ends were built up with acrylic cores, and the hardened cores were prepared for full crown restorations (Fig. 10-132). A rubber base impression

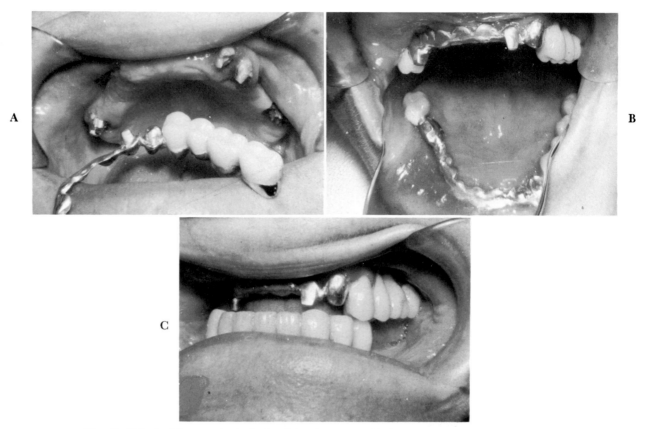

Fig. 10-130. A, The prosthesis is fitted in the mouth. B, The cemented prosthesis. C, The occlusion is carefully equilibrated.

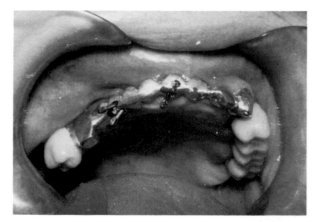

Fig. 10-131. Pin implants are slowly and carefully drilled through the previously prepared holes in the template.

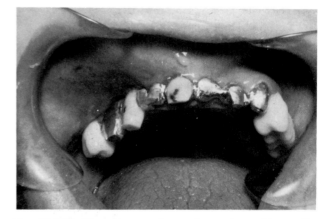

Fig. 10-132. The pins are fastened together with acrylic cores and the hardened cores are prepared for full crown restorations.

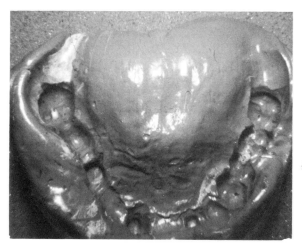

Fig. 10-133. A full arch rubber base impression is taken.

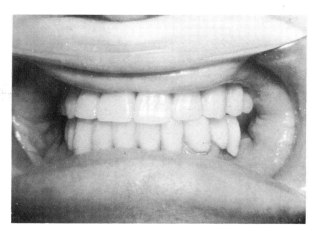

Fig. 10-134. The completed prosthesis.

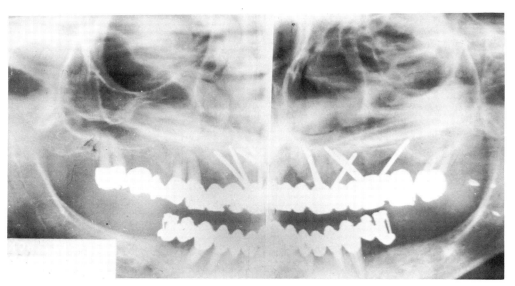

Fig. 10-135. Panorex showing pins crossing through template into bone. In these early cases teeth with infrabony pockets were sometimes retained (if they were not mobile) to offer support to the pins.

of the entire arch was taken (Fig. 10-133), as well as a wax interocclusal record of centric relation.

A one-piece, final fixed splint was fabricated from the master model and cemented permanently over the substructure (Fig. 10-134).

A Panorex of the completed case reveals the pins inserted through the template into bone (Fig. 10-135). Sometimes, as in this case, infrabony pocket reduction is done after the entire case is completed. Otherwise, the few remaining teeth, if previously treated periodontally, might not have enough hard

or soft tissue attachment left to maintain them long enough for the completion of a prefabricated prosthesis.

Case 15
A full arch restoration for a partially edentulous maxilla using internally threaded vent-plants and a template

The patient, a woman in her early fifties, had only three teeth remaining in her upper arch and all three were on the right side: a lateral, cuspid, and first bicuspid. The patient wore a removable pros-

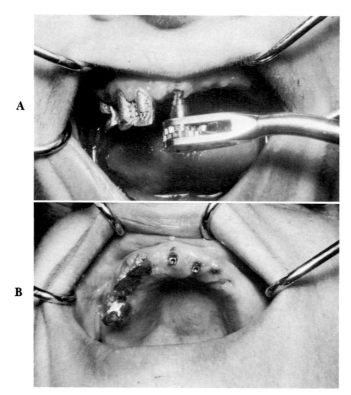

Fig. 10-136. A, A ratchet is used to screw in the vent-plant. Only three existing teeth prevail. **B,** Two internally threaded vent-plants are set into the bone. Their shafts barely extend out of the fibromucosal tissue.

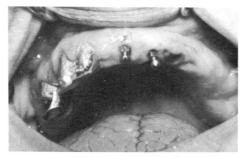

Fig. 10-137. Threadless screws are attached inside the internally threaded vent-plants with sticky wax.

thesis that constantly irritated her fibromucosal tissue, which became progressively thicker as the underlying alveolar bone resorbed.

The patient's jaw was carefully evaluated by x-ray studies, and internally threaded implants were chosen for the anterior implants and triplants for the posterior areas.

Because internally threaded vent-plants were to be used, they had to be inserted before the impression for the template was taken (Fig. 10-136). The

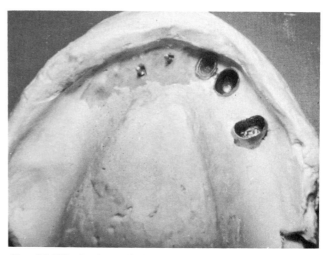

Fig. 10-138. A plaster index is taken picking up the three castings and the two threadless screws. Interchangeable implant shafts are placed inside the index and attached to the two threadless screws with wax.

threads of the set screws were trimmed away so that the screws could be easily inserted into and pulled out of the implants. Sticky wax was applied to the threadless screws, and they were set inside the implants with their heads protruding about 4 mm. (Fig. 10-137).

A wax interocclusal record and a plaster index, including the gold veneer crown castings and impressions of the implant shafts with their protruding screws, were taken. The set screws are used to facilitate laboratory procedures (Fig. 10-138). If the screws are to be used only to fasten the template to the implants, vertical posts to act as supporting pontics for the final prosthesis must also be included in the wax-up. Obviously, if the screws are to pass through the superstructure crowns down into the implants, the vertical posts are not needed.

The template was cast in gold and soldered to the veneer crown castings. The castings were then processed with acrylic facings. The finished substructure included the processed veneer crowns soldered together, the gold template attached to the crowns, and holes in the template corresponding to the hollow implant shafts that would allow passage of the set screws. A temporary acrylic splint was also fabricated at this time (Fig. 10-139).

The substructure was then placed in the mouth and the bite adjusted on the right side, where the soldered veneer crowns existed. The set screws were screwed through the template and into the implants until their heads were flush with the template (Fig.

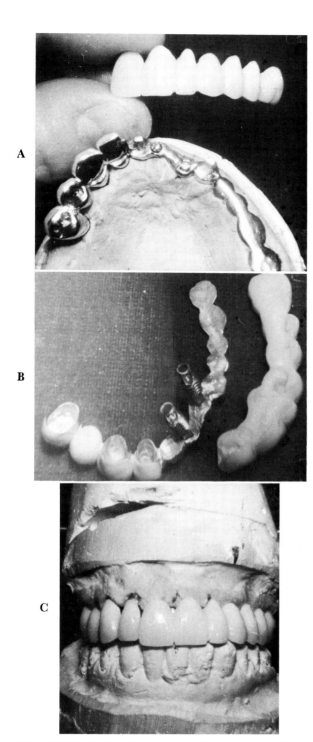

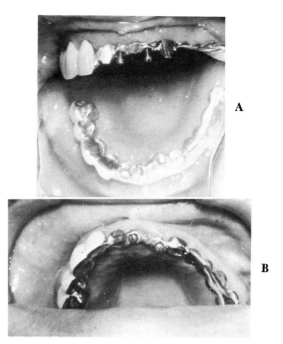

Fig. 10-140. A, The prosthesis is cemented over the three remaining teeth on the right side and the template is further secured with the set screws engaging the implants. **B,** The screws fit flush with the template.

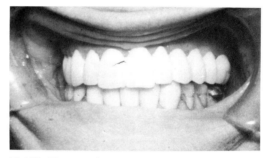

Fig. 10-141. The acrylic splint is temporarily cemented over the template.

Fig. 10-139. A, The first portion of the prosthesis is completed from the master stone model. It includes the scalloped template with two holes to accommodate the small set screws used to secure it to the implants. A temporary acrylic splint is also seen. **B,** Another view of the prosthesis shows how the set screws secure the implants to the template. **C,** The temporary acrylic splint should fit accurately to the template.

10-140). The temporary acrylic splint was also placed in the mouth over the template, and the occlusion was closely checked and adjusted (Fig. 10-141).

Everything was removed, holes were drilled for the triplants, and the substructure was cemented over the teeth with hard cement. The pin implants were then driven through the predetermined holes (Fig. 10-142). Excess length was cut off and the posts were built up with acrylic cores. When the acrylic hardened, the cores were prepared for crown restorations (Fig. 10-143).

The fixed partial denture was completed from

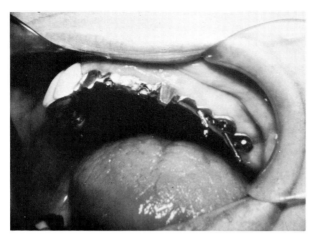

Fig. 10-142. Pin implants are then drilled obliquely through the holes previously made through the template.

the master stone model. The prosthesis, which had a lingual extension to lock into previously prepared deep-seated grooves on the lingual aspect of the upper right lateral and cuspid restorations, was then cemented in the mouth (Fig. 10-144).

A full series of intraoral radiographs is seen in Fig. 10-145. The finished case is shown on a cross-sectional film (Fig. 10-146). Fig. 10-147 compares the differences in bulk and size of the original removable prosthesis and the new fixed partial denture. Esthetically, the original tooth contours were duplicated.

If a removable substructure, as well as a removable superstructure, had been desired for this patient, the following steps would have been taken to construct the template. First, the post type implants would be inserted. Then the copings would be cemented permanently over the abutment teeth

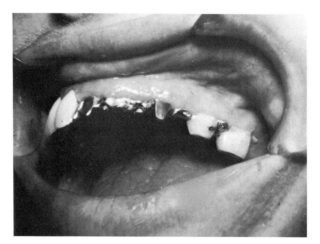

Fig. 10-143. Acrylic liquid and powder are used to lock the pins to each other.

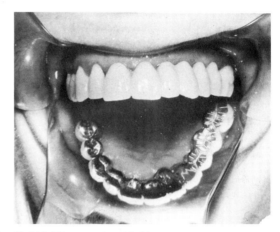

Fig. 10-144. The completed bridge.

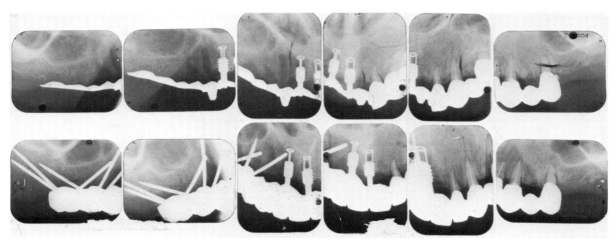

Fig. 10-145. A full series of intraoral radiographs of the completed case.

and another set of copings, with roughened surfaces, would have been cast and fitted over the smooth copings.

After the plaster index is taken and the master model articulated with the model of the opposing jaw, it should contain the roughened gold copings as well as the duplicate implant shafts. The template is then designed with a pencil on the master model. It should extend to the roughened gold copings that are nearest the edentulous space, and it should be scalloped so that it follows the labiolingual and interproximal contours of the tissue-bearing surfaces of the restorations.

The wax template should fit snugly around the duplicate implant shafts that protrude out of the stone model. The wax-up should contain accurate insets for housing the heads of the set screws. This

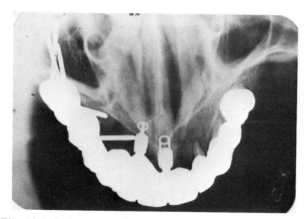

Fig. 10-146. A cross-sectional occlusal film radiograph.

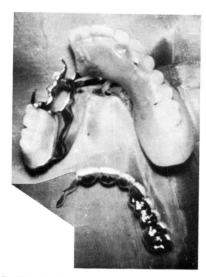

Fig. 10-147. The fixed prosthesis as compared to the large, bulky original removable prosthesis.

is easily accomplished by screwing the set screws through the wax template and into the hollow threaded duplicate implant shafts. By applying a little heat to the wax, a definite seat in it for the screw heads can be determined. The wax-up should also include a thin vertical bar, or strut, along its center buccolingually to act as a strengthening device. The peripheral borders of the wax-up should be rolled to avoid any sharp line angles that would irritate the fibromucosal tissue.

Case 16
A full arch restoration for long edentulous spans using a removable partial denture and template

Sometimes, in order to psychologically satisfy a patient, the dentist must proceed with a completely atypical approach. Of course, this is done only if the results will benefit the patient.

In this case, done over 7 years ago, the patient claimed she was on the verge of committing suicide over her loose-fitting removable denture. Although she was originally advised to have the flabby tissues covering the resorbed alveolar crest around her entire arch removed and to have a new full denture fabricated, she refused adamantly. She was willing to take her chances on obtaining added retention for a removable prosthesis by the use of implants. She agreed to have her excess soft tissue removed, and complete healing took place before the implantation procedure was undertaken.

Only two teeth remained in the maxilla, both of which were second molars with some mobility

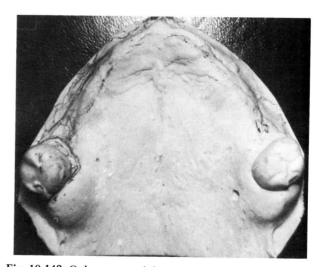

Fig. 10-148. Only two remaining teeth existed.

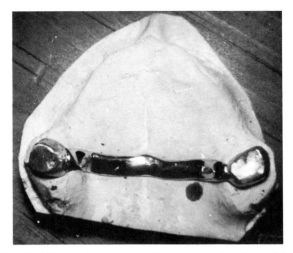

Fig. 10-149. Copings were splinted to each other with a connecting palatal bar.

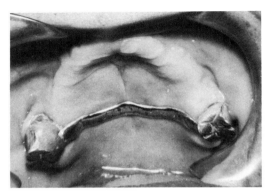

Fig. 10-150. Veneer castings were fabricated to fit over the two copings.

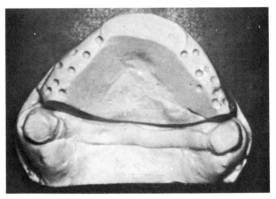

Fig. 10-151. A fast-setting stone bite rim was fabricated to facilitate an accurate interocclusal record of centric relation.

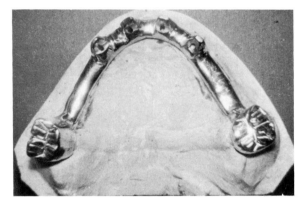

Fig. 10-152. Both veneer castings were connected to one another by means of a gold rigid template. Anteriorly, four protruding posts with internal threadings are seen.

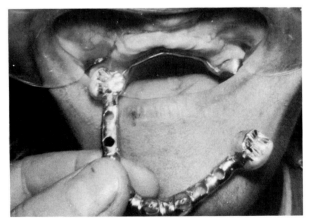

Fig. 10-153. Holes were made through the template for the pin implants.

(Fig. 10-148). To aid retention of these teeth, they were prepared for full crown coverage. Copings were made to fit over them, and then veneer crown castings were fabricated to fit over the copings. The copings were joined together with a wide palatal bar that fitted passively on the termination of the hard palate (Fig. 10-149). This bar was removable by the snapping on and off of female attachments soldered to the lingual surfaces of the copings. The copings and connecting palatal bar were placed over the two prepared molar teeth and cemented with hard cement. The veneer castings were then placed over the copings (Fig. 10-150). Because there was such a long expanse of soft tissue, a quick-setting stone tray was made directly in the mouth to get a more accurate bite. Grooves were cut on the occlusal surface of the stone model (Fig. 10-151), and

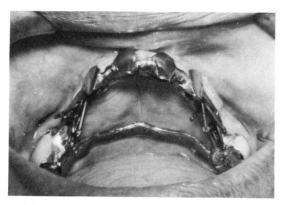

Fig. 10-154. The two crowns were cemented over the two gold copings and then the pin implants were drilled through the openings in the template into the bone.

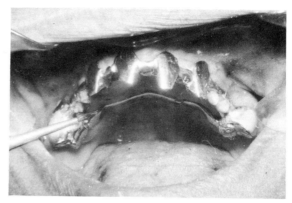

Fig. 10-155. The pins were fastened to one another using acrylic liquid and powder with the brush-on technique.

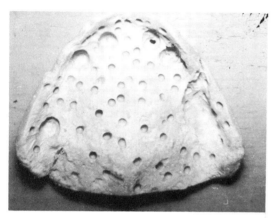

Fig. 10-156. A fast-setting stone impression tray was then made to fit over the restoration.

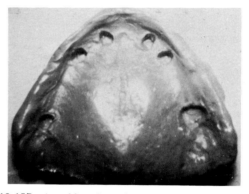

Fig. 10-157. A rubber base impression was taken of the entire maxillary template with the built-up acrylic cores, using the stone tray.

soft wax was placed over it for a wax bite. A plaster index of the entire maxilla, including the veneer castings, was taken.

From the articulated master stone casts, a horse-shoe template was waxed, cast, and then soldered to the polished molar castings. Acrylic facings were processed to the buccal surfaces of the two posterior castings. Anteriorly four vertical pontics, or pivots with internal threadings, were included in the template so that the removable prosthesis could be screwed into position if desired and could be removed only by the dentist (Fig. 10-152).

At the next visit, the template with the soldered veneer crowns was tried in the mouth and radiographed. It was then removed, and holes were drilled through the template in the areas where the pin implants were to be driven (Fig. 10-153).

After making sure that the two posterior crowns were in proper occlusion, the operator placed hard

cement inside them and cemented them over the two copings. All excess cement was removed when it hardened.

Carefully checking with intermittent x-rays, the operator slowly drove pin implants through the template at various angles to avoid the sinus and nasal vestibulum (Fig. 10-154). To avoid occlusal interference, the excess length of the pins was cut off. The terminating ends were then notched with a fissure bur to aid retention when being fused with cold cure acrylic (Fig. 10-155). The acrylic cores, when hardened, were trimmed, prepared, and polished. They were parallel to the anterior gold posts on the template.

Again, a stone model tray was fabricated directly in the mouth, trimmed, and made more retentive by drilling holes across its tissue-bearing surface (Fig. 10-156). It was then painted with Permalastic adhesive to make the rubber base impression of the entire maxilla adhesive to the model (Fig. 10-157).

A two-piece removable palateless denture with lingual set screws was fabricated. The set screws hold the denture securely in place and give the patient more confidence in the appliance. (The screws are not needed if the patient is satisfied without them.)

One of the pieces included processed acrylic teeth and a pink acrylic framework that fit flush with the tissues and gold copings. It was fabricated in order to build out the lips and fill out the face. The other

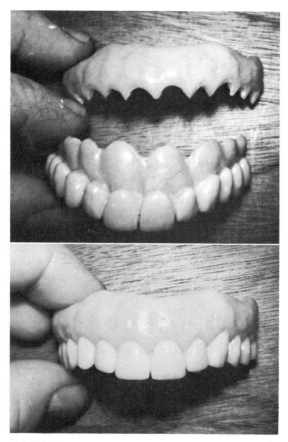

Fig. 10-158. The stent snaps over the underlying acrylic.

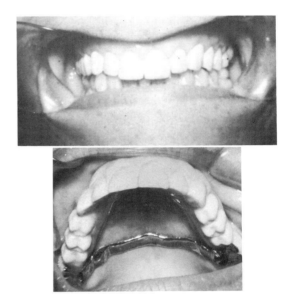

Fig. 10-159. The completed prosthesis in the mouth.

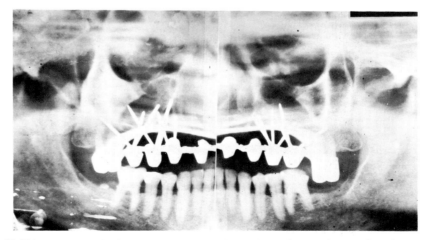

Fig. 10-160. Panorex of pin implants supported by the gold template and both remaining molars.

piece was a pink acrylic "stent" that snapped into place over the underlying pink acrylic framework and was removed by the patient to clean the underlying piece. The processed acrylic teeth were quite a distance below the tissue-bearing surfaces of the pink acrylic, which indicates how much bone has resorbed (Fig. 10-158).

The finished case worked out quite well for the patient, both physically and psychologically (Fig. 10-159). A Panorex of the completed case reveals the pin implants supported by the gold template and both remaining molars (Fig. 10-160).

Case 17
A full arch splint for a partially edentulous maxilla using a template and a one-dimensional triplant

Sometimes, because of anatomic anomalies, it is necessary to insert triplant pins along one plane rather than three. This naturally forms a weaker type of abutment but nevertheless works, providing a rigid full arch splint and template are made to join with the triplant, thus adding a great deal of support. When the operator faces such a situation, he is advised to simplify his problem, and incidentally provide greater security, by using the blade-vent.

This case, done before the invention of the blade-vent, shows a porcelain-baked-to-metal full arch prosthesis and template with superstructure attached. The template's pin holes are in a straight line rather than in the usual triangular or quadrangular configuration (Fig. 10-161).

After all necessary adjustments had been accomplished, the bridge was cemented over the prepared abutment teeth with hard cement (Fig. 10-162). When the cement hardened, all excess was removed.

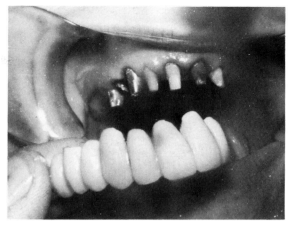

Fig. 10-162. The prosthesis is fitted over the prepared teeth.

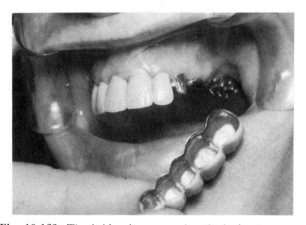

Fig. 10-163. The bridge is cemented and pin implants are drilled through the template.

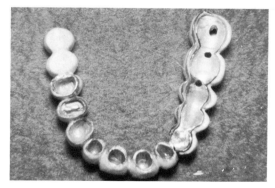

Fig. 10-161. A prefabricated porcelain-baked-to-metal fixed full arch denture including the scalloped template with three parallel holes made through it to accommodate the pins that are to be placed in a knife-edge ridge.

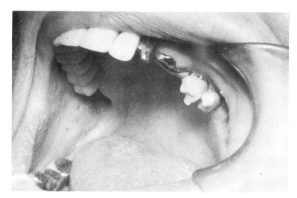

Fig. 10-164. The pins are locked to the template and to each other with acrylic.

The pin implants were driven through the template and the superstructure fitted over the protruding pins (Fig. 10-163). In such a situation, if the superstructure does not seat, the protruding portions of the pins must either be bent within the peripheral margins of the template or be cut shorter.

When the superstructure fitted with no impingement from the pins, the bridge was removed and the pins fused to one another with acrylic (Fig. 10-164). While the acrylic was still soft, the superstructure was fitted into position. Any impingement was caused by the soft acrylic, which was easily removed. When the acrylic hardened, the superstructure was cemented into position. Acrylic was used

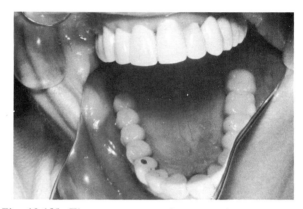

Fig. 10-165. The superstructure is cemented over the template with hard cement.

inside the crowns covering the acrylic cores, and oxyphosphate of zinc cement was used inside the crown that covered the gold coping (Fig. 10-165). Fig. 10-166 is a Panorex of the completed case.

Case 18
A roundhouse restoration using a three-part prosthesis, template, and a triplant

Sometimes, because of inconvenience or inability to parallel all the teeth in an arch as a result of their original positions, it may be beneficial to fabricate the bridgework in three separate sections rather than one. This case illustrates such a situation.

The remaining teeth were prepared (Fig. 10-167) and copings cast (Fig. 10-168). A wax interocclusal record of centric relation was made. An alginate (irreversible hydrocolloid) impression of the lower arch was taken, as well as a maxillary plaster index picking up all of the copings (Fig. 10-169).

From these records the prosthesis was fabricated in three sections (Fig. 10-170). Connecting with the right central and left central and lateral incisors were two copings with posts going into the two corresponding roots (Fig. 10-171). The two unilateral right and left posterior bridges were made to fit over the gold copings anteriorly. The right bridge had a molar crown supported by a molar tooth while the left bridge contained the template for the edentulous area (Fig. 10-172).

The anterior quadrant was cemented into posi-

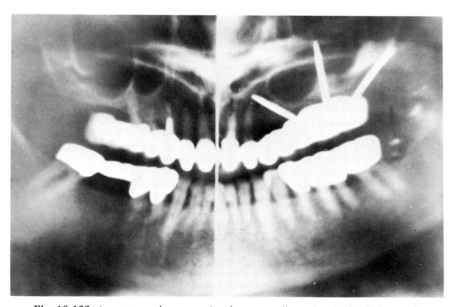

Fig. 10-166. A postoperative x-ray showing a one-dimensional tripodial spread.

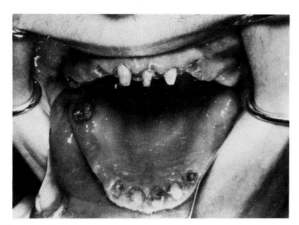

Fig. 10-167. A right central incisor, lateral incisor root, and second molar and a left central and lateral incisor and cuspid root are all that remain.

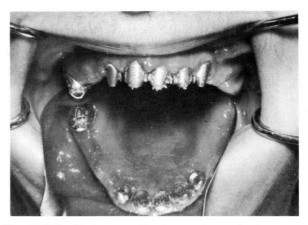

Fig. 10-168. Castings are fitted over the tooth abutments, and smooth-surfaced gold post thimbles are placed into the left cuspid and right lateral incisor roots.

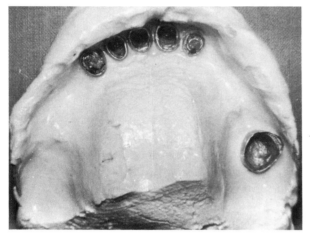

Fig. 10-169. A plaster index is taken.

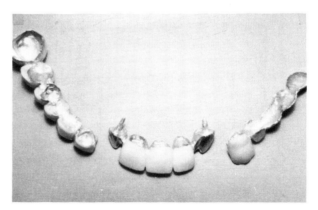

Fig. 10-170. The prosthesis is fabricated in three parts.

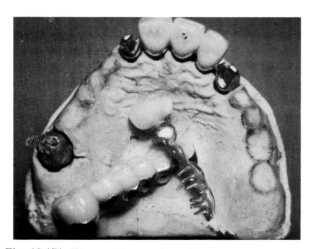

Fig. 10-171. The anterior quadrant includes the left cuspid thimble and the right lateral thimble, while the left posterior quadrant contains the scalloped template.

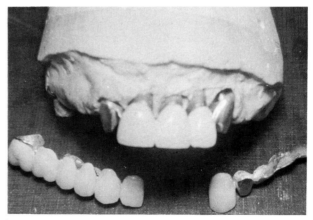

Fig. 10-172. The anterior quadrant seen on the master model and below it are the two posterior superstructures.

tion with hard cement (Fig. 10-173). The right posterior bridge was then cemented into position with hard cement, being supported anteriorly by the gold coping and posteriorly by the prepared molar tooth (Fig. 10-174).

The left quadrant was then cemented into position by placing oxyphosphate of zinc cement in-

side the cuspid crown only (Fig. 10-175). The pin implants were drilled through the template and trimmed (Fig. 10-176), and the pins were then fused with acrylic cores. Sometimes, as in this case, the three pins are fused together with two acrylic cores instead of one because of the influence of the anatomic landmarks on the pin placement. For ex-

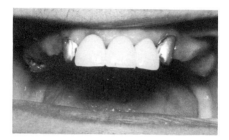

Fig. 10-173. The anterior quadrant is secured to the abutment teeth with oxyphosphate of zinc cement.

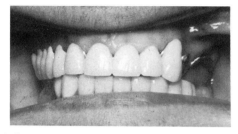

Fig. 10-174. The right posterior quadrant is cemented into position utilizing the lateral incisor thimble and molar tooth preparation as the abutments.

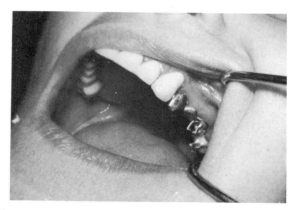

Fig. 10-175. The left posterior quadrant cemented into position.

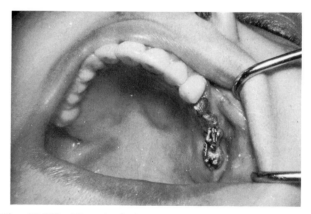

Fig. 10-176. The pin implants are drilled into the bone, passing through the template.

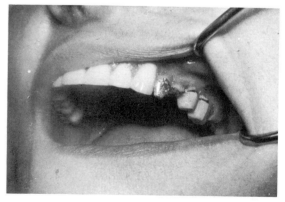

Fig. 10-177. The acrylic cores are built up to affix the pins together. They are then prepared for full crown restorations.

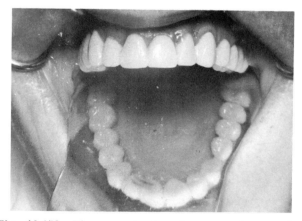

Fig. 10-178. The superstructure is cemented over the template.

ample, in order to avoid a low-flaring sinus floor, a pin may have to be so acutely angled that its protruding end may excessively extend along the template. It thus becomes necessary to make two acrylic cores instead of one in order to follow the contours of the template. In this manner the pins are still locked to one another to form a tripod, even though

one pin may be inside one core while the others are inside the second core. As long as these two cores are joined interproximally, the pins are secure.

When the cores hardened, they were prepared for full coverage restorations (Fig. 10-177). The superstructure was then fitted, adjusted, and cemented into position over the two acrylic cores and gold coping (Fig. 10-178). Fig. 10-179 shows the pins driven through the scalloped template and the superstructure cemented over the acrylic core and gold coping.

Case 19
A full arch prefabricated splint for a partially edentulous maxilla using vent-plants and bilateral triplants

One of the more practical applications of prefabricated splints is that the patient's own dentist can work him up to a point where the implantologist need only insert the implants. Thus a dentist inexperienced in the insertion of implants can do the bridgework construction and follow up, radiographically and clinically, the progress of the implants placed in his patient's mouth. This approach was used successfully on a 53-year-old male patient. His dentist, with guidance from Linkow as to design and articulation, made the prosthesis. The implants were then inserted and adapted to the bridge.

The patient only had two remaining teeth in the maxillary arch, a left central and left cuspid. These were prepared and covered with gold copings by his regular dentist (Fig. 10-180). A prefabricated full arch fixed denture was processed on a Hanau articulator (Fig. 10-181).

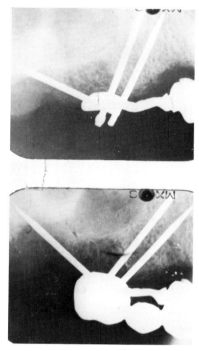

Fig. 10-179. Roentgenograms show the pins drilled through the template and the superstructure cemented over the pins.

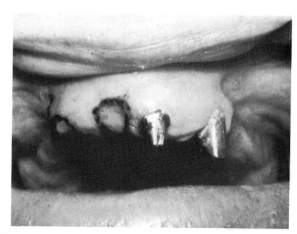

Fig. 10-180. Only two teeth remained in the entire arch.

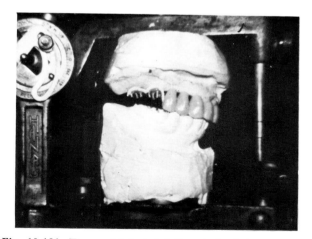

Fig. 10-181. The prefabricated full arch fixed denture was fabricated with the aid of a Hanau articulator.

Because the templates were designed without vertical posts to avoid interference with the acute angulation of the pin implants, the two posterior superstructures had to be affixed to the templates with acrylic rather than cement. The inner surfaces of the superstructures were processed with hundreds of tiny bubbles (Fig. 10-182), which helped lock the acrylic inside the crowns. The superstructures were cast to fit exactly over the templates.

The prosthesis was fitted over the two remaining teeth and, from the radiographs and palpation of the soft tissues, the areas for the vent-plants were reassessed. Only one implant was seated at a time. When proceeding in this manner, it is imperative to

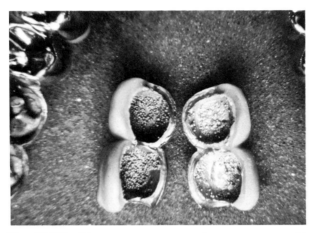

Fig. 10-182. The superstructure castings were cast with "masses" of tiny bubbles in order to secure the acrylic.

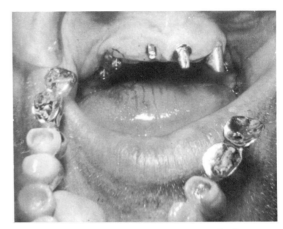

Fig. 10-183. The vent-plants were set into the bone one by one, and the tissue-bearing surfaces of the pontics were opened to accommodate the protruding shafts.

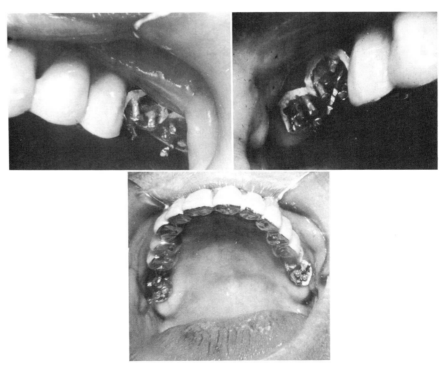

Fig. 10-184. After the bridge was cemented, pin implants were drilled through the template between the vertical mushroom-like pin heads. The ends of the pins were cut short so that they would not interfere with the fit of both superstructures.

try the prosthesis over each implant and to hollow out its corresponding pontic before going on to the next implant.

After all the vent-plants were seated (Fig. 10-183) and the bridge with its hollowed pontics fitted properly over them, the operator had two choices. He could have fashioned acrylic lumens by placing cold cure acrylic within the hollowed pontics and repeatedly seated over Vaseline-covered implant shafts. On the other hand, he could have used interchangeable gold copings over the implant shafts,

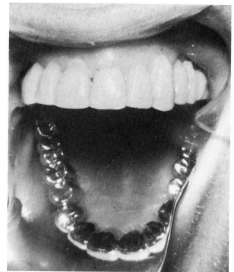

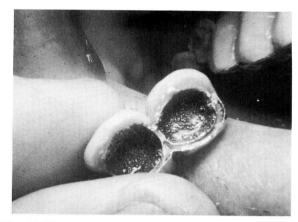

Fig. 10-185. The pins were fastened with acrylic on both sides and the superstructures were cemented over the acrylic cores. In this case, acrylic was used inside the superstructure to secure them.

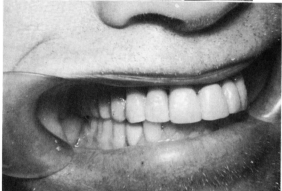

Fig. 10-186. The completed case.

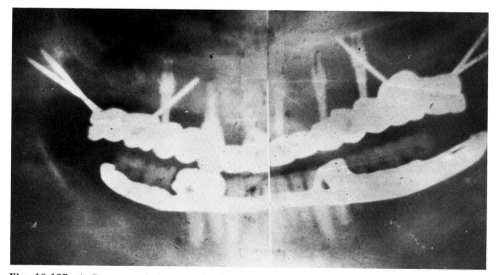

Fig. 10-187. A Panorex of the completed case showing the vent-plants and the tremendous spread of the tripodial pins, which were used to avoid the broad and low-flaring maxillary sinus.

as was done in this case. The gold copings were placed over the implant shafts and the bridge placed over them. Larger hollows were made in the pontics to avoid impingement. Cold cure acrylic was placed inside the hollowed pontics and the bridge set into position, allowing the acrylic to set inside the mouth. The bridge was removed with the gold copings attached to its tissue-bearing surface. All excess acrylic was trimmed and polished, and the bridge was cemented in place with oxyphosphate of zinc cement.

The triplant pins were then drilled through holes previously made in the bilateral posterior templates (Fig. 10-184). The pins were fastened together with a minimum amount of acrylic to avoid impingement from the superstructures, which were cemented with a loose mix of acrylic (Fig. 10-185). The finished prosthesis was thus supported by the two teeth, four vent-plants, and the two triplants (Fig. 10-186). A Panorex radiograph clearly shows the implant's placement (Fig. 10-187).

Case 20
A full arch splint for a partially edentulous maxilla using internally threaded vent-plants with a screw-on superstructure

Sometimes a screw-on type of fixed partial denture may be preferred instead of the routine type of cemented bridge. If such a prosthesis is desired, it is essential to protect remaining natural teeth against future decay with some form of gold copings. These copings, soldered together, will act as a meso-structure, or internal framework, to which the superstructure can be screwed. The screws holding the superstructure to the mesostructure may be placed through the occlusal surfaces of the superstructure or obliquely angled through the superstructure, as in the following case.

A 52-year-old man with an extremely powerful bite had broken a few of the anterior maxillary teeth off his removable partial denture (Fig. 10-188). His remaining teeth showed rampant caries (Fig. 10-189).

Because his cuspid teeth were so far apart, two internally threaded vent-plants were advisable for the central incisor region.

The remaining teeth in the maxillary arch were prepared for full crown restorations, and all necessary plaster indices and a wax interocclusal record of centric relation were taken. From these, acrylic transfer copings were made and fitted in the mouth (Fig. 10-190). These were picked up with a full mouth plaster index (Fig. 10-191), and from pre-

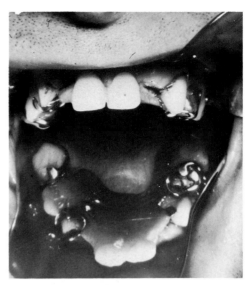

Fig. 10-188. A broken removable partial denture with two lateral incisor teeth missing from it is all that the patient had been wearing.

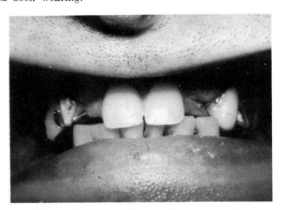

Fig. 10-189. The poor condition of the remaining teeth is clearly evident.

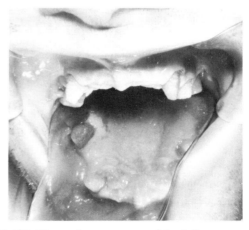

Fig. 10-190. The teeth were prepared for full crown restorations, and acrylic transfer copings were fitted over them.

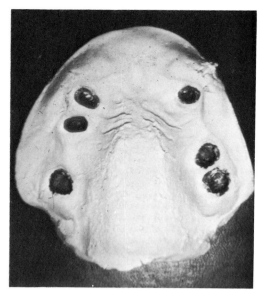

Fig. 10-191. A plaster index was taken, picking up all of the copings.

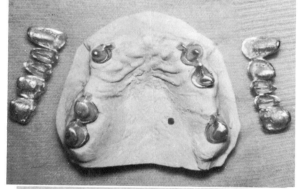

A

B

Fig. 10-192. A, Two mesostructures are seen on the master stone model. Flanking the mesostructures are the two cast superstructures. B, The superstructures are fitted over the mesostructures.

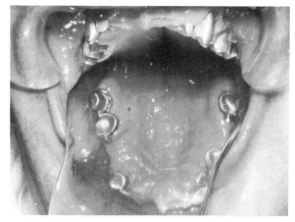

Fig. 10-193. The mesostructures are fitted in the mouth over the prepared teeth.

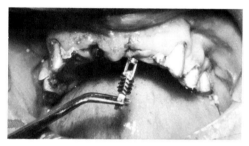

Fig. 10-194. Internally threaded vent-plants are screwed into the incisor regions.

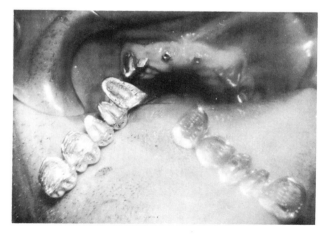

Fig. 10-195. The superstructures are fitted over the mesostructures for the final impression, which was taken 1 week after the implants were inserted.

viously taken wax occlusal records and opposing jaw impressions the master stone model was articulated. A gold mesostructure consisting of smooth surfaced copings with high interproximal solder walls and veneer crown superstructures were cast (Fig. 10-192).

At the next visit, the copings comprising the mesostructure were fitted over the prepared abutment teeth (Fig. 10-193). Two internally threaded ventplants were then screwed into the right and left maxillary central incisor regions until only about 1 mm. of their shafts protruded out of the fibromucosal tissue (Fig. 10-194). The veneer crown superstructures were then placed over the mesostructures (Fig. 10-195) and a wax interocclusal record of centric relation and a full mouth plaster index were taken(Fig. 10-196).

The master stone model was then made. Duplicate internally threaded implant posts were used as part of the mesostructure framework for the completion of the superstructure (Fig. 10-197). Obliquely-set channels were made in various strategically located portions of the mesostructure and superstructure wax-ups, and female internally threaded inserts were placed into the wax patterns before the wax frameworks were cast.

The full arch gold framework was tried in the mouth, and all necessary adjustments were accomplished (Fig. 10-198).

The gold was highly polished and the acrylic

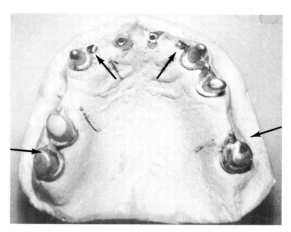

Fig. 10-197. The master stone model. Oblique channels were made at strategic areas in the mesostructure *(arrows)*. (From Linkow, L. I.: Maxillary endosseous implants, Dent. Concepts **10**[1]:14-24, 1966.)

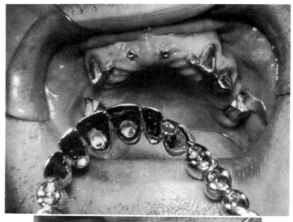

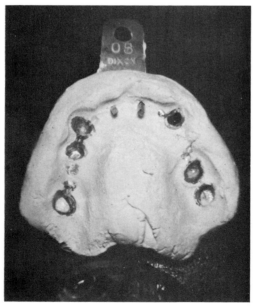

Fig. 10-196. A plaster index picks up the superstructure and mesostructure. Also seen are two duplicate implant shafts.

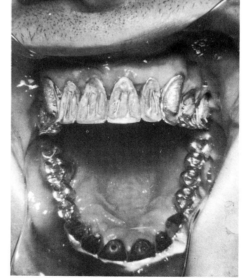

Fig. 10-198. The soldered full arch denture is tried in position.

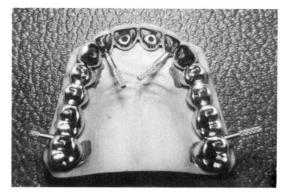

Fig. 10-199. The case is processed in acrylic and gold and includes small set screws that secure the superstructure to the mesostructure. (Courtesy Herman W. Goodman Dental Laboratories, Inc.)

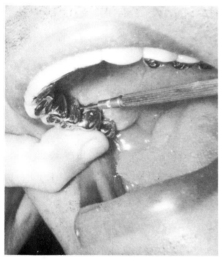

Fig. 10-200. With specially designed screwdrivers, the small set screws secure the superstructure to the underlying mesostructure.

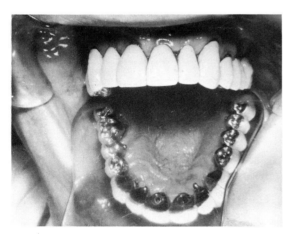

Fig. 10-201. The superstructure in place.

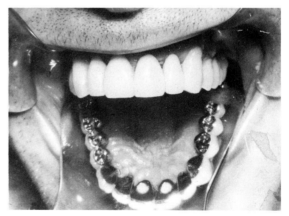

Fig. 10-202. Acrylic was mixed and placed over the holes made inside the two central incisors to further lock the set screws to the prosthesis.

facings were processed to the labial and buccal surfaces. Set screws were screwed through the obliquely set channels of the superstructure and into the mesostructure (Fig. 10-199).

On the following visit the mesostructure was placed over the teeth and the superstructure attached to the mesostructure by screwing the set screws into place with a specially designed screwdriver (Fig. 10-200). After all adjustments were made and the prosthesis fitted properly, both the superstructure and mesostructure were removed.

The teeth, the inside of the mesostructure, and the superstructure were thoroughly dried and the mesostructure was then carefully cemented over the abutment teeth with oxyphosphate of zinc cement. To make sure that the mesostructure was seated properly, the superstructure was immediately placed over the mesostructure for a few moments. However, before placing the superstructure over the mesostructure, the unset cement around the mesostructure crowns was wiped off to prevent the superstructure from sealing to it.

When the cement hardened, all excess was removed. Some form of soft temporary cement was placed inside the dry superstructure crowns, and the superstructure was seated firmly into position (Fig. 10-201). When this cement hardened, the set screws were fastened through the central incisor crowns and into the mesostructure, and cold cure acrylic was placed over the set screws, covering the implants so that they would not loosen (Fig. 10-202). If the bridge ever needs to be removed, the acrylic can be drilled out to expose the heads of the set screws.

The remaining portions of the prosthesis were

then fastened to the mesostructure with the obliquely directed set screws. The bite was once again balanced (Fig. 10-203), and a postoperative radiograph of the implants was taken (Fig. 10-204).

Case 21
A full arch reconstruction with a single anterior tooth remaining using a double rail template with triplants

The double rail template (a modification of Lew's single rail template) was fabricated on a master stone cast obtained from an original elastic impression (Fig. 10-205). It was inserted (Fig. 10-206) using oxyphosphate of zinc cement inside the coping for the remaining tooth. The triplant pins were driven through the predetermined holes (Fig. 10-207). After all the pins had been seated, a soft

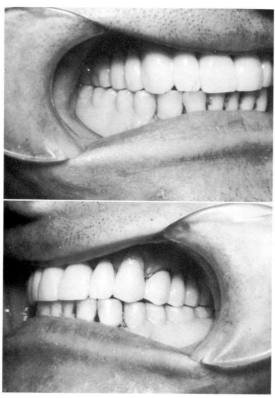

Fig. 10-203. Occlusion on both sides of the arch was carefully balanced.

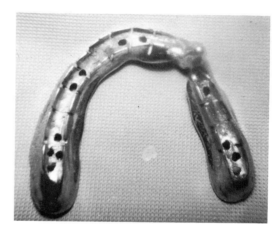

Fig. 10-205. Double rail template on stone model.

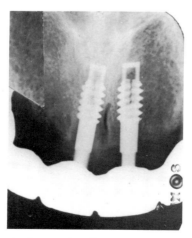

Fig. 10-204. An intraoral radiograph reveals the two internally threaded vent-plants.

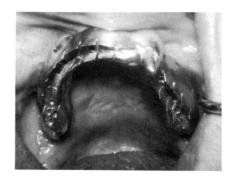

Fig. 10-206. The template was fitted in position using the one remaining tooth as a guide.

mix of acrylic was pushed between the peripheral rails of the template, thereby locking the terminal protruding portions of the pins. The hardened acrylic was trimmed flush with the occlusal rims of both rails (Fig. 10-208).

An elastic impression was taken of the entire template with an occlusal bite record to complete the palateless denture (Fig. 10-209). (The denture also could have been prefabricated from the original gold double rail template, since the acrylic was not intended to extend beyond the occlusal borders of the double rails. If done in this manner, the technician merely had to fill in the space between both rails with stone or plaster before fabricating the denture.)

The palateless denture was placed over the rail template (Fig. 10-210) and had good retention be-

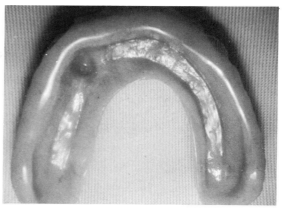

Fig. 10-209. A full arch palateless removable denture was fabricated to fit accurately over the rail template.

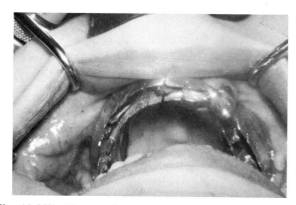

Fig. 10-207. The template was cemented over the one remaining tooth, and pin implants were drilled through the template.

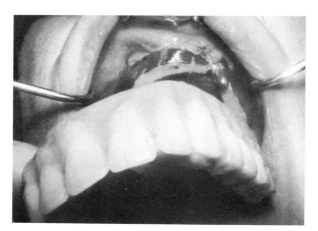

Fig. 10-210. The removable appliance is fitted.

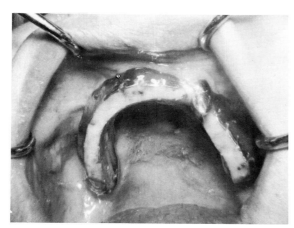

Fig. 10-208. The pins were secured to one another and to the double rail by fast cure acrylic. When the acrylic hardened, it was carefully trimmed flush with the occlusal peripheral borders of both rails.

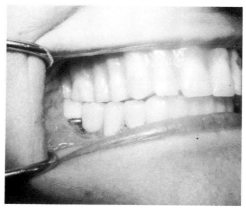

Fig. 10-211. The articulation must be accurately balanced.

cause of frictional grip (Fig. 10-211). Although such a template may be successful, its shape tends to obscure the outline of the bone and make implant insertion tricky. Also, it is unnaturally wide bucco-lingually.

THE EDENTULOUS MAXILLA

Only one other type of implantation—the single tooth restoration—has given more problems than a full arch of implants for the edentulous maxilla. The difference in long-term stability between restorations for the completely edentulous maxilla and those for the maxilla with as few as one or two remaining teeth has been great. The inclusion of some type of stress-distributing support, such as a connecting bar or template, has improved the prognosis.

The rehabilitation of the maxillary dental arch may be accomplished with the use of one type of implant, such as the vent-plant, spiral-screw, or blade, or by the combination of triplants with post type implants. Triplants alone will not work for more than a short while. The final prosthesis can be either a complete full arch fixed splint or a palateless removable denture with some form of internal clip bar, Gerber type attachments, or Ceka attachments.

The choice of implants can be determined through a careful radiographic examination of the bone available in relation to anatomic obstructions, such as the nasal vestibulum and the maxillary sinuses. For example, if the nasal vestibulum is dropped very low and extends distally close to the anterior wall of the maxillary sinus on both sides, then the only osseous structure available for utilization in the anterior region would be the nasal septum, which is usually quite thin. In this area a narrow vent-plant with a hollow threaded shaft or a combination of single pin implants could be used. Posteriorly, either triplants are used to circumvent the maxillary sinus or, preferably, blades are used distal to a low-flaring sinus in the maxillary tuberosity. Wherever possible the pin implants should be used in conjunction with a metallic template. However, when not enough alveolar bone is available, implants must be contraindicated.

The factors determining the choice of a fixed or removable appliance should be considered carefully. The most important one is the amount of bone resorption, especially in the area of the anterior labial plate. If a profile view of the patient reveals a great deal of labial plate resorption, making the anterior portion of the lower jaw—with or without teeth—

appear more protrusive, it would be impractical to construct a fixed bridge unless it is fabricated to a Class III relationship. Otherwise too much torque would result from the extreme flaring of the anterior teeth of a fixed restoration. If this is ignored and the incisal edges are fabricated to contact those of the lower incisal teeth and the gingival tissue-bearing surfaces would contact the resorbed labial and alveolar crest surfaces of the maxilla, the teeth would create a tremendous amount of torque on the underlying implants as a result of the extreme labial flare. In such situations, a removable, palateless type denture should be used. Some other factors influencing the choice of a removable or fixed denture are the presence of a full complement of mandibular teeth and possible detrimental habits, such as bruxism, tongue thrusts, and pencil or pipe biting.

A fixed full arch denture for a completely edentulous maxilla should be fabricated whenever possible of all-acrylic fused to thin gold copings so that the overall weight of the prosthesis is as light as possible. The acrylic also minimizes trauma. A porcelain-baked-to-metal fixed denture or an acrylic veneer crown fixed denture may be used, providing there is enough deep, dense bone to adequately place and secure enough implants. A lower partial or full denture opposing the maxillary restorations, rather than a full complement of natural teeth, also influences the choice of material for restoring the maxillary arch. The importance of good articulation, especially when using a fixed restoration, cannot ever be overemphasized.

In order to establish the rationale for present-day procedures, the first few cases will involve failures and the reasons for them.

Case 22
A full arch removable palateless denture for the endentulous maxilla using triplants with Teflon cylinders

Triplants alone were used in this case. After intraoral and extraoral radiographs were taken to evaluate the sites, an elastic impression of the entire maxilla and an alginate (irreversible hydrocolloid) impression of the opposing jaw were taken. A denture base plate with a wax rim was fabricated from the maxillary cast. It was muscle trimmed with compound material and lined with Opotow. The wax rim was softened, and a wax interocclusal record of centric relation and vertical dimension was made.

A complete wax-up palateless denture was fabricated from the articulated casts and tried in the

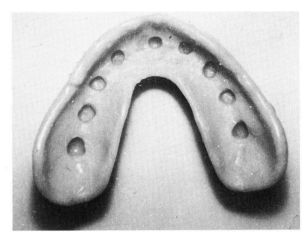

Fig. 10-212. A prefabricated palateless denture with predetermined holes to accommodate the pin implants is seen.

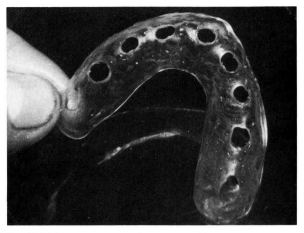

Fig. 10-213. A colorless palateless acrylic template with its holes corresponding to the holes made inside the denture was also prefabricated. (Courtesy I. Lew.)

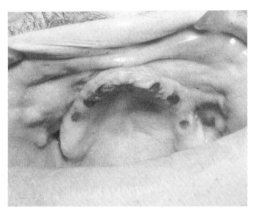

Fig. 10-214. Indelible pencil marks were made through the openings in the colorless acrylic template while it was seated in the mouth. These markings were transferred to the fibromucosal tissue. (Courtesy I. Lew.)

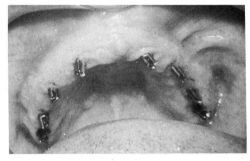

Fig. 10-215. Pin implants in series of three's were driven through the marked areas and into the bone. Their ends were then bent parallel to one another and their excess length removed. (Courtesy I. Lew.)

mouth for esthetics and proper bite. When these were satisfactory, the denture was processed (Fig. 10-212). The teeth were made of acrylic instead of porcelain. Holes were made inside the denture to coincide where the terminal ends of the triplant pins were to extend out of the fibromucosa. A clear, colorless acrylic template was also processed (Fig. 10-213). This too had predetermined holes that coincided with the areas for the triplant pin insertions and with the holes inside the denture.

The template was then placed in the mouth and the location of the holes marked with indelible pencil (Fig. 10-214). The template was removed, and the pins were driven through the marked areas. (Alternately, the template could have been left in position while the pins were driven through.) Roentgenograms were taken with the insertion of each pin.

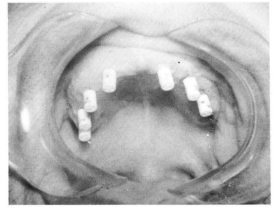

Fig. 10-216. The pins were affixed to one another by placing Teflon cylinders (exhibiting three parallel holes along their entire internal structures) over them with the aid of acrylic. (Courtesy I. Lew.)

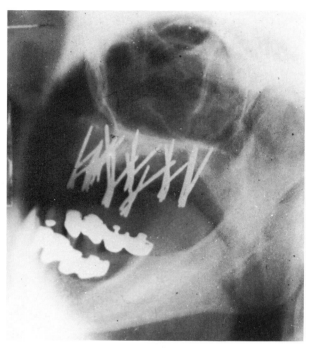

Fig. 10-217. A postoperative lateral plate roentgenogram shows the eight sections of triplants in position. (Courtesy I. Lew.)

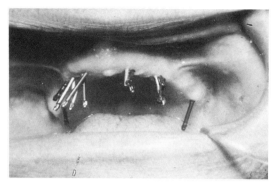

Fig. 10-218. Pins were driven in various directions through the soft tissue and into the bone.

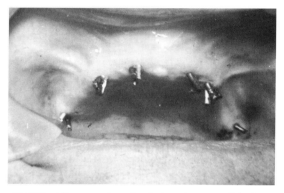

Fig. 10-219. All excess length of the pins was disked away.

The pins were then bent so that their ends were parallel with one another, and the excess length was cut away (Fig. 10-215). Teflon cylinders, each containing three parallel holes, were then filled with acrylic and placed over the pins to lock them together as individual tripods (Fig. 10-216). The denture was then fitted into position and a postoperative radiograph taken (Fig. 10-217).

The case rapidly failed for a number of reasons that still prove valid. Triplants do not hold up, especially where no teeth or post implants are present to support them. Nothing sticks to Teflon, and therefore the pins loosened. The series of triplants also should have been supported by a full arch connecting bar to reduce the buccolingual movements of the implants.

Case 23
A full arch splint for the edentulous maxilla using triplants with acrylic cores

Attempting to prolong the duration of a restoration supported only by triplants, numerous variations were tried: The implant pins were made longer so that they could be driven deeper into the bone and made more divergent from each other. Broader angulation of the protruding pin heads and fastening of the pin heads with acrylic resin, eliminating the Teflon, was accomplished. Here the ends of the pins, instead of being bent parallel to each other, were left extended in their diverging positions (Fig. 10-218).

The pins were then notched and cut short so that there would be no occlusal interferences (Fig. 10-219). Using the brush-on technique the pins were securely locked with one another with acrylic liquid and powder. After hardening, the acrylic cores were prepared for full crown restorations (Fig. 10-220). A full arch splint fabricated with all acrylic-over-gold thimbles was then cemented over the prepared acrylic cores (Fig. 10-221). Radiographs reveal the finished case (Fig. 10-222). This case, and others done in this manner, lasted a few months longer than those done using the method presented in Case 22. However, none of the cases exceeded 14 months' duration. By that time the pins had loosened substantially enough to warrant removal of the entire

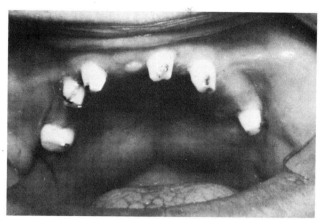

Fig. 10-220. The pins were locked to each other with acrylic. The pins were left diverging at their ends rather than making them parallel to each other. The cores were then prepared for full crown restorations.

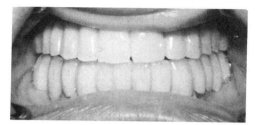

Fig. 10-221. The completed prosthesis.

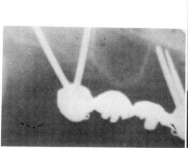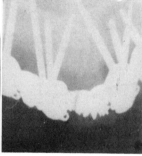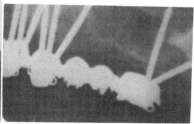

Fig. 10-222. Roentgenograms of the completed case show pins circumventing the maxillary sinus and nasal vestibulum.

restoration. Surprisingly, most of these restorations were able to be "pulled out" in one piece with all of the pins still attached and still diverging from one another.

Case 24
A full arch palateless removable denture for the edentulous maxilla using triplants and an early template design

It is now known that pin or post type implants in an edentulous maxilla must be combined with a template, which helps distribute stress and stabilize the implants. It also keeps the wet acrylic used for fastening the triplant pin heads together away from the soft tissues, thereby preventing tissue burns or irritations caused by the acrylic. Here an early template is used with triplants.

First the usual sets of impressions of the edentu-

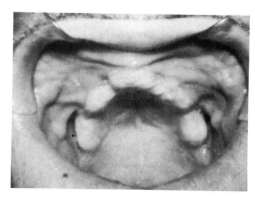

Fig. 10-223. The edentulous maxilla shows a very shallow ridge.

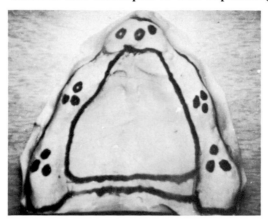

Fig. 10-224. An outline for the template was made directly on the master stone model. (From Linkow, L. I.: Maxillary endosseous implants, Dent. Concepts **10**[1]:14-24, 1966.)

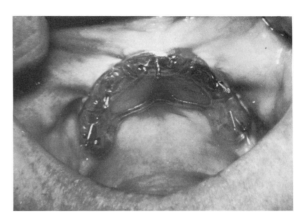

Fig. 10-225. The template was held in position while the pins were individually driven through the holes.

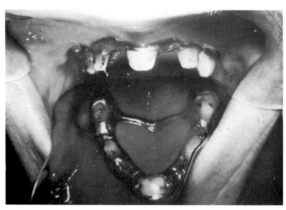

Fig. 10-226. The pins were secured to the template and the template was secured to the fibromucosal tissue by fastening the pins with cold cure acrylic.

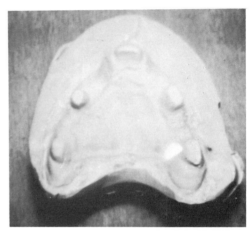

Fig. 10-227. The master stone model was poured from an elastic impression.

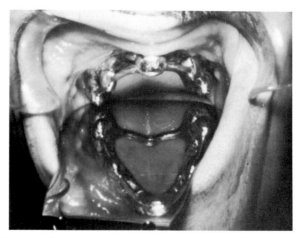

Fig. 10-228. A mesostructure framework consisting of five gold copings joined together with a connecting bar.

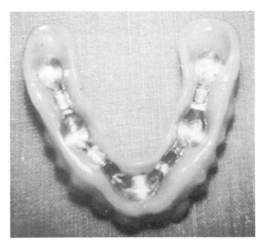

Fig. 10-229. The completed palateless denture with internal clip bars which secured it to the connection bar of the mesostructure. (From Linkow, L. I.: Maxillary endosseous implants, Dent. Concepts **10**[1]:14-24, 1966.)

lous maxilla were made (Fig. 10-223), then the template was designed on the master stone model (Fig. 10-224). The finished template with holes for the implants was coated with a denture adhesive and placed over the fibromucosa. While the template was secured with one hand, the pins were inserted through the holes (Fig. 10-225).

The pins were affixed together with acrylic and the hardened acrylic cores prepared for full crown restorations (Fig. 10-226). An elastic impression material was used to take an impression of the prepared acrylic cores. A wax interocclusal record of centric relation was made, and the master stone model was poured (Fig. 10-227). A one-piece full arch mesostructure that included copings for the acrylic cores soldered together with a connecting bar was then waxed and cast. It was fitted in the mouth over the acrylic cores (Fig. 10-228).

Another elastic impression was taken of the entire maxilla, and the connecting bar mesostructure was picked up with the impression. From these a

palateless denture with internal clip bars was fabricated (Fig. 10-229).

The connecting bar mesostructure was then cemented with hard cement over the acrylic cores. The palateless denture was once again placed in the mouth and rearticulated for any occlusal adjustments (Fig. 10-230).

Case 25
A fixed full arch denture using mixed implants and a template

After numerous attempts to use triplants as the only implant design in the edentulous maxilla, it became obvious that triplants could not hold up without some other type of support. Templates were tried, and although they prolonged the life of the prosthesis a few months by reducing the types of motion that tend to dislodge an implant, they could not adequately compensate for a basic flaw in the triplant. Unlike post type implants and the blade-vent, which becomes tightly bound by bone that

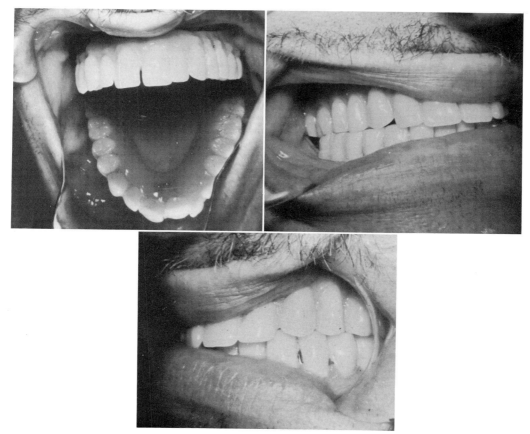

Fig. 10-230. The finished case.

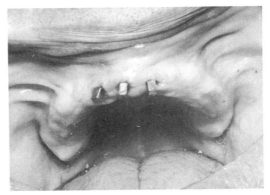

Fig. 10-231. Three vent-plants are placed in the incisor region.

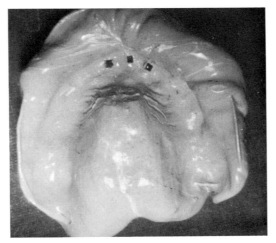

Fig. 10-232. A full arch rubber base impression is taken.

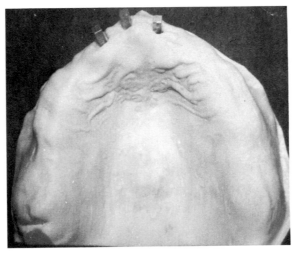

Fig. 10-233. A master model, which includes three duplicate implant shafts, is poured.

may grow through the implant, the triplant pins merely rest in bone. Unlike the tightly integrated connective tissue in and around a post type implant or a blade-vent, the connective tissue around a triplant pin merely forms a sleeve into which the pin slips, an action aided by the slight rocking that occurs during normal motions of the jaws. Although the template tends to reduce this rocking, the triplant can never be used as really more than an internal brace. This became obvious when triplants were combined with other implants and the restoration endured longer.

This case and those following it indicate the evolution of the mixed implant rationale. In the first cases all the implants, no matter what design, were inserted simultaneously. Operative difficulties were alleviated by inserting the post type implants

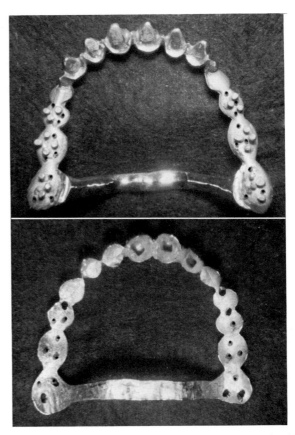

Fig. 10-234. A scalloped template is fabricated. It should include a posterior palatal connecting bar and vertical mushroom pin heads with predetermined holes through the template. It should also include a number of pontics for the support of the superstructure. The peripheral borders should be rounded so as not to injure the soft tissue. It should have a polished undersurface.

before making the template, as illustrated by the following case.

Three anterior vent-plants were screwed into the alveolar bone (Fig. 10-231), and an elastic impression was taken of the entire maxilla, including the three implant shafts (Fig. 10-232). (A full mouth plaster index including the three protruding implant shafts—with or without interchangeable gold copings —could also have been taken.)

A master stone model with three duplicate implant shafts was prepared (Fig. 10-233), and a scalloped gold template was fabricated from the stone cast. The template included vertical extensions anteriorly, an improvement that eliminates the need for the gold coping connecting bar shown in the previous cases, and mushroom-shaped protrusions in the triplant areas for inclusion in the acrylic cores. These help bind the triplants to the template. Holes were then made between the mushroom-shaped protrusions to accommodate the triplant pins (Fig. 10-234). These holes were determined by taking radiographs while the template was in the mouth.

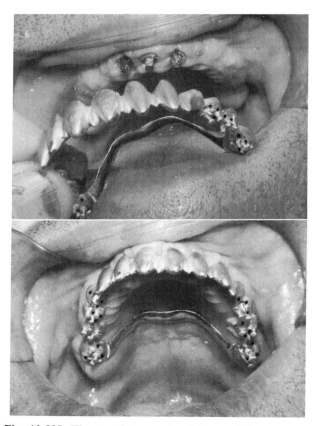

Fig. 10-235. The template was fitted into position.

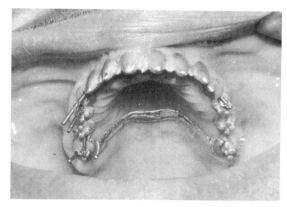

Fig. 10-236. Pin implants were then drilled through the template.

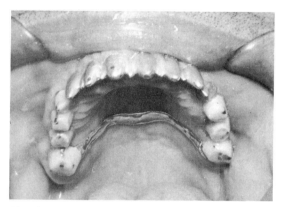

Fig. 10-237. Acrylic cores were built up to secure the pins and then prepared for full crown restorations.

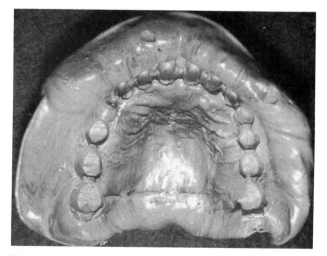

Fig. 10-238. A full arch rubber base impression was then taken.

The template was cemented over the three protruding vent-plant posts with hard cement (Fig. 10-235). The pin implants were slowly drilled through the predetermined holes, avoiding the antrum and avoiding perforation of the buccal and palatal plates of bone (Fig. 10-236). The pins were fastened together and to the mushroom-shaped protrusions with acrylic and locked to the gold template. The acrylic cores were then trimmed and prepared for crown restorations (Fig. 10-237).

An elastic impression of the entire maxilla was taken (Fig. 10-238), as well as a final wax interocclusal record of centric relation. A temporary anterior acrylic splint, made at the same time that the template was fabricated, was placed over the anterior portion of the template and secured with temporary cement (Fig. 10-239).

At the final visit the acrylic-over-gold full arch splint was cemented with hard cement over the template (Fig. 10-240).

Case 26
A full arch fixed denture for the edentulous maxilla using mixed implants with a template

Well-placed post type implants proved to be far more retentive over a period of time than did the pin implants. As techniques improved, more and more post implants and fewer and fewer pins were used. Combination of the two types of implants was acceptable only when the bulk of the support came from the post type implants, as in the following case using internally threaded vent-plants.

There was adequate bone anteriorly to insert five vent-plants (Fig. 10-241). These were inserted one by one (Fig. 10-242) until their ends were al-

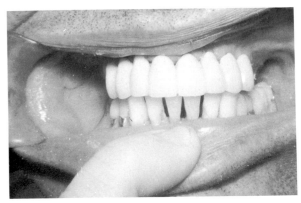

Fig. 10-239. A temporary anterior acrylic splint was fitted with soft cement.

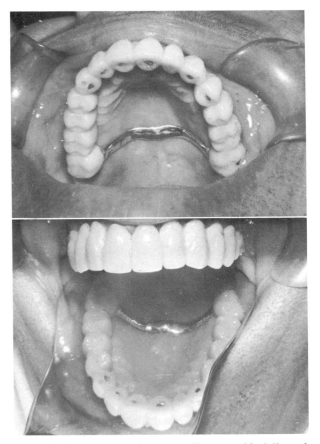

Fig. 10-240. The completed acrylic-over-gold full arch fixed denture.

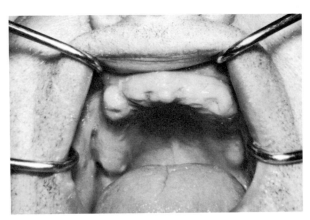

Fig. 10-241. An edentulous maxilla.

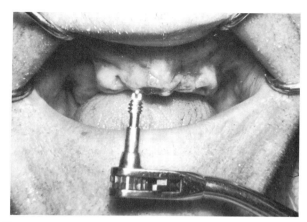

Fig. 10-242. The first vent-plant was screwed into position.

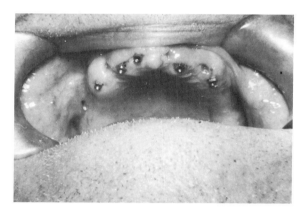

Fig. 10-243. Five internally threaded vent-plants are seen in proper position.

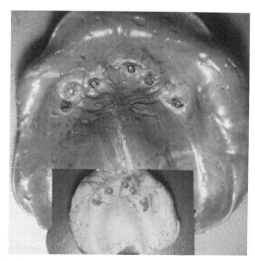

Fig. 10-244. A full arch rubber (top) or plaster impression (bottom) was taken.

most flush with the tissue covering the alveolar crest (Fig. 10-243). A full mouth plaster impression was taken, and duplicate hollow threaded shafts were included (Fig. 10-244). A master stone model was poured, from which a metal template was fabricated (Fig. 10-245). This was to be held in place by passing small set screws through the template into the internal threads of the implants. The design provided for recessing the small set screws into the

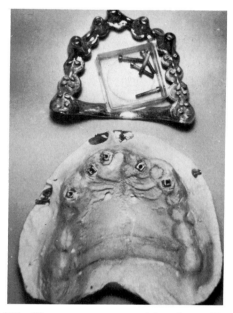

Fig. 10-245. The master stone model and maxillary template are seen. The small set screws that secured the template to the implants are also seen.

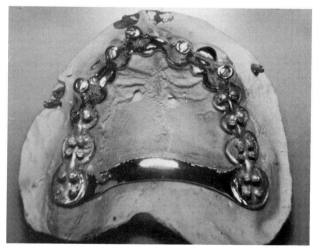

Fig. 10-246. The template was screwed into the internal threads of the duplicate implant shafts on the master stone model.

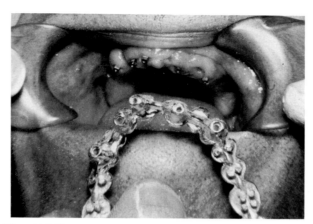

Fig. 10-247. The template was then fitted in the mouth. (From Linkow, L. I.: Prefabricated endosseous implant prostheses, Dent. Concepts 10[3]:2-10, 1967.)

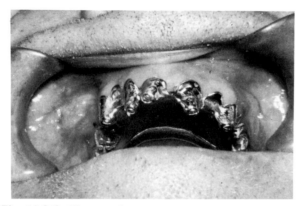

Fig. 10-248. The template was secured to the implants by screwing the small set screws through it.

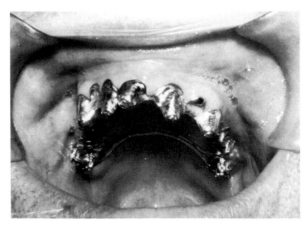

Fig. 10-249. Posteriorly, pin implants were driven through the predetermined holes in the template to avoid the low floor of the maxillary sinus.

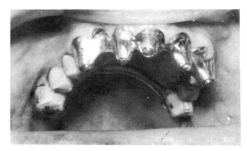

Fig. 10-250. The pins were secured to each other with acrylic cores that were prepared for full crown coverage.

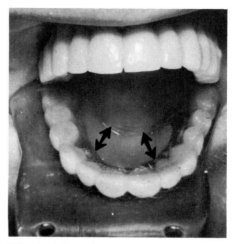

Fig. 10-251. A full arch acrylic-over-gold fixed denture was then cemented over the template with a temporary form of cement. Arrows mark the palatal border of the template.

vertical extensions of the template so that they were flush with it (Fig. 10-246). The template was tried in the patient's mouth (Fig. 10-247), and the small set screws were inserted through the template and into the internal threads of the implants (Fig. 10-248).

The triplant pins were then drilled posteriorly through predetermined holes in the template and the excess length cut away (Fig. 10-249). The terminal ends of the pins were joined with quick cure acrylic, and the hardened acrylic cores were then prepared for full crown preparations (Fig. 10-250).

An elastic impression of the maxilla and a wax interocclusal record of centric relation were taken. The full arch acrylic-over-gold splint was processed and cemented into position with a hard cement (Fig. 10-251). A Panorex reveals the entire case (Fig. 10-252).

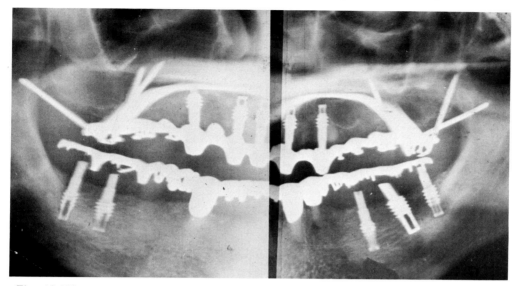

Fig. 10-252. A postoperative Panorex reveals the five vent-plants, two posterior triplants, scalloped template, and posterior palatal connecting bar. Notice also that this patient had lower vent-plants that he had been using successfully for 3 years previous to the upper reconstruction. Since the lower posterior pontics were constructed mostly of acrylic, only the gold occlusal surfaces are seen.

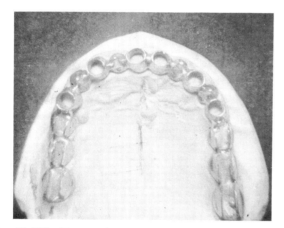

Fig. 10-253. The scalloped "tube template" with double rails on both posterior quadrants.

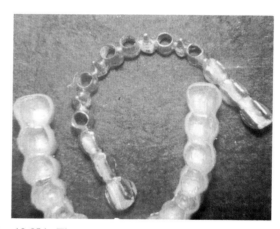

Fig. 10-254. The superstructure was cast and processed at the same time that the template was done.

Case 27
A full arch fixed denture for the edentulous maxilla using the tube template and mixed implants

The tube template, designed by Linkow, is scalloped, allowing soft tissue invagination between the interproximal embrasures and providing greater surface for a frictional grip of the denture. Its buccolingual width approximates the outline of the natural teeth. Because the tubes open directly to the mucosa, it is easier to insert post type implants.

The hollow tube template was fabricated from the master cast poured from the elastic impression taken of the edentulous maxilla (Fig. 10-253). An opposing jaw alginate (irreversible hydrocolloid) impression was also taken and, because the bite was accurate enough, the superstructure—in this case, a full arch fixed denture—was fabricated at the same time that the template was cast (Fig. 10-254). Using a denture adhesive cream on the tissue-bearing side, the template was placed into position on the soft tissue (Fig. 10-255).

To start implant insertion, round or spear-point burs were drilled through the hollow tubes into bone. Various sized helical burs replaced the initial burs

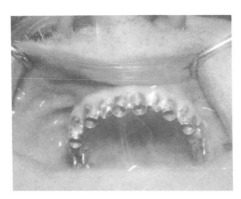

Fig. 10-255. The template was fitted over the edentulous fibromucosal tissue with the aid of a denture adhesive.

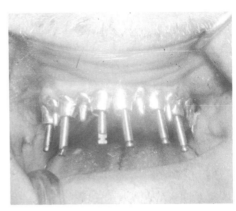

Fig. 10-256. The burs were used with the template in place.

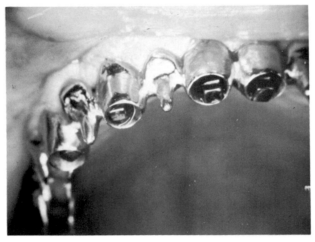

Fig. 10-257. The implants were screwed into position. Their ends should not extend beyond the occlusal rims of the tubes.

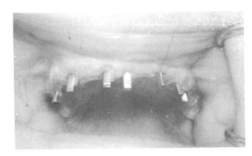

Fig. 10-258. The vent-plants are seen to be closely parallel to one another.

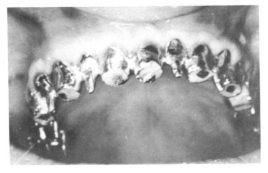

Fig. 10-259. The template was locked to the protruding vent-plant shafts with a mix of cold cure acrylic resin.

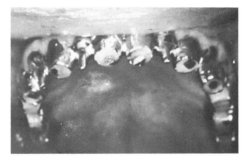

Fig. 10-260. Pin implants were then drilled through the double railed portion of the template that existed posteriorly on both sides and secured to it with acrylic. All excess acrylic was carefully trimmed so it did not extend occlusally beyond any portion of the occlusal rims of the template.

and were drilled to the desired depth (Fig. 10-256). Radiographs were taken during the entire procedure.

The vent-plants were then screwed through the template, using the tubes as their guides (Fig. 10-257). Once they were halfway in the bone, the template was removed to facilitate carefully inserting each implant to its proper depth (Fig. 10-258).

Quick cure acrylic was placed inside the template tubes, and the template was placed over the Vaseline-coated protruding implant posts. Before the acrylic completely set, the template was removed and left outside the mouth to harden. All excess acrylic on the tissue-bearing side of the template was removed, and the template was smoothed and polished. The resulting square-shaped holes inside the acrylic were widened to ease seating the template over the posts. The occlusal and incisal surfaces of

the acrylic were also trimmed and polished flush to the occlusal rims of the tubes.

The template was replaced in the mouth and checked to see if it fit without any impingement from the protruding implant shafts. Posterior radiographs were taken to determine where to make the holes for the triplant pins. The template was removed to make the holes. Then the post type implant's protruding shafts and their corresponding holes in the acrylic were thoroughly dried. Oxyphosphate of zinc cement was placed inside the holes and the template held firmly in position (Fig. 10-259).

The pin implants were drilled through the prepared holes in the posterior area of the template (Fig. 10-260), and they were then locked together and to the template with acrylic.

A full maxillary impression, including the entire template, was taken with an elastic impression ma-

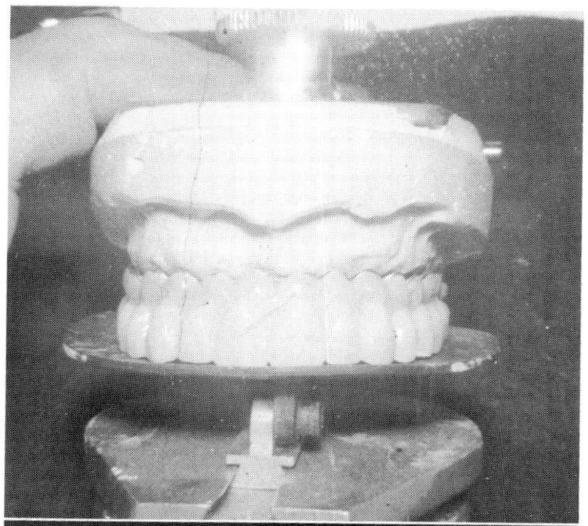

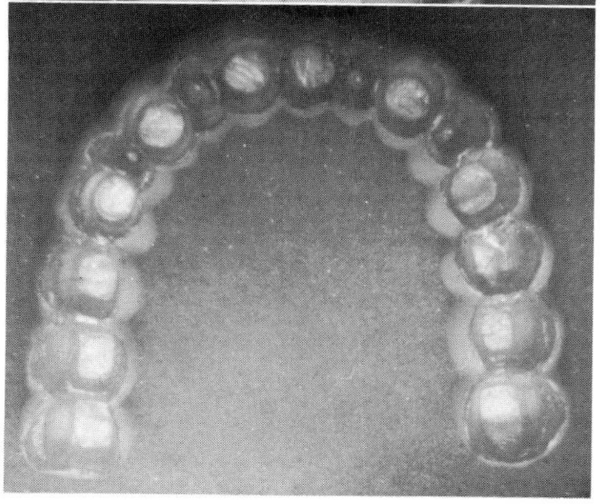

Fig. 10-261. A, The superstructure was carefully balanced on a specially designed occlusal template (Zelnigher), which is adaptable to any three-dimensional articulators. The occlusal planes on both posterior quadrants are geometrically parallel to each other. **B,** The internal side of the superstructure.

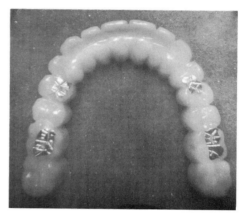

Fig. 10-262. A few gold occlusal stops are sometimes included to slow down the occlusal "wearing down" of the acrylic.

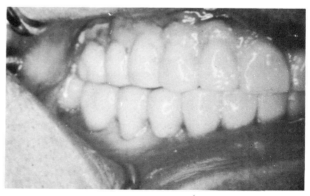

Fig. 10-263. The balanced completed prosthesis.

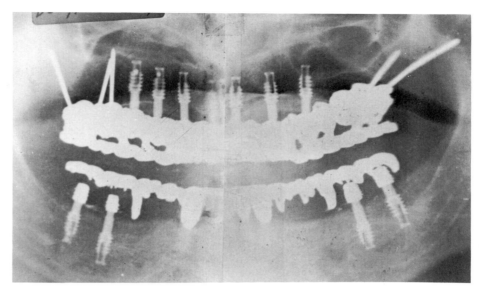

Fig. 10-264. A Panorex shows the seven vent-plants, triplant, and biplant. The lower jaw was also reconstructed with four vent-plants.

terial, and a final wax registration of centric relation was made. From these registrations and with the use of a specially designed Zelnigher articulator, the full arch fixed denture was processed (Fig. 10-261). Because the teeth were fabricated with acrylic occlusal surfaces, gold stops were made in a few of the occlusal surfaces to reduce wear on the acrylic (Fig. 10-262). The finished prosthesis was then cemented into place (Fig. 10-263). Temporary cement was used in case any implant ever needed attention. If such a situation arises, the operator can remove the bridge and drill away the acrylic covering the involved implant with a vulcanite bur.

The mixed implants supporting the prosthesis, their placement, and their relationships are clearly visible in Fig. 10-264.

Case 28
A full arch removable palateless denture for the edentulous maxilla using the internally threaded vent-plant, triplants, a template, and a mesostructure with surface-breaker attachments

Two other advances in improving the long-term stability of a full arch denture for the edentulous maxilla were combining a template and triplants with an internally threaded vent-plant and the soldering of "surface-breaker" attachments to the mesostructure.

A hollow threaded vent-plant was screwed into the nasal septum (Fig. 10-265). Care was taken to angle

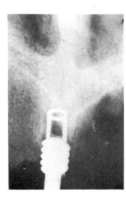

Fig. 10-265. An internally threaded vent-plant was screwed into the center of the anterior maxillary process.

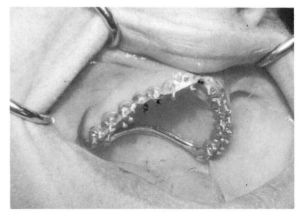

Fig. 10-266. The scalloped template was secured to the vent-plant by the small set screw. The pin implants were then drilled through predetermined holes in the template.

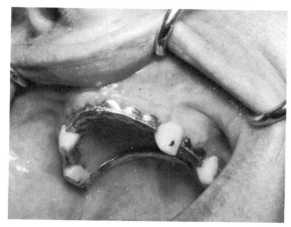

Fig. 10-267. The pins were secured with acrylic cores that were then prepared for full coverage restorations.

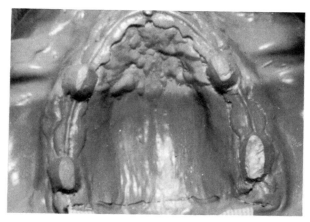

Fig. 10-268. A full arch rubber base impression was taken.

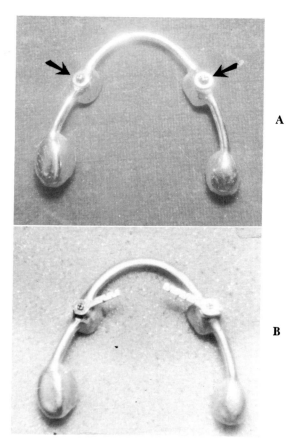

Fig. 10-269. A, A superstructure consisting of four gold copings connected to each other with a connecting bar. Soldered to the two anterior copings *(arrows)* were Ceka male attachments. (From Linkow, L. I.: Maxillary endosseous implants, Dent. Concepts 10[1]:14-24, 1966.) B, The two female attachments are seen attached to the male attachments. The female attachments will be processed to the palateless denture.

it from the alveolar crest in a palatolingual direction to engage the septum. If it had been placed perpendicular to the alveolar crest, the chances of its entering the vestibulum would have been great. The hollow threaded vent-plant was inserted until slightly over 1 mm. protruded into the oral cavity.

A full arch maxillary impression in plaster was taken. A duplicate hollow threaded shaft was put in the plaster index and a master stone model was poured, allowed to set, and then separated from the plaster index. The hardened stone model contained the duplicate shaft in its proper position.

An outline of the scalloped template was marked directly on the stone model with a pencil. In those situations where fixed dentures are contemplated, this outline is planned by using properly

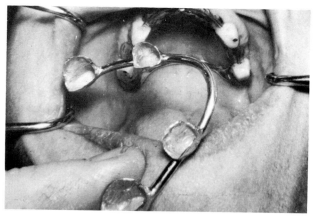

Fig. 10-270. The superstructure is tried in position. (From Linkow, L. I.: Maxillary endosseous implants, Dent. Concepts 10[1]:14-24, 1966.)

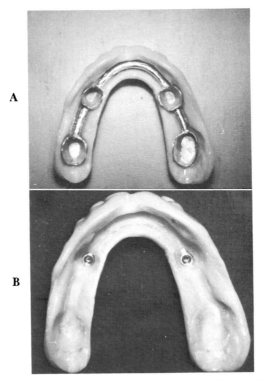

Fig. 10-271. **A,** A palateless denture was fabricated to fit the gold superstructure. **B,** The palateless denture with the two female Ceka attachments. (From Linkow, L. I.: Maxillary endosseous implants, Dent. Concepts **10**[1]:14-24, 1966.)

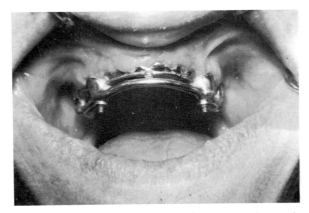

Fig. 10-272. The superstructure was then cemented over the acrylic copings with hard cement.

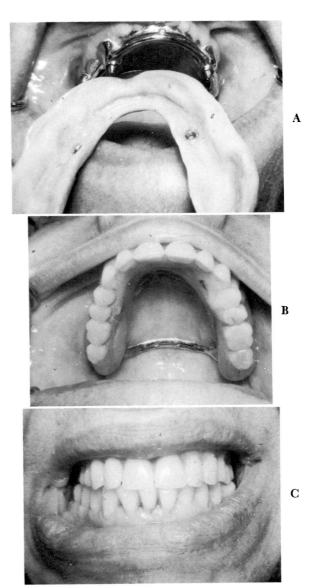

Fig. 10-273. **A,** The denture was fitted. **B,** The palate was completely exposed, giving the patient a great deal more satisfaction. **C,** The finished palateless denture snaps on and off with ease of manipulation. It must be carefully balanced. (From Linkow, L. I.: Maxillary endosseous implants, Dent. Concepts **10**[1]:14-24, 1966.)

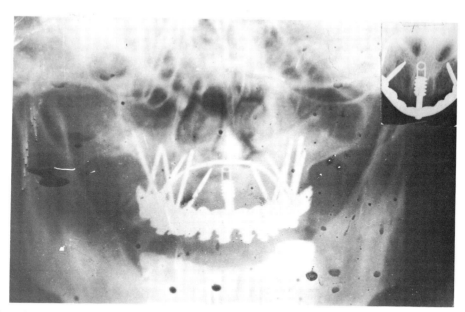

Fig. 10-274. A posteroanterior roentgenogram shows the pin implants as well as the anterior vent-plant.

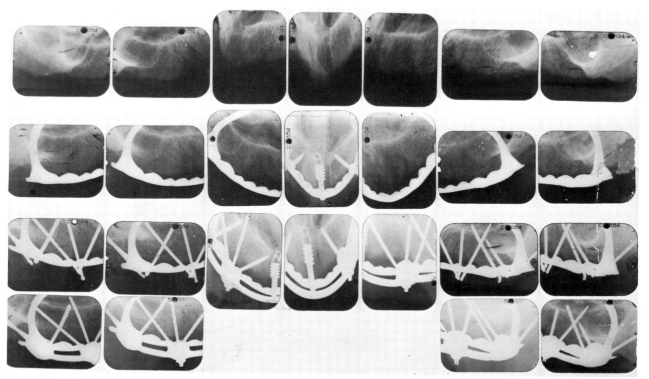

Fig. 10-275. A complete series of preoperative and postoperative x-rays reveals clearly the direction and depth of all the implants.

contoured and sized denture teeth positioned on the master model. If a removable prosthesis is to be used, the template need not be scalloped.

The template was tried in the mouth, held in position by screwing the small set screw through the template into the internally threaded vent-plant (Fig. 10-266). This template contained a palatal connecting bar to distribute some of the forces from one side of the arch to the other, a small vertical central strengthening strut throughout its entire length, and mushroom-like posts in the areas of the various pin holes. Although Vitallium was also suitable, this template was cast in gold and was extremely thin in order to be lightweight. Its peripheral borders were also rolled.

Triplant pins were driven through predetermined holes in the template and built up with acrylic cores, which were then prepared for full crown restorations (Fig. 10-267). A full arch elastic impression was taken (Fig. 10-268), and a connecting bar mesostructure with soldered copings was fabricated (Fig. 10-269).

The mesostructure was tried in the mouth (Fig. 10-270). An accurate wax interocclusal record of centric relation was made, picking up the mesostructure. The mesostructure was returned to the master model and articulated with the lower jaw. A palateless removable denture with female Ceka attachments was processed (Fig. 10-271), although Gerber or internal clipbar attachments also could have been used.

On the final visit, the mesostructure was cemented permanently to the acrylic cores (Fig. 10-272). The removable denture was fitted and balanced (Fig. 10-273). A postoperative radiograph shows the triplants posteriorly, the vent-plant anteriorly, and the template and posterior palatal bar (Fig. 10-274). Intraoral radiographs summarizing the entire case are seen in Fig. 10-275.

CHAPTER 11 Endosseous blade implants

As versatile as the post type and pin implants are, there are many situations in which their use is difficult or impossible, and, unfortunately, these situations are present in many patients. For example, in some cases problems have arisen with post type implants in long edentulous spans. The resistance of the implant, or implants, against lateral forces was not great enough. Neither post type implants nor triplants can be used in many partially or totally edentulous maxillae because of narrow or shallow ridges.

Experience has shown that one of the architectural features essential to good retention is the width of the implant. This is particularly true when it comes to resisting lateral forces. Increasing the diameter of a post type implant or diverging the legs of a triplant even more was clearly difficult or impossible. Such an increase would obviously threaten the cortical plates of bone and frequently lead to per-

foration. A new design approach was therefore needed.

With the idea in mind of creating an implant that incorporated the good features of previous implant designs and deviated from those features that limited their use in a good many sites, Linkow designed the blade implant, or blade-vent. Originally conceived for narrow ridges and long edentulous spans, its success in the past 3 years has been so remarkable that the blade is now Linkow's choice implant for most endosseous implant intervention procedures.

Description

The blade-vent has a wedge-shaped body surmounted by a narrow neck whose uppermost part is broadened to bear the prosthesis (Fig. 11-1). The wedge, which tapers from the top toward the bottom, is very narrow buccolingually, never exceeding 1½

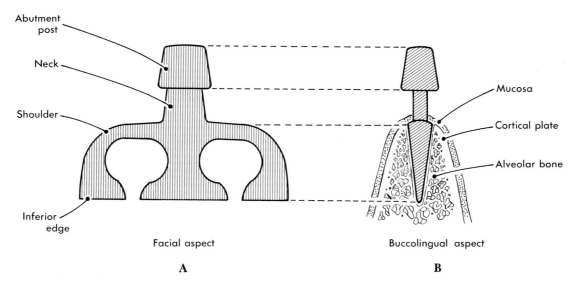

Facial aspect

A

Buccolingual aspect

B

Fig. 11-1. A, The facial aspect of the blade. **B,** Buccolingual aspects of blade implant illustrating the wedge principle.

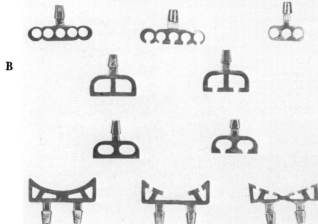

Fig. 11-2. A, Various blade implants. **B,** The shape of blade-vents may be changed to suit the site. The far left implant in each row is the basic implant; others in the row are variations.

mm. in thickness. Its anteroposterior dimension is quite broad and contains holes of various sizes and shapes (Fig. 11-2). These holes are much larger than the spaces in post type implants, thus enhancing bone deposition.

The shoulder of the wedge must be set 1 or 2 mm. below the cortical plates at the alveolar crest. If the alveolar crest is shallow, the supero-inferior aspect of the wedge may be shortened. Shortening the implant in this manner does not reduce its retentive potential because retention is based on the width, not the depth, of the implant. Thus, if the landscape of a particular site is unusual, the operator can sketch an appropriate blade shape directly on the radiograph and have it made to order.

Atop the wedge is the narrow neck that will extend upward through the tissues and into the oral cavity where it becomes thicker to form the post. The length of the neck is variable. The operator may choose that length most appropriate to the problems of a particular site. If the implant can be buried very deep, a long neck is needed to reach the oral cavity. If the fibromucosa is particularly thick and the operator chooses not to thin it before the implant intervention, the long-necked blade implant can be used. If a short post is required to ensure occlusal harmony, a short-necked implant may be selected. The neck may also be easily bent so that the implant may be set most advantageously into bone, with the prosthesis-bearing portion parallel to other abutments.

Basic insertion techniques

The blade-vent is easy to insert; this is one of its chief advantages. Briefly, neighboring teeth are prepared as abutments. Then the bone is exposed and a slot prepared for the implant. The implant is set in the slot, tapped into place, and the tissues sutured closed over the site. Details of this summary and variations in the basic procedure follow.

1. The mucoperiosteal tissues should be incised directly over the center of the alveolar crest, down to the bone, with a sharp scalpel (Fig. 11-3). The incision should be slightly longer than the antero-posterior length of the blade and made cleanly and evenly. Cross incisions are not used because they complicate healing.

2. The soft tissues should be carefully retracted with a periosteal elevator and must be completely separated from the bone. Tearing or destroying peri-osteal tissue during retraction will result in healing by secondary, rather than primary, intention. This will cause undue pain and bone resorption.

3. When the bone is clearly exposed, a groove is made with a No. 700L tapering fissure bur (Fig. 11-4). This extends through the cortical plate and deeper into the medullary bone. The depth of the groove should be the same as the blade itself. The groove must be made evenly (Fig. 11-5). Its length should never be shorter than the actual anteropos-terior length of the blade measured at its widest dimension (Fig. 11-6). It can be made slightly longer

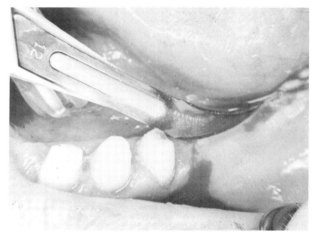

Fig. 11-3. Incising the tissue. (From Linkow, L. I.: The blade vent, a new dimension in endosseous implantology, Dent. Concepts **11:**3-18, 1968.)

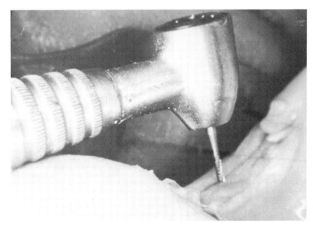

Fig. 11-4. Making the groove. (From Linkow, L. I.: The blade vent, a new dimension in endosseous implantology, Dent. Concepts **11:**3-18, 1968.)

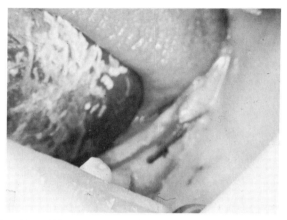

Fig. 11-5. The groove should be sharp and even. (From Linkow, L. I.: The blade vent, a new dimension in endosseous implantology, Dent. Concepts **11:**3-18, 1968.)

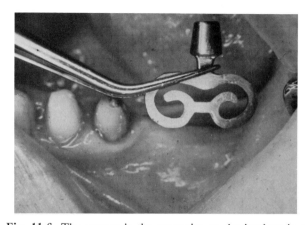

Fig. 11-6. The groove is the same size as the implant in a mesiodistal relationship and should be as deep as the blade portion of the implant.

with no problems encountered. The buccolingual width should not be wider than the implant, because the uppermost part of the blade must be wedged between both cortical plates of bone slightly below the alveolar crest. The wedge principle works better when the superior portion of the blade is firmly held by thick cortical bone rather than by the softer bone beneath the cortical layer. In many instances, the overhanging cortical bone can be swedged over the shoulders of the implant.

4. The implant is set in the prepared groove (Fig. 11-7) and tapped further into the bone with a mallet and an inserting instrument (Fig. 11-8). Because the implant is wedge-shaped, it becomes tight-

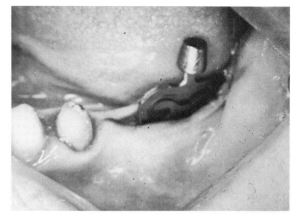

Fig. 11-7. The implant is placed inside the groove.

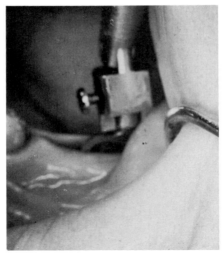

Fig. 11-8. The implant is gently tapped to the desired depth with an inserting instrument and mallet.

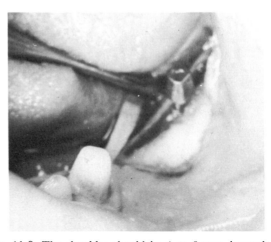

Fig. 11-9. The shoulder should be 1 to 2 mm. beneath the cortical plate.

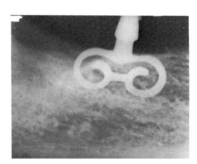

Fig. 11-10. A radiograph showing the blade implant as it is tapped into the bone.

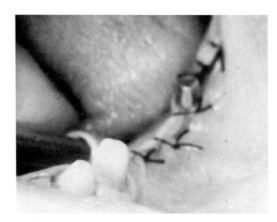

Fig. 11-11. The site is closed with simple surgical ties.

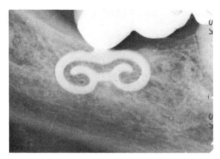

Fig. 11-12. A final radiograph is taken prior to final cementation of bridge.

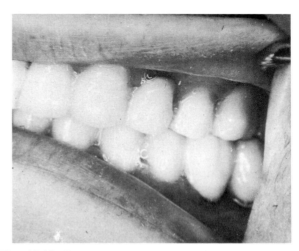

Fig. 11-13. The final prosthesis is checked and balanced.

er as it is tapped deeper. It compresses the alveolar bone flanking it on its buccal and lingual surfaces, reducing the bone's porosity and making it denser. There is little danger of compressing the bone too much because of the honeycombed character of the alveolar bone. When the shoulders of the implant rest from 1 to 2 mm. below the cortical plates, the implant has been inserted deeply enough (Fig. 11-9). A radiograph is taken to confirm this (Fig. 11-10).

5. Two or three interrupted sutures are all that are needed to close the incised edges of the soft tissues (Fig. 11-11). The tissues must cover the entire superior portion of the blade—both the anterior and posterior shoulders and the neck portion of the blade.

6. The temporary splint is seated over implant and prepared tooth abutments (not required).

7. The sutures are removed 4 to 5 days later, and the final prosthesis is fitted and checked carefully for good occlusion and soft tissue adaptation. The site is again x-rayed with the prosthesis in place

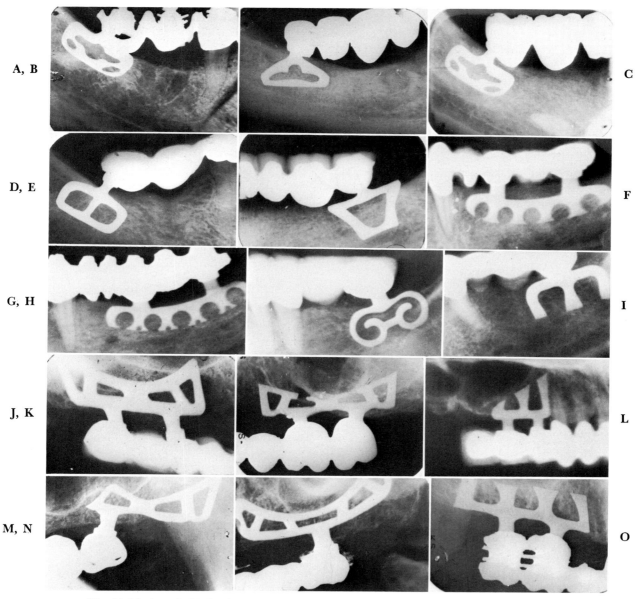

Fig. 11-14. A to I, Blades for free-end saddle areas. **J to O,** Blades for maxillary sinus areas.

(Fig. 11-12). Final cementation occurs, and the occlusion is once again checked and balanced (Fig. 11-13).

In certain situations, such as in a mandible with extremely dense bone, it may be difficult to tap the entire blade into the bone until its shoulders are slightly below the alveolar crest. In order to minimize the trauma caused by hard tapping, the implant should be removed with forceps and the groove sufficiently deepened with the bur. The implant is then replaced and lightly tapped to the desired depth. In such situations, as soon as the experienced operator gets the feel of the bone, he will immediately drill about 5 or 6 mm. deep to avoid removing and replacing the blade. Generally the depth of the groove is proportional to the density of the underlying cancellous bone. The denser the bone, the deeper the slit. However, Linkow firmly suggests that the groove always be made the same depth as the blade portion of the implant to be used, or even deeper.

If a blade implant is not absolutely firm after its final placement, it should be removed and replaced with a thicker implant. Careful evaluation will determine whether the second implant should be different in design, with a longer as well as a thicker body. If a longer implant is desirable, the groove must first be lengthened to fit the new blade. A loose implant should always be substituted. Besides being undesirable for healing reasons, it will cause pain and discomfort.

If either shoulder does not seat evenly so as to maintain the post of the implant in a vertical position and parallel to other abutments, either the implant can be removed or the protruding post can be prepared with a tapering diamond stone to make it parallel to the other abutments. The offending area should be slightly deepened with a No. 700L tapering fissure bur until the blade can be seated properly.

Simple interrupted sutures should be used to approximate the incised tissues. Mattress sutures are not necessary, as they are around the posts of subperiosteal implants, because healing over the blade implant is usually rapid and uneventful.

When a blade is contemplated around the curvature of an arch, such as in a cuspid area, the trench or groove must be curved to follow the center of the ridge. Before the blade implant is inserted, it must be bent to exactly fit the curved groove; otherwise, it could fracture or break off a piece of the surrounding bone as it is tapped into place.

Advantages

The blade implant has a number of distinct advantages, both in design and in insertion.

1. It offers far more resistance to lateral and occlusal forces than any other types of endosseous implants. This is because the body of the blade intimately contacts more alveolar bone than does a screw or pin type implant. Purely from a mechanical point of view, the average blade contacts more bone than does a large three-rooted molar. This can play

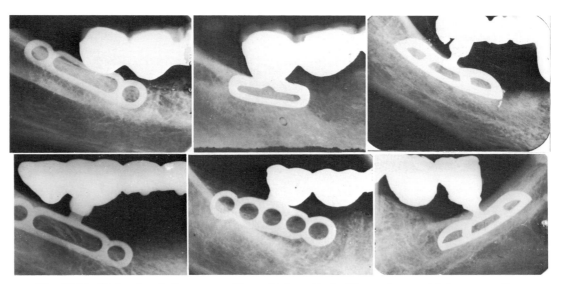

Fig. 11-15. Blades for shallow areas. (From Linkow, L. I.: The endosseous blade, a new dimension in oral implantology, Rev. Trim. Implant., Nov., 1968.)

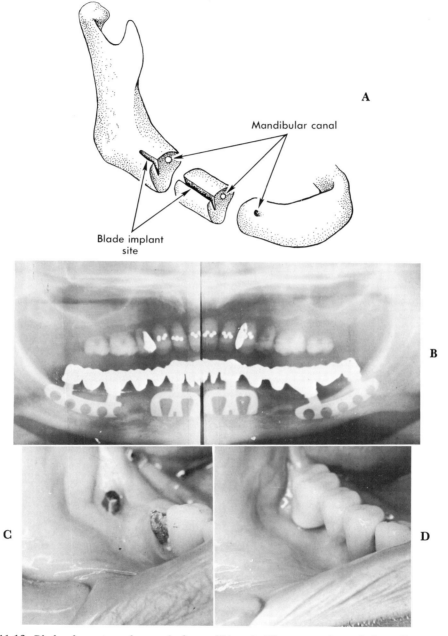

Fig. 11-16. Blades for extremely resorbed mandibles. A, The groove is made buccally to the mandibular canal. B, The right posterior implant in this case was set buccally to the mandibular canal. C, Here a blade was set near the external oblique ridge to avoid perforating the mandibular canal. D, The finished case, a unilateral partial fixed porcelain-baked-to-metal prosthesis.

an important role in resisting periodontal breakdown. Because the blade is broad, it cannot be swiveled on its axis as can any post type implant.

2. The openings in the blades are much larger than those of the screw. Whereas such large openings would weaken a post type implant, they have little effect on the strength of the wide body of the blade. The large openings allow a freer flow of blood carrying bone-rebuilding materials. Thus bone reconstruction is enhanced and retention of the implant improved.

3. Because the buccolingual width of the implant is quite narrow, the span between the alveolar bone walls is very short. Thus less bone needs to be regenerated to bind the implant. This means faster healing of the area where bone was depleted. Furthermore, the wedging of the blade into the viscoelastic environment of the bone appears to greatly stimulate osteogenesis.

4. A minimum amount of alveolar bone is sacrificed when surgically implanting the blade.

5. The threat of endangering anatomic landmarks, such as the mandibular canal with its contents and the maxillary sinus with its schneiderian membrane, can be reduced by shaping the blade to its site (Fig. 11-14). As long as a broad body is incorporated into the design, the implant may be manufactured or trimmed accordingly. The adverse consequences of perforating a maxillary sinus are also minimized by the blade's insertion technique. Because the blade is tapped into the bone and is broad and smooth, it merely pushes up the schneiderian membrane, rather than perforating it. Thus no pathway is created for drainage of the sinus' contents.

6. Because retention does not rely upon how deeply the implant is buried, as is the case with post type implants, blade-vents may be used in more sites. The broad anteroposterior length of the blade gives it stability. Thus in shallow areas a shallow blade may be used (Fig. 11-15). In extremely resorbed mandibles, blades have been successfully implanted buccally to a nearly dehiscent inferior alveolar nerve (Fig. 11-16).

7. There is very little opportunity for epithelial invagination below the shoulders of the blade because the mucosa, its underlying tissues, and the periosteum are completely incised down to the bone, retracted, and kept harmlessly away while the blade is implanted. Thus epithelial tissue cannot be pushed down into the implant site to form epithelial inclusions, such as can occur when using an implant that does not require soft tissue retraction.

Afterward uncomplicated healing may take place as a result of the minimal amount of surgical trauma to the soft tissues. The healed soft tissues are extremely closely adapted, more so than those surrounding any other type of implant (Fig. 11-17).

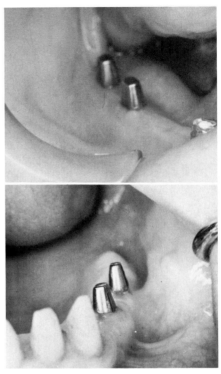

Fig. 11-17. The soft tissues heal more firmly around the posts of a blade implant than around those of any other type of implant. This is a result of the blade's greater stability in bone.

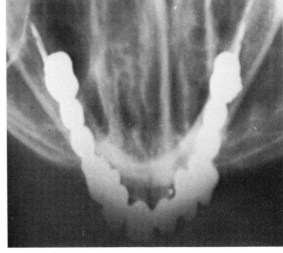

Fig. 11-18. This radiograph clearly shows the suitability of the blade implant for knife-edge ridges.

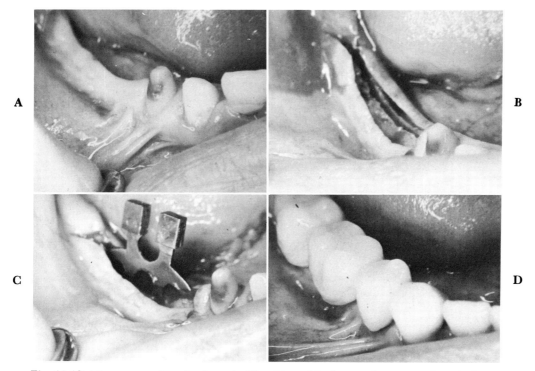

Fig. 11-19. The narrow ridge implant. **A**, The ridge with the anterior prepared tooth. **B**, The exposed bone with the groove made. **C**, The implant in the groove. **D**, The completed prosthesis.

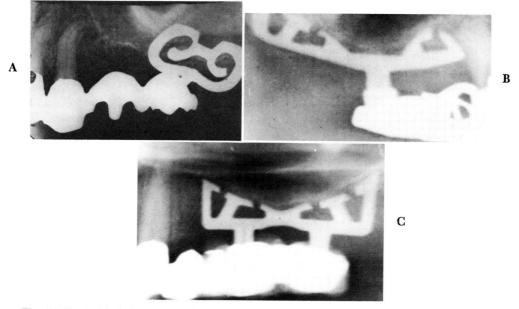

Fig. 11-20. **A**, Blade for the maxillary tuberosity area. (From Linkow, L. I.: The endosseous blade, a new dimension in oral implantology, Rev. Trim. Implant., Nov., 1968.) **B and C**, Two other cases showing the distal ends of the blades in the tuberosities and the mesial ends below the antrum.

8. Determining the most advantageous position for the implant is much easier because the underlying bone is always exposed during insertion. In the case of a post type or pin implant, the bone is usually not viewed directly because the tissues are not necessarily retracted. Thus the implant may

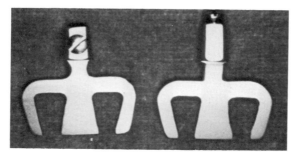

Fig. 11-21. Horizontal and vertical set screws inside the posts may give added stability in affixing the prosthesis. (Courtesy Park Dental Research Corporation.)

terminate out of the bone rather than well within it.

9. In porous areas, such as the maxillary tuberosity, the blade implant is by far the most advantageous because of its width. Several screw type implants have actually fallen into and through porous areas, thereby injuring vital structures. However, the anteroposterior width of the blade with its characteristic wedge design becomes an extremely strong abutment where it is wedged into the porous bone. Therefore it is almost impossible to drive a blade deeper than its superoinferior height, no matter how porous the bone may be.

10. A blade implant can be placed into a knife-edge ridge. No other type of implant can be used in such a ridge without perforating the cortical plates of bone flanking the ridge (Figs. 11-18 and 11-19).

11. It is not absolutely necessary to splint a blade implant immediately after its insertion, as must be

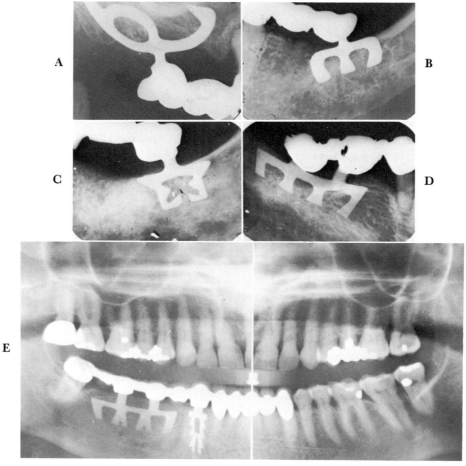

Fig. 11-22. A to D, For dense bone the apical end of the blade should be open. **E,** A Panorex showing open-ended blades for dense and deep bone.

done with a screw or pin implant. Because the blade post is smooth and tapered, it is less irritating to the tongue, cheeks, and lips. However, although not essential, it is sometimes better to splint the blade and to place it in immediate function.

12. When the maxillary sinus is too low and too broad, a blade may be tapped into the maxillary tuberosity to act as a posterior abutment. Although this area is very porous, the blade is extremely retentive (Fig. 11-20).

13. The post of the blade implant provides greater retention for the various types of prostheses. This is because of the larger size and greater length of the blade's post. Also, the head of the post may be manufactured at any angle to the implant's shoulders. This permits seating the blade most advantageously in bone in any direction, yet ensures that the alignment of the post head follows that of the arch of the jaw. Some blades have a post whose head is rotated 180 degrees.

14. The heads of the posts are coordinated in size and shape. This permits using interchangeable prefabricated gold or plastic copings. Because the posts are also tapered, the copings can be slipped on and off more easily. Compare these features with the nonstandardized acrylic cores built around pins and with the paralleling problems resulting from the small square shaft of any post type implant.

For added retention of the prosthesis, the posts are also manufactured with either vertical or horizontal set screws (Fig. 11-21).

15. Making the abutment posts parallel with other artificial or natural abutments is easier with the blade. Buccolingual parallelism is very simply achieved by bending the neck before tapping the blade into bone. Mesiodistal parallelism can be achieved by grinding *after* insertion because the implant is so securely held by bone. In situ grinding of another type of implant is impossible, unless the post can be firmly supported by pliers.

16. The various designs serve specific purposes. For example, when extremely dense alveolar bone is anticipated, a blade whose inferior border is not continuous should be used (Fig. 11-22). Because the

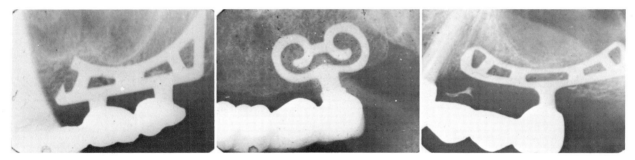

Fig. 11-23. Blades with more secondary struts are used in porous areas.

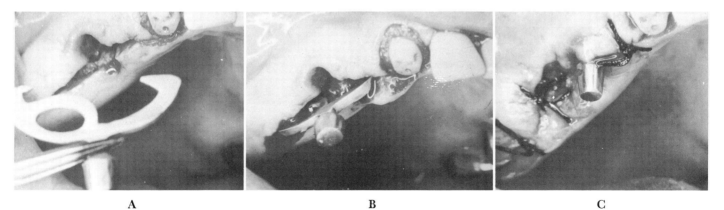

A   B   C

Fig. 11-24. The blade for an open socket. A, The blade extends anteriorly and posteriorly in unaffected bone beyond the socket. B, The blade in the groove. C, The correctly seated blade and tissues sutured over the blade.

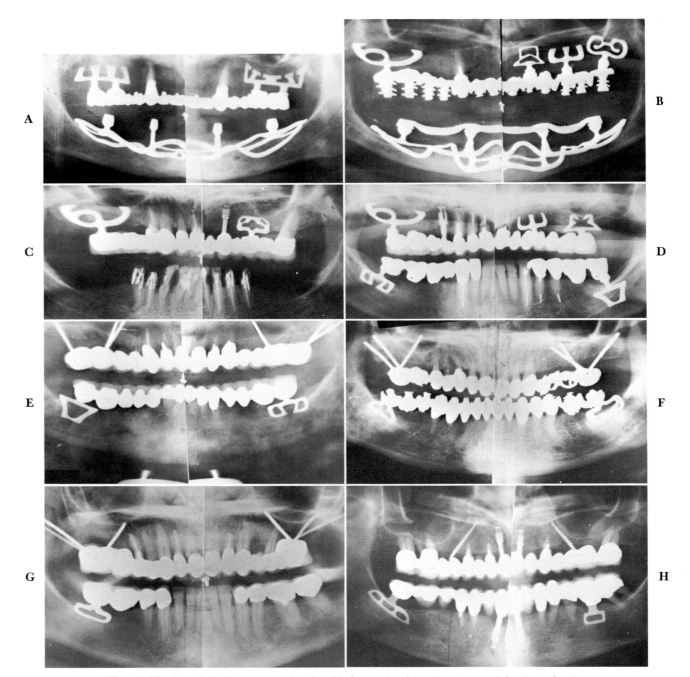

Fig. 11-25. A and B, Two cases showing blades used with other types of implants in the maxilla with opposing subperiosteal mandibular implants. (From Linkow, L. I.: The blade vent, a new dimension in endosseous implantology, Dent. Concepts 11:3-18, 1968.) C and D, Mixed mandibular and maxillary endosseous implants. (From Linkow, L. I.: The endosseous blade, a new dimension in oral implantology, Rev. Trim. Implant., Nov., 1968.) E to G, Blades in the mandible opposing tripods in the maxilla. H, Mandibular blades and vent-plants opposing narrow-ridge implants and vent-plants. (From Linkow, L. I., and Weiss, J. L.: The endosseous blade: a progress report, Prom. Dent., No. 5, 1969.)

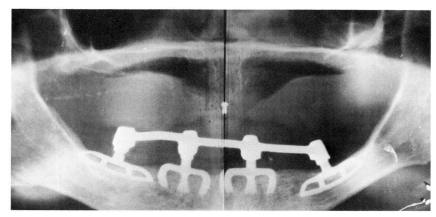

Fig. 11-26. Four blades, splinted with a connecting bar mesostructure, provide more than adequate support for a removable denture.

border is interrupted, less malleting pressure is needed to tap the implant to its desired depth. Also, less bone is sacrificed than when using a blade with a continuous border. Accordingly, areas of greater porosity require blades with more secondary struts to provide greater contact surface and support (Fig. 11-23).

17. Whereas most other types of implants are contraindicated for an open socket, the blade-vent is ideal. Because of its length, its most mesial and distal ends extend beyond the socket and can be embedded in bone (Fig. 11-24). If there is not enough flanking bone and the bone below the socket is deep, a specially designed blade can be driven below the socket. Or, if there is enough bone around the socket, a curved blade may follow the socket's contour.

18. The blades adapt themselves excellently in combination with other types of screw and pin implants in the same mouth (Fig. 11-25).

19. Because the blades are so self-retentive, there is no need for a template. The additional support and stress-distributing properties of a template would be superfluous with blade implants, whereas with triplants a template is essential.

20. Blades are the strongest design to date for the support of a removable prosthesis. If a removable prosthesis is desired, the blades' protruding posts are splinted with a fixed dolder bar, which will serve as a mesostructure (Fig. 11-26).

SHORT EDENTULOUS SPANS

The blade has been very successfully used in single tooth restorations, in restorations for free-end saddle areas, and as supports in areas flanked by

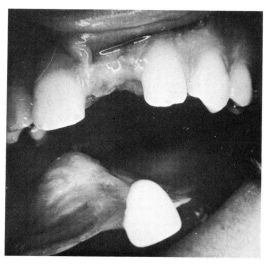

Fig. 11-27. A missing left maxillary central incisor originally restored with a removable prosthesis.

teeth. Because the design is adaptable, the implant may be fashioned to suit the particular demands of the site.

Case 1
A single tooth blade implant for the maxilla

Although other single tooth implants cannot be left unsplinted immediately after insertion, the prognosis with a blade implant seems to be much more hopeful. Also, unlike screw and pin implants, the restoration does not have to be prefabricated for a blade-vent.

In this case a restoration for a left central maxillary incisor was planned (Fig. 11-27). The fibromucosal tissue was incised and reflected to expose the underlying bone, which was grooved with the No. 700L tapering fissure bur. Because the single tooth blade is much longer than usual (Fig. 11-28), the groove was made 9 to 10 mm. deep (Fig. 11-29). This was done so that only a small amount of force would be necessary to tap the implant to its proper depth. The blade was then carefully tapped into position (Fig. 11-30). After the tissue had completely healed, an impression for the crown was taken with elastic.

During the waiting period from implant insertion to crown cementation, the patient wore a temporary acrylic jacket. The crown was fabricated with lingual gold rest seats (Fig. 11-31) and cemented into position (Fig. 11-32). A postoperative x-ray shows the implant and crown braced against the lingual surfaces of the neighboring teeth by the gold rest seat (Fig. 11-33).

Case 2
A unilateral mandibular restoration

The following sample case is typical of unilateral restorations using a single blade-vent. The area was first x-rayed to diagnose the feasibility of using an endosseous implant and to choose an appropriate implant. Then the anterior tooth that was to be used as the abutment was prepared for a full crown preparation. The casting was then fitted at the next visit (Fig. 11-34).

The implantation procedure began by incising the fibromucosal tissue over the implant site. (The

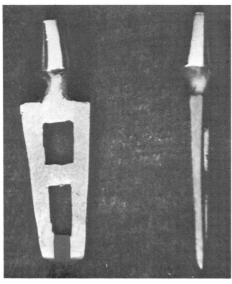

Fig. 11-28. A facial and profile view of the single tooth blade. Note length.

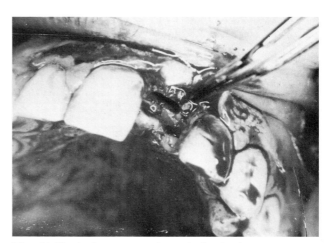

Fig. 11-29. A deep groove is made in the bone.

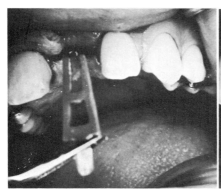
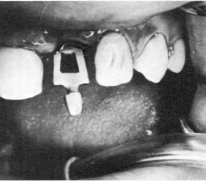
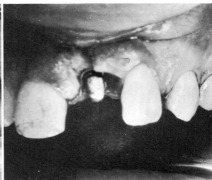

Fig. 11-30. Inserting the implant.

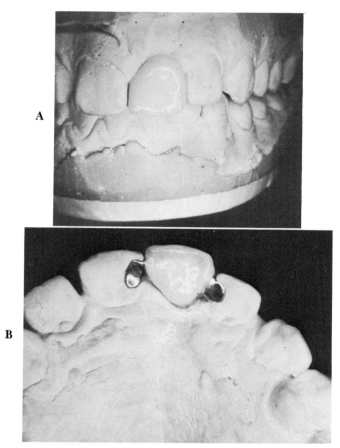

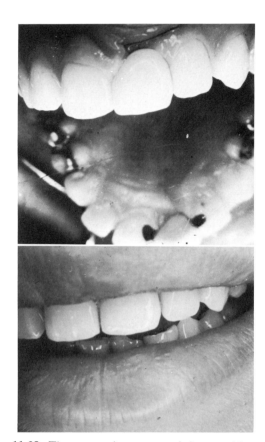

Fig. 11-31. A single tooth restoration. A, Labial view showing slight overlapping of interproximal surface. B, With two gold lingual rests.

Fig. 11-32. The restoration cemented into position.

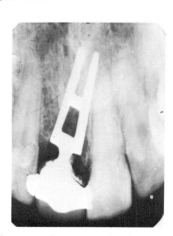

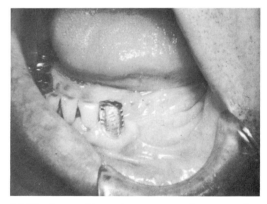

Fig. 11-33. Postoperative x-ray showing completed case.

Fig. 11-34. A cuspid casting over tooth preparation.

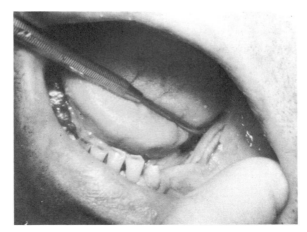

Fig. 11-35. Groove made at implant site.

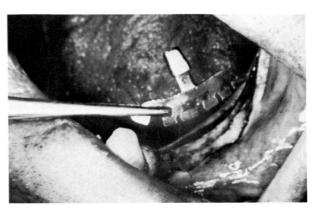

Fig. 11-36. Implant set in groove.

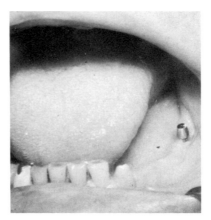

Fig. 11-37. The healed implant site.

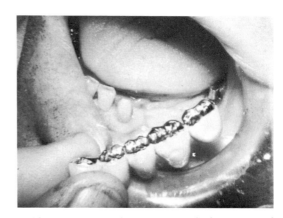

Fig. 11-38. The fixed partial denture ready for cementation.

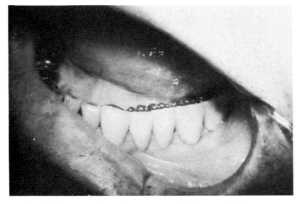

Fig. 11-39. The bridge is cemented into position.

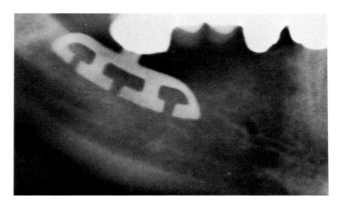

Fig. 11-40. Radiograph of completed case.

incision should be at least 10 mm. longer than the mesiodistal dimension of the blade and must go straight down to the bone.) A thin groove was made through the cortical plate and down 5 or 6 mm. into the underlying cancellous bone with a No. 700L tapering fissure bur. The tissues were cleanly reflected away from the bone with a periosteal elevator (Fig. 11-35). With the alveolar ridge in clear sight, the operator can confirm his x-ray diagnosis as to its true shape.

The blade was then placed into the prepared groove (Fig. 11-36). The implant should be snug and sit so that its abutment post is parallel to the prepared tooth. If it is loose it should be substituted with a thicker blade. If the post is not parallel, further drilling of the post is necessary.

Once the implant was in correct position, it was tapped further into the bone until its shoulders were slightly below the cortical plates. The site was then closed with sutures, and a temporary splint was placed over the implant and natural tooth abutments.

In about a week the patient was recalled. Since the tissue over the implant site had healed nicely (Fig. 11-37), impressions were taken for the fixed partial denture.

A gold coping was placed over the implant post and—together with the veneer casting on the cuspid—was picked up with the plaster index. The fabricated bridge was tried in position (Fig. 11-38). After all necessary occlusal adjustments were accomplished, the bridge was cemented with oxyphosphate of zinc cement (Fig. 11-39). A final radiograph reveals the bridge and implant (Fig. 11-40).

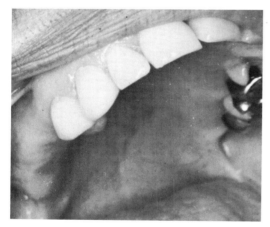

Fig. 11-41. The edentulous site.

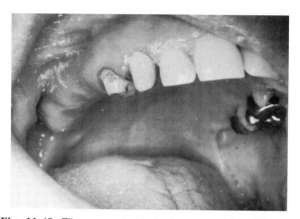

Fig. 11-42. The two anterior teeth prepared for full crown restorations.

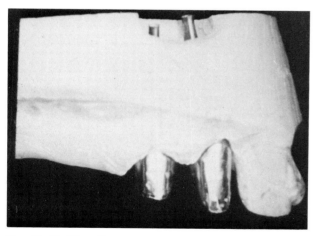

Fig. 11-43. The dies on master stone cast.

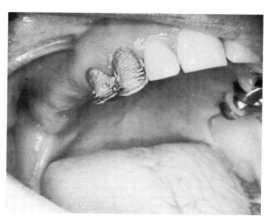

Fig. 11-44. Castings over prepared abutment teeth.

Case 3
A unilateral maxillary posterior restoration

In most unilateral implant restorations, a posterior implant in the cancellous bone of the maxilla usually does not give the same amount of support as when used in the more dense bone of the mandible. With the blade implant, however, maxillary unilateral cases have achieved the same degree of success as mandibular unilateral cases.

In this sample case (Fig. 11-41), the anterior abutment teeth were prepared for full crown restorations (Fig. 11-42). Impressions were taken of them, as well as a wax bite, plaster index, and alginate impression of the opposing jaw, for the fabrication of the master models and dies (Fig. 11-43).

At the next visit the castings were fitted over the prepared abutment teeth (Fig. 11-44), and all final gingival and occlusal adjustments were accomplished.

The castings were removed and the implant inserted (Fig. 11-45).

When the tissues around the abutment post had completely healed (Fig. 11-46), final impressions and a wax interocclusal record of centric relation were taken for the fabrication of the fixed partial denture (Fig. 11-47). The prosthesis was cemented into position with hard cement (Fig. 11-48) and a final radiograph taken (Fig. 11-49, *A*). Fig. 11-49, *B* and *C*, shows two other cases supported by blades that avoid encroachment of the maxillary sinus.

Case 4
Bilateral mandibular and unilateral maxillary restorations

Patients with bilaterally missing posterior teeth can be restored in very much the same manner as patients with unilaterally missing teeth. Basically, all

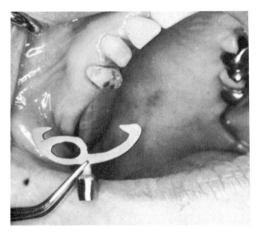

Fig. 11-45. Implant is placed into groove.

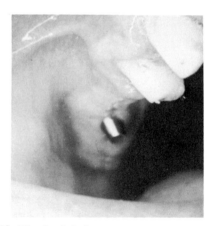

Fig. 11-46. The healed site.

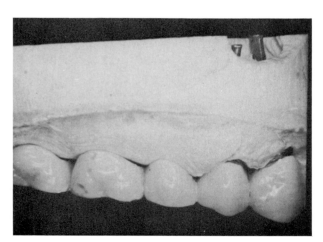

Fig. 11-47. The completed prosthesis.

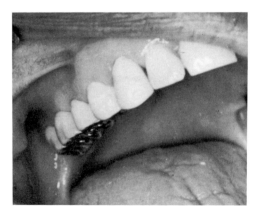

Fig. 11-48. The bridge cemented in place.

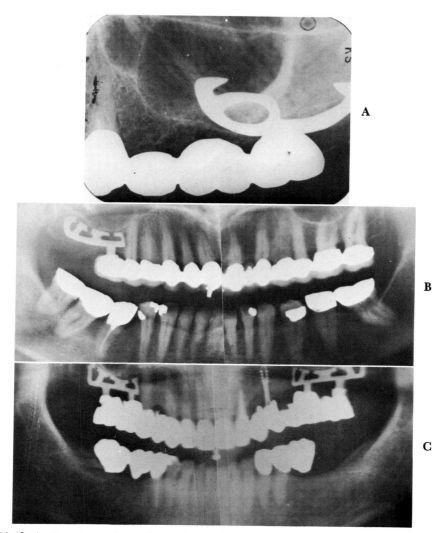

Fig. 11-49. A, A postoperative radiograph reveals the anterior portion in the maxillary sinus. Because no complications occurred, the implant probably rests below the schneiderian membrane. (From Linkow, L. I., and Weiss, J. L.: The endosseous blade: a progress report, Prom. Dent., No. 5, 1969.) B and C, Clear view of how the blades are used to avoid the maxillary sinuses.

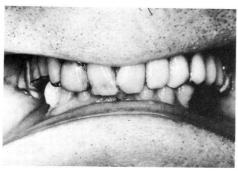

Fig. 11-50. Malpositioned and poorly occluded teeth.

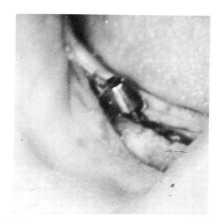

Fig. 11-51. The right mandibular implant in place.

of the abutment teeth must first be prepared, and their castings should be fitted and soldered together prior to the implant insertion. Advance fabrication is extremely important, even though the blade implant is so much more stable than a screw. To prevent complications, the time elapsing between implant insertion and final cementation of the fixed partial denture must be minimized.

This patient's teeth were unattractive and in poor condition (Fig. 11-50). His remaining mandibular teeth were prepared for full crown restorations. After the castings were fitted over the abutment teeth and all occlusal adjustments made, local anesthesia was given, one side at a time. The first blade was inserted in the right mandibular molar area (Fig. 11-51) and the second in the left (Fig. 11-52). The sites were then sutured closed (Fig. 11-53), and a prefabricated temporary splint lined with a soft tissue conditioner was placed over the abutment teeth and implant posts (Fig. 11-54).

To provide ample abutment support, a double-posted blade implant was placed into the alveolar

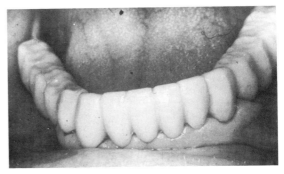

Fig. 11-54. The temporary acrylic splint.

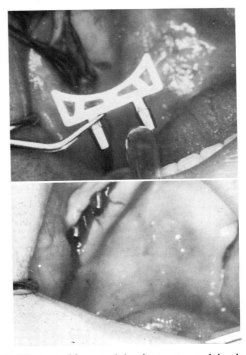

Fig. 11-55. A double-posted implant was used in the maxilla.

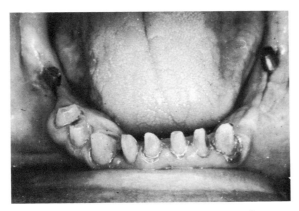

Fig. 11-52. Both mandibular implants are seated.

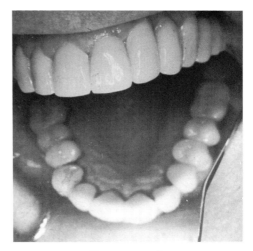

Fig. 11-56. Final maxillary restoration.

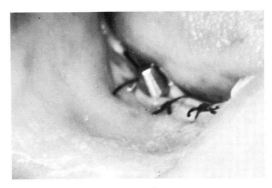

Fig. 11-53. The site sutured closed.

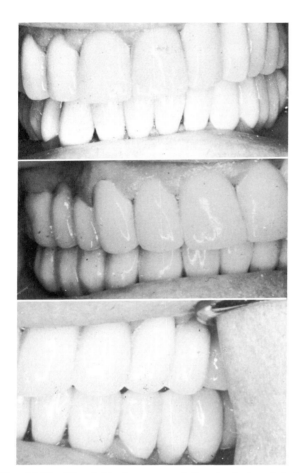

Fig. 11-57. The finished case carefully checked and balanced.

bone in the right posterior maxillary molar area (Fig. 11-55). The natural teeth and implant abutments were then splinted (Fig. 11-56). The final prosthesis was seated with hard cement and the occlusion carefully checked and balanced (Fig. 11-57).

A final Panorex shows the mandibular and maxillary blade-vents in the bone (Fig. 11-58).

LONG EDENTULOUS SPANS

Many problems encountered in supporting a bridge for a long edentulous span have been alleviated by the use of the blade implant. The blade's uniquely wide mesiodistal dimensions provide the kind of resistance needed against lateral forces. Also, because two prosthesis-bearing posts can surmount the same blade, the support is increased without complicating operative procedures by the necessity of introducing two implants.

Case 5
Simultaneous upper and lower blade implantations

The following case is that of a 50-year-old woman who needed implants in both arches. A full arch restoration was determined for each jaw, and all of her teeth were prepared for full crown coverage (Fig. 11-59). Various impressions were taken, including bites and opposing jaw impressions.

A single maxillary implant with two abutment posts was placed into a groove prepared in the left posterior quadrant (Fig. 11-60); the site was then sutured (Fig. 11-61). Another blade was similarly inserted in the long edentulous span on the right

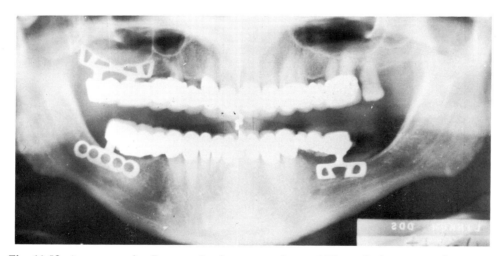

Fig. 11-58. A postoperative Panorex. Implants were also used bilaterally in the posterior areas of the mandible.

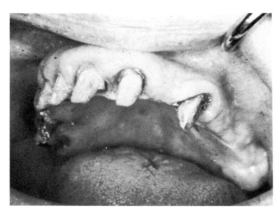

Fig. 11-59. Remaining maxillary teeth prepared for full crown restorations.

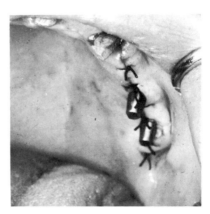

Fig. 11-61. The site sutured closed. Note even spacing between both natural and implant abutments.

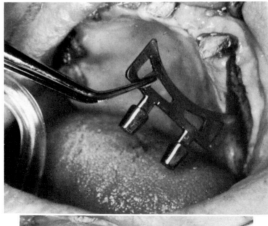

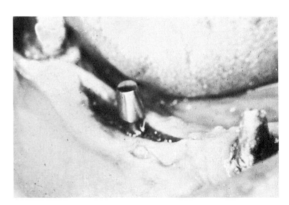

Fig. 11-62. The mandibular blade centered between natural abutments.

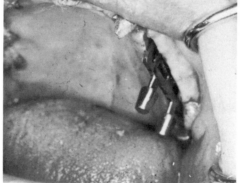

Fig. 11-60. A double-posted blade was used in the fairly long span to produce ample support.

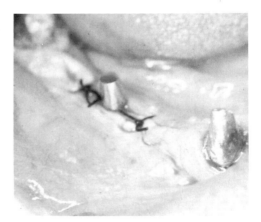

Fig. 11-63. The mandibular site closed with simple sutures.

side of the mandible between the cuspid and the wisdom tooth (Fig. 11-62), and the site was closed with simple surgical ties (Fig. 11-63).

Less than 1 week later the tissue around the implants was almost entirely healed (Fig. 11-64). Both upper and lower porcelain-fused-to-metal full arch dentures were temporarily inserted so that the patient could test them for pain resulting from pontic impingements on the soft tissues. This is very important, since sometimes the pain experienced from impingement is far worse than any pain produced by a faulty implant.

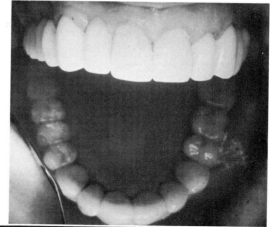

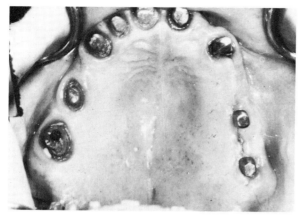

Fig. 11-64. The implant site 5 days later. Considerable healing has taken place.

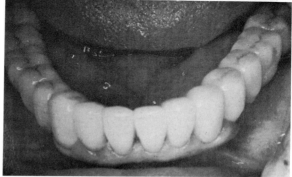

Fig. 11-65. Upper and lower restorations cemented in place.

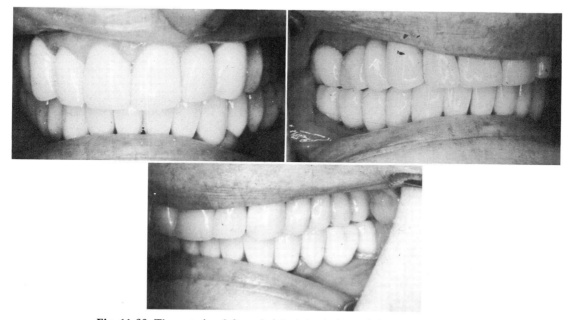

Fig. 11-66. The anterior, left, and right lateral views of the completed case.

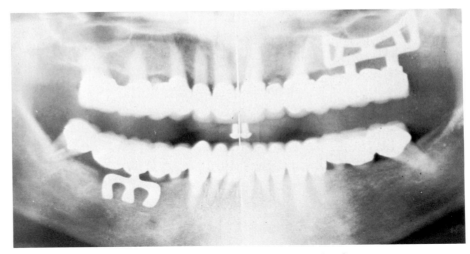

Fig. 11-67. The final Panorex of the completed case.

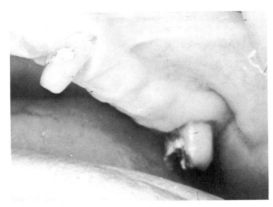

Fig. 11-68. The edentulous span between cuspid and second molar.

After the prostheses were worn for about 5 days, they were removed and the tissues checked for any pontic impingement. All necessary adjustments were made. The teeth and the two full arch prostheses were then thoroughly cleansed and dried before final cementation. A final check was made of the occlusion (Fig. 11-66), and a Panorex of the entire jaw was taken (Fig. 11-67).

Case 6
A full arch splint for a maxilla with long edentulous spans

Only four of this patient's teeth remained: two maxillary cuspids and two molars. For additional support of a full arch restoration, a blade was diagnosed to be placed between the left cuspid and second molar (Fig. 11-68). The tissue was incised and

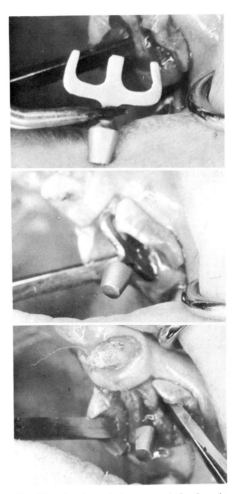

Fig. 11-69. The implant being seated in its site. (From Linkow, L. I.: The blade vent, a new dimension in endosseous implantology, Dent. Concepts 11:3-18, 1968.)

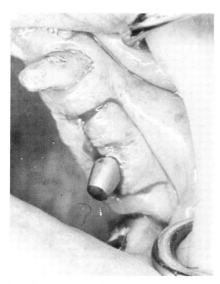

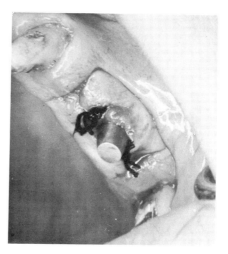

Fig. 11-70. Tissues approximated over the site. Vertical incisions should be avoided as they do not heal as rapidly as a single horizontal incision. (From Linkow, L. I.: The blade vent, a new dimension in endosseous implantology, Dent. Concepts 11:3-18, 1968.)

Fig. 11-71. The sutures should be closely adapted to the post. (From Linkow, L. I.: The blade vent, a new dimension in endosseous implantology, Dent. Concepts 11:3-18, 1968.)

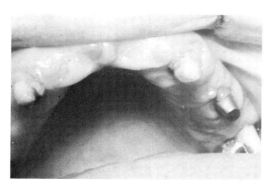

Fig. 11-72. The implant site after only 5 days.

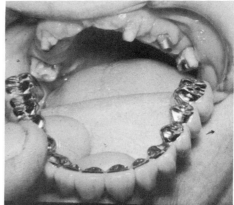

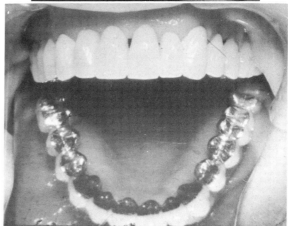

reflected to expose the underlying bone, and a groove was made in the bone to correspond in depth with the blade. The blade was then placed into the groove and tapped into the cancellous bone until its shoulders were buried (Fig. 11-69). The soft tissues were brought together (Fig. 11-70) and sutured (Fig. 11-71). Since this was one of the earlier blade cases, vertical incisions were also used. Only horizontal incisions are done today, since delayed healing usually accompanies the vertical incisions.

Five days later the sutures were removed (Fig. 11-72), and all necessary impressions and bites were taken to complete the full arch fixed denture. During the following visit the final prosthesis was temporarily seated (Fig. 11-73). When complete healing had taken place, it was affixed with hard cement and the occlusion checked (Fig. 11-74).

Fig. 11-73. The full arch acrylic-and-gold prosthesis being cemented in position. The final prosthesis should be seated only temporarily until the tissues look smooth and tightly adapted to the underlying bone and implant post.

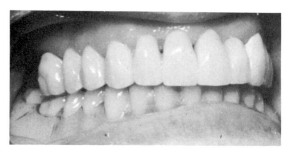

Fig. 11-74. After complete healing, the prosthesis was affixed with hard cement.

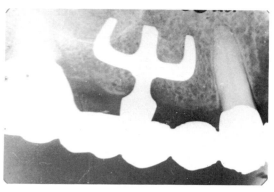

Fig. 11-75. An x-ray of the completed case. Because this maxilla was unusually dense, an open-ended implant was used. (From Linkow, L. I.: The blade vent, a new dimension in endosseous implantology, Dent. Concepts **11**:3-18, 1968.)

A periapical radiograph reveals the depth to which the blade was seated (Fig. 11-75).

Case 7
Stabilizing periodontally involved teeth with blade implants

No other implant is as useful for supporting periodontally involved abutment teeth as is the blade-vent. Because its mesiodistal length makes it impossible to rotate in its site, it has greater immediate stability than either post or pin type implants. In this case five periodontally involved teeth were helping to support a poorly functioning removable appliance (Fig. 11-76). The old crown restorations were removed and the remaining teeth were reprepared (Fig. 11-77). Impressions of them were taken for fabricating metal copings for porcelain bridgework.

Three blade-vents were determined for supports. To insert each, the mucoperiosteal tissue was carefully incised and reflected. Each blade was set in its groove and tapped into its respective position in the bone (Fig. 11-78).

The castings with their already soldered pontics were set over the prepared abutment teeth, and the tissues around the three implants were sutured (Fig. 11-79). Aluminum shells of the proper size were festooned to fit over the implant posts. Compound stick wax was softened and placed inside each shell, and impressions of the posts were taken. The shells were then trimmed and placed back over the implant posts (Fig. 11-80). A wax interocclusal record of centric relation and full mouth plaster index were then taken of the upper arch, picking up the

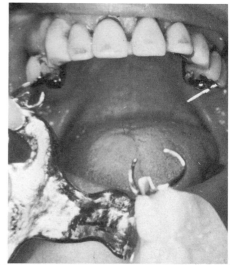

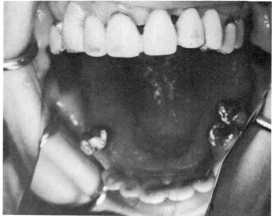

Fig. 11-76. Preoperative views of periodontally involved teeth that helped support a removable appliance.

three aluminum shells and the metal framework (Fig. 11-81).

By the next visit the tissue around each implant post had completely healed (Fig. 11-82). The completed restoration, a full arch fixed porcelain-fused-to-metal full arch denture, was then cemented into position with hard cement (Fig. 11-83). A final Panorex shows the completed upper case (Fig. 11-84). The lower had not been treated as yet. If this case were to be done today, either annealed No. 1 copper tube impressions with the compound or one of the elastic type impressions such as silicone or hydrocolloid would be used for the implant post impressions. It is extremely important not to cool the compound tube impressions while in the mouth, since some of the material would lock around the narrower neck of the implant, preventing the removal of the impression. Instead, while the compound is still soft, it is taken off and placed back on the implant post a few times, which eliminates the "drag."

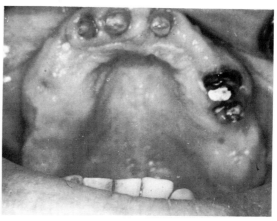

Fig. 11-77. After periodontal therapy, the teeth were prepared.

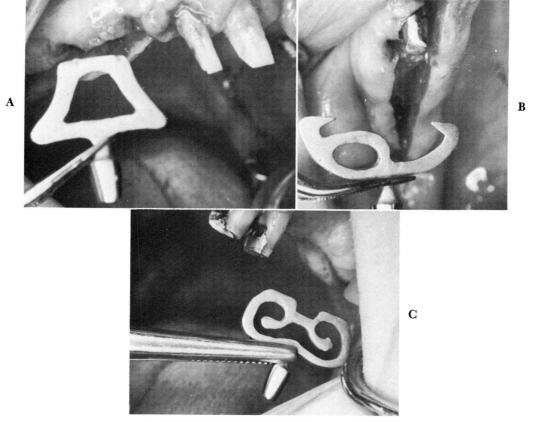

Fig. 11-78. A, The bicuspid implant being placed into the groove. B, Another implant was placed distally in the molar region. C, Another implant was placed in the edentulous area on the opposing side.

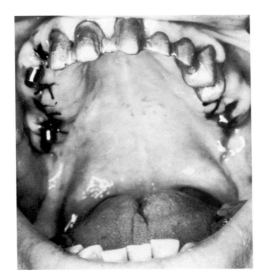

Fig. 11-79. After all the implants were seated, the tissues were sutured closed. Soldered gold copings attached to the required number of pontics are fitted over the prepared teeth.

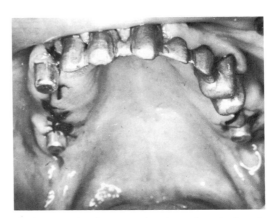

Fig. 11-80. The aluminum shells trimmed and placed over the implant posts with soft compound.

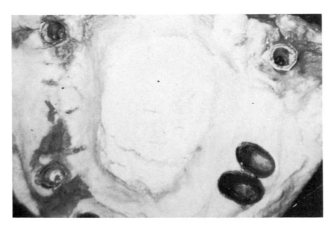

Fig. 11-81. The plaster index.

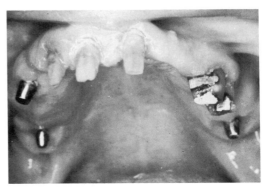

Fig. 11-82. The healed implant sites and the healing tissue around the prepared teeth.

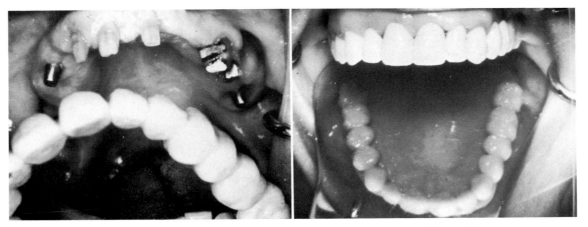

Fig. 11-83. A full arch porcelain-fused-to-metal prosthesis cemented in position.

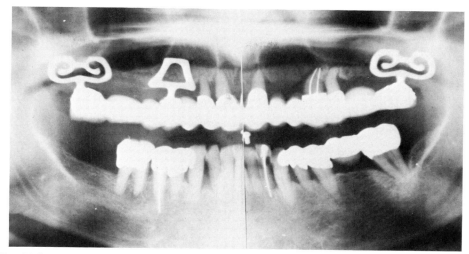

Fig. 11-84. A Panorex of the completed upper restoration. This was a referred patient who requested that only the upper arch be reconstructed. Today, since we know the true value of the blades, the anterior teeth would be extracted and replaced by two more blade implants.

Case 8
Blade implants combined with the nonparallel pin technique

It is sometimes neither necessary nor advantageous to prepare all remaining anterior teeth for full crown restorations, particularly when they are caries-free and esthetically acceptable. Instead, the anterior quadrant of teeth can be splinted to full coverage restorations in both posterior quadrants by using a gold splint that passes behind the teeth and that is held in position by pins pushed horizontally through the anterior teeth into the splint.* A case in point was done on a woman patient in her late forties.

The remaining posterior teeth on both sides of the arch were prepared for full crown restorations. A wax interocclusal record of centric relation was made and compound tube impressions, a plaster index, and opposing jaw alginate (irreversible hydrocolloid) impressions were taken.

From intraoral periapical x-rays, the most advantageous location between the incisal edges and the height of the pulp horns for perforating the four anterior teeth were then determined. These sites were marked on the teeth with indelible pencil.

The enamel of the anterior four teeth was perforated labially, with an obliquely angled No. ½ carbide round bur. A long-shanked Splint-mate system R3 round bur in a contra-angle was then used to

---
*Splint-mate system, Whaledent, Inc., New York, N.Y.

complete the perforation through each tooth. A Splint-mate system E4 end-cutting bur was used to align and enlarge the apertures enough to accept the positioning pins (Fig. 11-85). A shallow hole approximately ½ to ¾ mm. wide was countersunk into the cingulum area of each incisor tooth with a No. 6 round bur to help retain and seat the lingual gold castings.

To make an impression for fabricating the gold splint, any well-fitted stock perforated tray with a labial cut-out allowing for clearance of the positioning pins could have been used. The tray was loaded with an elastic impression material. Just before inserting it in the mouth, the positioning pins were pushed out labially so that their intraoral extensions were flush with the lingual surfaces of the anterior teeth (Fig. 11-86). Immediately after the loaded tray had been set over the anterior quadrant of teeth, the positioning pins were pushed lingually until their intraoral extensions contacted the lingual surface of the tray (Fig. 11-87). After the impression hardened, the pins were withdrawn from the teeth in a labial direction and the tray was removed. The positioning pins were then reinserted into the impression material, and it was sent to the laboratory (Fig. 11-88). The small perforations in the teeth were sealed with temporary cement before the patient was dismissed.

On the following visit, the anterior splint was tried in the mouth by positioning it from the lingual aspect. The two cuspid and posterior veneer crown restorations were fitted, articulated, and balanced

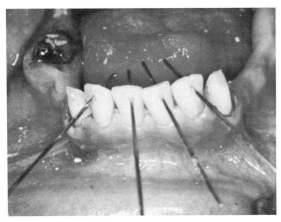

Fig. 11-85. Nonparallel pins inserted labially above the pulp horns.

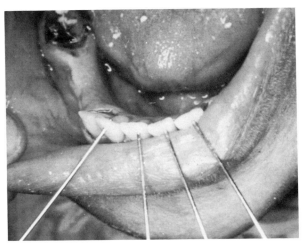

Fig. 11-86. The pins should be adjusted so that they fit flush with the lingual aspects of the anterior teeth.

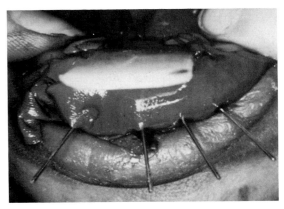

Fig. 11-87. An elastic impression is taken with a specially prepared tray.

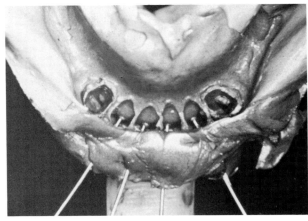

Fig. 11-88. The pins are reinserted in the rubber impression after the impression is removed from the mouth.

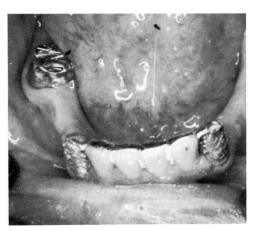

Fig. 11-89. The lingual casting as well as the veneer crown restorations were fitted and articulated.

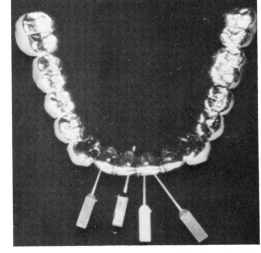

Fig. 11-90. The finished prosthesis with the plastic-headed screws in position.

(Fig. 11-89). Once these were satisfactory, the splint and the temporary cement in the holes in the teeth were removed.

Color-coded, plastic-headed screw threads were inserted labially through the teeth and screwed in until they perforated the lingual surface of the gold splint. They were then backed out labially until they did not extend beyond the lingual surfaces of the splint. A full lower plaster index was taken, including only the lingual surface of the splint. The tray had a labial cut-out so that the color-coded screws could be removed before the set cast was taken out of the mouth. The plaster index included both the crowns and the splint.

The castings and splint were soldered together and once more tried in the mouth. The prosthesis was then processed (Fig. 11-90). This case was unusual in that the bridge was processed before implant insertion. Prefabricated bridges are no longer necessary when using blades as the abutments.

An incision was made in the left posterior quadrant for the implant (Fig. 11-91). The blade was inserted in the grooved bone (Fig. 11-92) and tapped into position. The site was then closed (Fig. 11-93). A lumen was made in the corresponding pontic and the prosthesis was fitted in position.

Five days later the prosthesis was taken off in order to remove the sutures. Final adjustments were

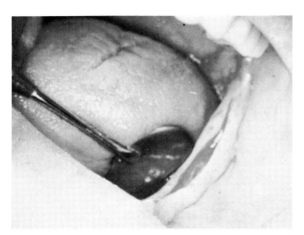

Fig. 11-91. The tissue covering the implant site was incised to expose the underlying bone.

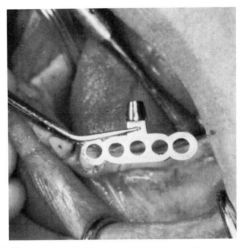

Fig. 11-92. A long shallow implant was used because of the lack of bone.

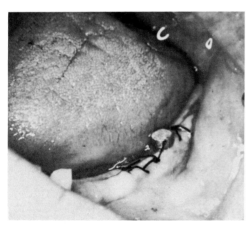

Fig. 11-93. The sutured site.

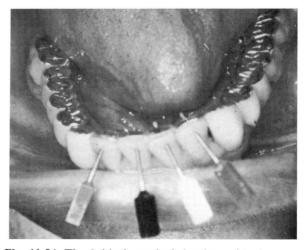

Fig. 11-94. The finished prosthesis in place with the screws inserted.

made and the case was ready for final cementation. (During this procedure it was imperative to use a slow-setting cement.)

The teeth were dried thoroughly and the cement applied to the lingual surfaces of the teeth and to the splint, as well as to the interiors of the full crown restorations. The prosthesis was then inserted into position. Next, the plastic-headed screws were coated with cement by dipping them with a rotating motion. The screws were then inserted through the labial surfaces of the anterior teeth. Although these screws are interchangeable, they were used in the same order as before to avoid minor complications. The screws were inserted by hand until each metal head on the screw engaged the labial surface of the teeth (Fig. 11-94). The cement was removed after it set. The plastic heads protruding from the labial surfaces and the projecting pins on the lingual side were then removed with a standard carbide bur. The surfaces were then polished smooth (Fig. 11-95). For maximum esthetic value, the labially exposed

pins could have been indented and the holes filled with silicate or acrylic materials.

A periapical intraoral radiograph shows the blade in position (Fig. 11-96), while the articulation is seen in Fig. 11-97.

Case 9
Aiding bone regeneration in an implant case with plaster of Paris

The addition of plaster of Paris to open sockets appears to encourage more rapid bone regeneration. The calcium salts in plaster seem to have an affinity for the bone-forming cells in the periosteum and endosteum. In orthopedic surgery, experimental and clinical studies on the use of plaster of Paris have been done by Bahn, Bonnerot, Calhoun, Gourley, Lebourg, Blackledge, Greene, Arnold, Biou, Pelletier, Radentz, Collings, and Tarsoly.

Dreesman in 1892 was one of the first to report on plaster of Paris implants. In a report in 1964 by Bell, plaster of Paris was found to show the most

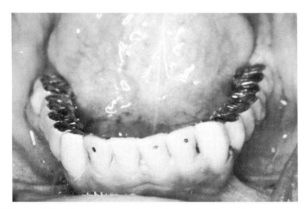

Fig. 11-95. After cementation, the projecting pins were cut flush with the teeth.

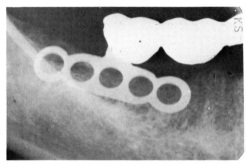

Fig. 11-96. The blade in position. Although the implant is shallow, its extreme mesiodistal width ensures retention.

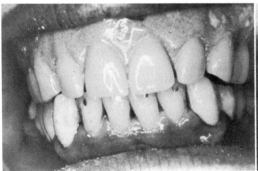
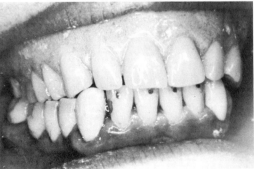

Fig. 11-97. The completed case articulated.

rapid resorption over ten other implant materials.

Some investigators claimed plaster of Paris, when in closed sterile wounds, showed little osteogenic capabilities. However, further investigators have described plaster of Paris to be of great value not only because of its osteogenic potential but also as a space filler that reduces the chances of secondary infection by discouraging epithelial invagination into the sockets and permitting connective tissue regeneration.

Also, although still no substantiation has been shown, it is believed that plaster of Paris releases calcium and phosphorus ions that participate in bone metabolism. All investigators agreed that there were no adverse inflammatory responses to plaster of Paris implants when used in tissue wounds.

Most cases reported on the use of plaster of Paris, including almost one hundred by Linkow, have shown little or no postoperative swelling or pain and no secondary infections. Plaster of Paris seems to

have a resorption characteristic that is compatible with the rate of new tissue replacement.

Although it is still not completely known, the length of time required for the complete resorption of plaster of Paris in a surgical wound from radiographic interpretation was from 3 to 5 weeks, according to Bier.

This next case illustrates a dental application.

The patient, a healthy 55-year-old woman, was suffering from a complete breakdown of her upper and lower dentitions, which were supported with two full arch porcelain-baked-to-metal splints. Large radiolucent areas appeared beneath the apices of all her lower teeth (Fig. 11-98), and a great deal of mobility and gingival recession were evident (Fig. 11-99).

With great care the entire lower bridge was disked away from the remaining teeth. These teeth were all so loose that they could be extracted with a slight tug of the fingers. However, even though there was a

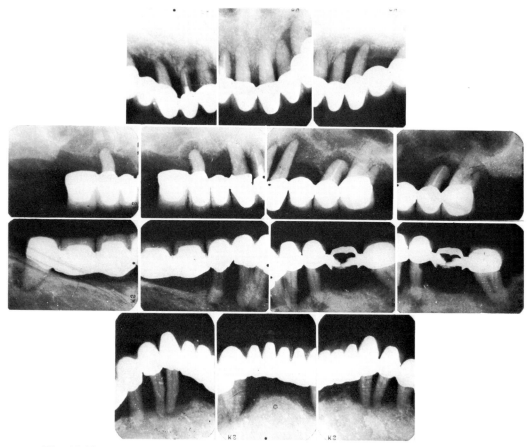

Fig. 11-98. Preoperative radiographs. Note extreme bone loss in mandible and maxilla.

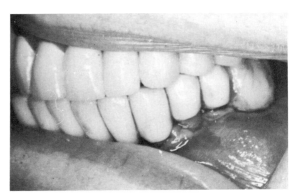

Fig. 11-99. The original bridge still in place. Note recession and poor condition of gums.

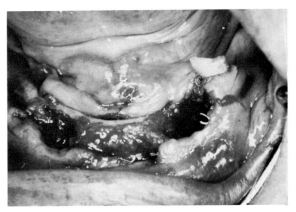

Fig. 11-100. The massive holes were created by removing granulation tissue from the open sockets.

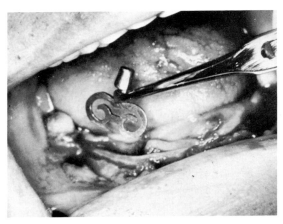

Fig. 11-101. An implant was placed in the unaffected bone in the right molar region.

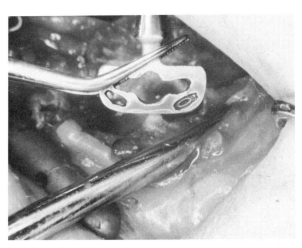

Fig. 11-102. Likewise, another blade implant was placed in the left molar region, in the area of the original pontics.

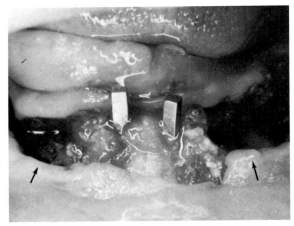

Fig. 11-103. Two vent-plants were inserted anteriorly. Note the massive bone loss *(arrows)* flanking both vent-plants.

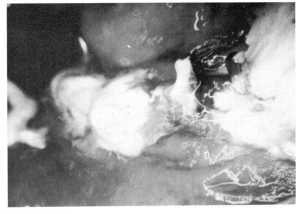

Fig. 11-104. Sterile plaster of Paris was poured into the open sockets.

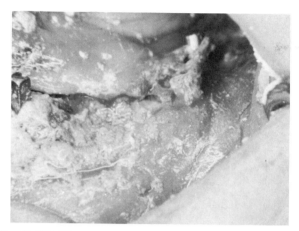

Fig. 11-105. The excess plaster of Paris was removed, while the remaining plaster was allowed to harden.

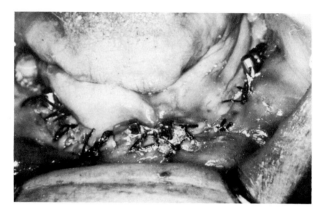

Fig. 11-106. The tissues were sutured closed.

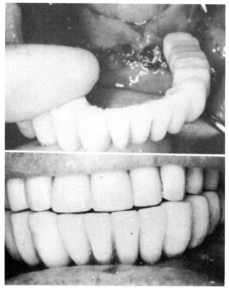

Fig. 11-107. A temporary acrylic splint was immediately placed over the implant abutments. The right posterior molar also helped support the splint.

radiolucent area at the apex of the lower second right molar, the tooth was temporarily saved because it was firmer than the others.

The extraction sites were so inflamed with granulation tissue that after all the tissues and denuded bone had been curetted, each of the sockets blended, leaving a few tremendously massive craters between the buccal and lingual plates of bone (Fig. 11-100).

Three ledges of undisturbed alveolar bone remaining between the large sockets—where the pontics of the original bridge were located—were utilized

as implant sites. Blades were placed in the right molar (Fig. 11-101) and left molar regions (Fig. 11-102), and two vent-plants were inserted into the anterior central incisor region (Fig. 11-103).

Quick-setting plaster of Paris powder, sterilized in dry heat for 30 minutes, was mixed with a sterile saline solution until it was the consistency of sour cream. It was then slowly poured into the large open sockets (Fig. 11-104). While the plaster was still soft (Fig. 11-105), the tissues were tied together with .000 surgical thread (Fig. 11-106). A temporary acrylic splint, cold cured from an original alginate impression of the former bridge, was immediately placed over the abutments (Fig. 11-107) and ground into proper occlusion. It can be noted here that oral antibiotics can be mixed with the plaster of Paris, which can act as a medicinal vehicle. As the plaster of Paris is resorbed, the antibiotic granules are released.

At the next visit the sutures were removed (Fig. 11-108). Gold copings were placed over the anterior vent-plants, and properly fitted aluminum shells were placed over the posterior blade implants (Fig. 11-109). A wax interocclusal record of centric relation, a full lower plaster index, and an upper alginate impression were taken. Duplicate implants were placed inside the plaster index to ensure accurate placement and alignment of the implants in the master stone cast (Fig. 11-110). A one-piece gold superstructure was then cast and fitted in the mouth over the implants and remaining molar tooth (Fig. 11-111). A final wax bite was taken. To get a close adaptation of the tissue-bearing surfaces of the forthcoming porcelain prosthesis, the gold superstructure

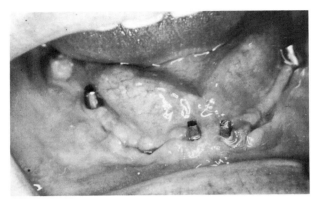

Fig. 11-108. Within 10 days the tissues had healed sufficiently over the bone and sockets to remove the sutures.

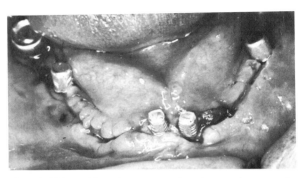

Fig. 11-109. Gold copings were placed over the vent-plants and No. 1 aluminum shells over the blades.

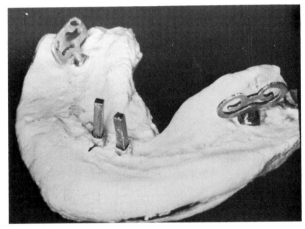

Fig. 11-110. Duplicate implants were placed into the copings, which had been picked up in the plaster index.

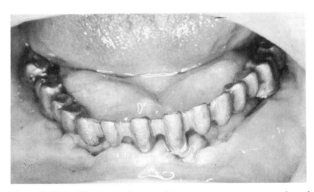

Fig. 11-111. The one-piece gold superstructure was placed over the abutments.

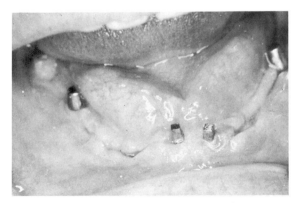

Fig. 11-112. The soft tissue as it appeared 2½ weeks after surgery.

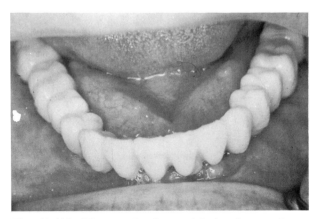

Fig. 11-113. The completed porcelain-fused-to-metal prosthesis cemented in position.

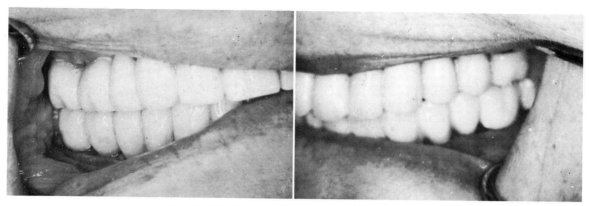

Fig. 11-114. The occlusion was carefully balanced.

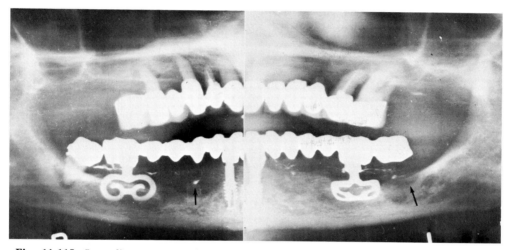

Fig. 11-115. Immediate postoperative x-ray. Note large areas of bone resorption *(arrows).* The remaining molar, although abscessed, was asymptomatic and immobile and was therefore retained to help stabilize the prosthesis during healing.

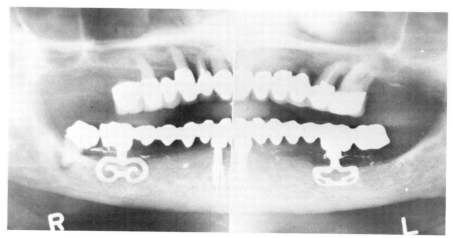

Fig. 11-116. Postoperative x-ray 6 months later. The extensive filling-in of bone is clearly evident. Because the implants were now able to provide full stability for the prosthesis, the molar was removed shortly after this picture was taken and the cantilever on the left side was also removed.

was picked up with an accurate alginate impression. As for tissue healing, it was continuing uneventfully (Fig. 11-112).

The processed lower full arch porcelain-fused-to-metal splint was affixed with hard cement (Fig. 11-113). All spot-grinding necessary for perfect occlusion was done (Fig. 11-114).

A comparison between an immediate postoperative Panorex (Fig. 11-115) and one taken 6 months later (Fig. 11-116) shows an impressive amount of bone rehealing. Needless to say, the patient was delighted with her restoration.

Case 10
A full arch restoration for a maxillary knife-edge ridge

The true knife-edge ridge develops in the maxilla rather than the mandible. When a knife-edge ridge is seen in the mandible, it is usually the unresorbed mylohyoid ridge. The true ridge crest has resorbed

to a flatter, and many times concave, surface buccal to the mylohyoid ridge. The situation is camouflaged by the mucoperiosteal tissue over the bone and cannot be realized readily until the soft tissues have been incised and retracted.

In the maxilla, however, the alveolar bone resorbs in a buccopalatal or labiopalatal direction. Therefore the knife-edge of the ridge is the true ridge. Here too the situation is often camouflaged as a result of the extreme thickness of the fibromucosal tissue over the ridge.

Because of the tendency of the mucoperiosteum to camouflage the bone's morphology, it is now considered imperative to incise and retract the tissues in order to expose the underlying bony ridge, no matter what type of implant is contemplated. This not only avoids perforating the cortical plates, it also ensures that no epithelium will be pushed down to the artificial socket and proliferate there.

This case, accomplished on a 52-year-old woman,

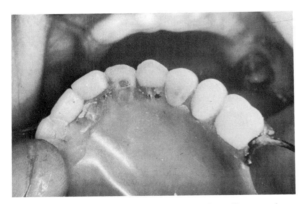

Fig. 11-117. The patient had been unhappily wearing a removable prosthesis.

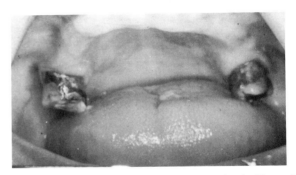

Fig. 11-118. Only two molar teeth remained. Note the thickness of the fibromucosal tissue, which often camouflages the morphology of the underlying maxillary ridge.

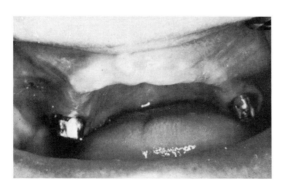

Fig. 11-119. Both molar teeth were prepared for full crown restorations.

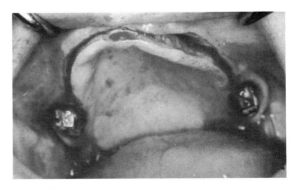

Fig. 11-120. The incision was made from molar to molar along the crest of the ridge.

will dramatically demonstrate that whereas knife-edge ridges were formerly contraindicated for implant procedures, they can now be utilized for the blade implants.

The woman had a poorly functioning removable prosthesis for many years (Fig. 11-117). Only the two teeth remaining in the upper arch, which were the second molars on each side, supported the denture

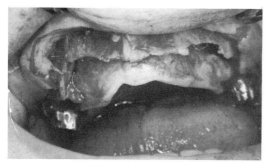

Fig. 11-121. Once the thick tissues were retracted, the degree of knife-like resorption was evident.

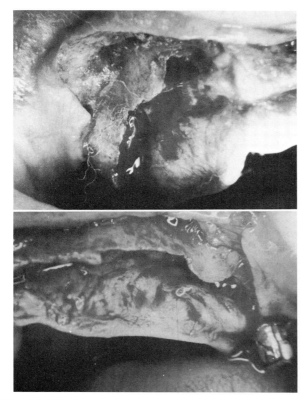

Fig. 11-122. These close-ups of the lateral views of the ridge are characteristic examples of why it is important to expose the bone before implant insertion.

(Fig. 11-118). These were prepared for full crown restorations, maintaining the same vertical dimension with temporary crown forms placed over them (Fig. 11-119).

At the next visit, two metal cast copings were tried over the molars for fit and accuracy. These were then removed and the operation proceeded. The maxilla was anesthetized by infiltration anesthesia on the labial, buccal, and palatal surfaces, using lidocaine (Xylocaine) 1:100,000. An incision was made along the crest of the soft tissue ridge from the mesial proximal surface of each of the two molar teeth (Fig. 11-120). The tissues covering the buccal, labial, and palatal surfaces of the bone were reflected

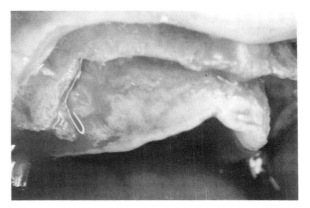

Fig. 11-123. Approximately 3 mm. of the ridge was reduced to widen the occlusal table.

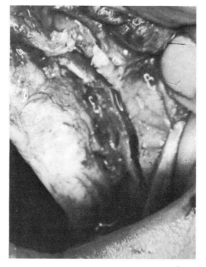

Fig. 11-124. Grooves were made in the flattened ridges.

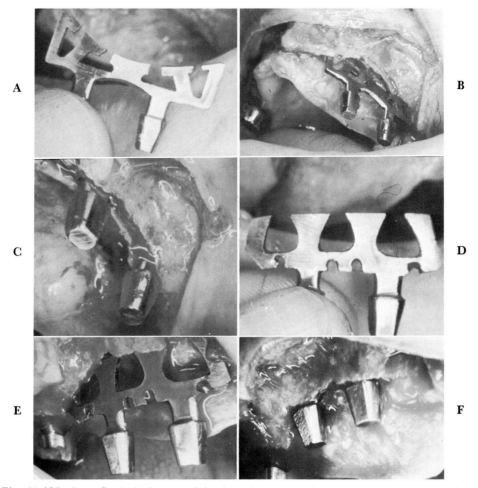

Fig. 11-125. A to C, A double-posted implant, bent to conform to the groove of the ridge, was inserted on each side. This is the left implant. D to F, The right implant, grooved accordingly, was inserted. Because of its unique design, a single blade may be used in the area rather than several post type implants.

to expose enough of the bone to determine the mode of approach (Fig. 11-121).

The alveolar bone had resorbed to a tremendously sharp knife-edge ridge around the entire arch (Fig. 11-122). In its current state, it was impossible to place any type of implant in such a ridge. However, a re-evaluation of the intraoral and extraoral radiographs indicated that there would still be enough alveolar bone height from the floor of the antrum to the knife-edge ridge if the table were flattened by removing 2 or 3 mm. of the sharp edge of the ridge. Therefore the ridge was filed shorter and rounded, automatically making the crest thicker buccopalatally (Fig. 11-123).

A narrow groove was made with extreme care on each side of the arch with a No. 700L fissure bur to bisect the buccopalatal width of the alveolar crest. The two grooves were also curved to follow the arch (Fig. 11-124). Two long, double-posted blade implants were bent to conform to the curved grooves, inserted, and tapped into the bone (Fig. 11-125). The incised tissues were sutured closed (Fig. 11-126).

A temporary acrylic splint fabricated from an alginate impression taken of the patient's old denture was cold-cured in the mouth, trimmed, and cemented into place with one of the soft tone conditioners (Fig. 11-127).

Six days later the sutures were removed (Fig. 11-128). Two gold copings were placed over the molar crown preparations, and acrylic copings were

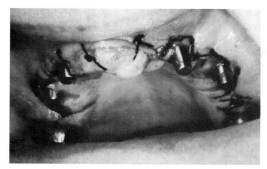

Fig. 11-126. The tissues were sutured over the implant.

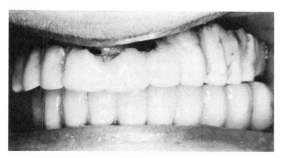

Fig. 11-127. A cold cure acrylic splint made from the patient's old denture was used for temporary stability.

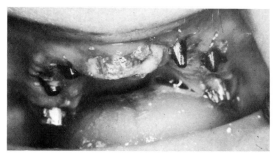

Fig. 11-128. Six days later the tissues had healed sufficiently around the implants to allow removal of the sutures. The inflammation of the anterior soft tissues was caused by the impingement from the ill-fitting temporary splint.

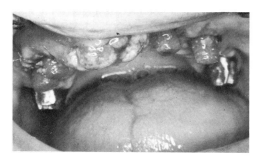

Fig. 11-129. In order to finish the prosthesis as rapidly as possible, the copings were fitted at this very same visit.

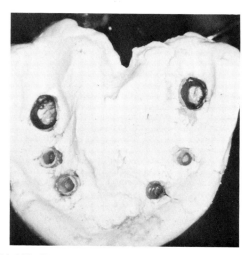

Fig. 11-130. The plaster index with the copings included.

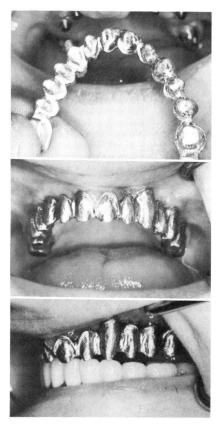

Fig. 11-131. Five days later (11 days postoperatively) the one-piece metal casting was fitted over the abutments.

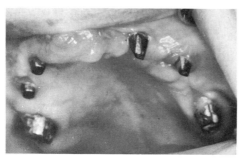

Fig. 11-132. The healed tissues 21 days postoperatively.

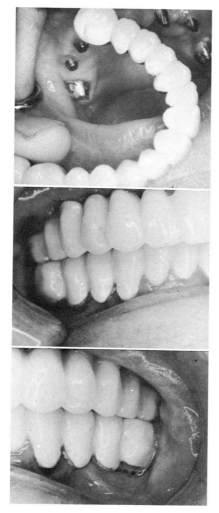

Fig. 11-133. The biscuit-baked prosthesis was tried. All necessary occlusal and esthetic changes were done during the final glazing process of the porcelain.

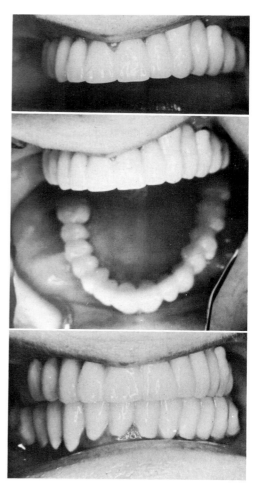

Fig. 11-134. The final prosthesis cemented in place.

placed over the implant posts (Fig. 11-129). A wax interocclusal record of centric relation was made, followed by a full upper plaster index that included the gold and acrylic copings (Fig. 11-130). An alginate (irreversible hydrocolloid) impression of the teeth in the opposing dental arch was also taken.

At the next visit a one-piece metal casting, which included the six copings and all of the metal pontics, was fitted over the implant posts and tooth abutments (Fig. 11-131). All necessary gingival and occlusal adjustments were made. A final wax interocclusal record of centric relation was taken.

At this point if any discrepancy exists between the tissue-bearing surfaces of the pontics and the underlying soft tissues, an Opotow* paste mix is placed over the shy surfaces of the pontics and the frame-

*Manufactured by Opotow Dental Manufacturing Co. Brooklyn, N. Y.

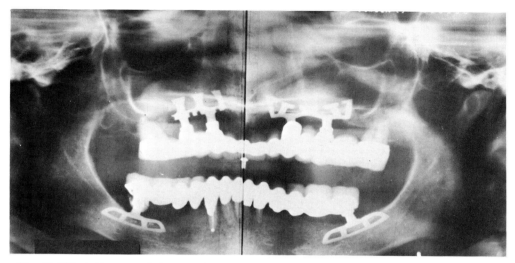

Fig. 11-135. A Panorex of the completed case. Although there are only two blades, each spans an area previously occupied by four teeth. The obvious stability against lateral dislodgment is evident.

work is once again replaced. After it sets, the entire framework is picked up with a full mouth alginate (irreversible hydrocolloid) impression, and a new master stone model is poured and articulated for the completion of the prosthesis.

By the next visit the tissue was completely healed (Fig. 11-132). The case was tried while still in the "biscuit bake" stage and any necessary adjustments were made (Fig. 11-133).

The final visit consisted of cementing the prosthesis with hard cement (Fig. 11-134) and last-minute spot-grinding. The final Panorex illustrates the extreme versatility and usefulness of blade implants (Fig. 11-135). It is Linkow's firm opinion that placing the blades into such a narrow ridge actually widens it by the wedge action of the blades. A blood clot forms that differentiates into fibrous tissue that eventually fills in with bone by intramembranous bone formation. The implants, when placed into proper function, continue to stimulate the bone to continue its osteogenic activities. Dozens of knife-edge ridges similar to this case have been restored in this manner and are all still functioning successfully.

THE EDENTULOUS MANDIBLE

Restoring an edentulous jaw with endosseous implants, even prior to the evolution of the blade variety, has been more successful in the mandible than in the maxilla. Mandibular bone is much denser and the thick cortical plate along the alveolar crest

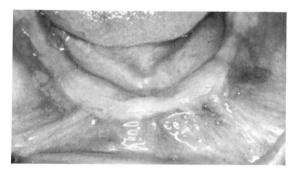

Fig. 11-136. The edentulous mandible.

provides an ideal brace for the shoulders of the blade. The law of gravity also favors lower implant cases as compared with upper ones.

The major considerations in inserting blades in the edentulous mandible are determining the most appropriate implant sites and creating grooves of the proper depth and width so that the blades can be tapped into the bone with a minimum of trauma.

The following sample case is typical of most blade implant restorations for the mandible.

Case 11
A typical restoration for an edentulous mandible

First, radiographs were taken to determine the height of alveolar bone above the mandibular canals and mental foramina. Based upon studies of these, four blades of the proper design and size were selected.

The edentulous ridge was injected with bilateral nerve blocks as well as infiltration anesthesia (Fig. 11-136). An incision was made along the crest of the ridge from retromolar pad area to retromolar pad area. The tissues were reflected to expose the bone. The groove for the first blade was made in the right molar area and the implant was set into it and tapped in until its shoulders were buried between the existing cortical plates (Fig. 11-137).

The second groove was made in the cuspid-bicuspid area. (If it is necessary to curve the groove in this area to follow the crest, the implant can be

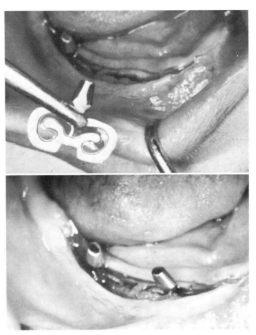

Fig. 11-137. Because there was not enough alveolar bone above the mandibular canal, a narrow blade was inserted. Careful evaluation of the x-rays before implant insertion helped ensure the appropriate blade.

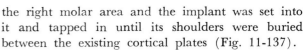

Fig. 11-138. Because more bone existed anteriorly, a blade longer in its superior and inferior dimensions was used.

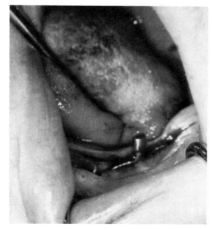

Fig. 11-139. Because there was not enough room to place double-headed blades that were wider anteriorly and posteriorly, four smaller single-headed blades were used.

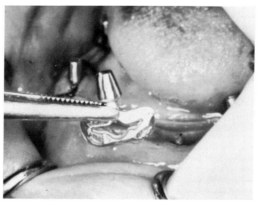

Fig. 11-140. A curved blade was used to follow the contour of the bone in the left cuspid region.

easily bent with pliers to conform to it.) The implant was slightly curved, set in its groove, and tapped into position (Fig. 11-138). The left posterior blade was inserted (Fig. 11-139), and then the left anterior blade was appropriately curved and tapped to its proper depth (Fig. 11-140).

The tissues were adapted and sutured with simple surgical ties (Fig. 11-141). When the sutures were removed (Fig. 11-142), the patient's old denture was hollowed out, lined with a soft tissue reliner, and used as a temporary splint until the final prosthesis could be fabricated (Fig. 11-143).

Impressions were taken with the necessary bite registrations for the fabrication and completion of the full arch fixed denture. In this case the final prosthesis was acrylic over gold, with six gold occlusal stops (Fig. 11-144). It was cemented into position with hard cement (Fig. 11-145). The teeth were carefully and accurately spot-ground in the mouth for final balancing.

A Panorex shows the edentulous mandible with four blades supporting the full arch fixed denture (Fig. 11-146, *A*).

It should be noted that the implants used in this

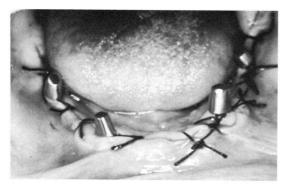

Fig. 11-141. The tissues were sutured over the implants.

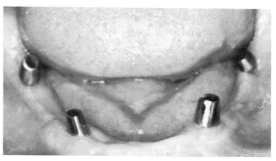

Fig. 11-142. The excellent healing around each implant post is evident 2 weeks postoperatively. Note also the lack of parallelism, which resulted from the fact that these earlier types of blades were cast in cobalt-chrome, which could not be bent. Also, the hardness of the metal made it extremely difficult to parallel the posts with grinding stones. In spite of this, note the excellent condition of the tissues around each post.

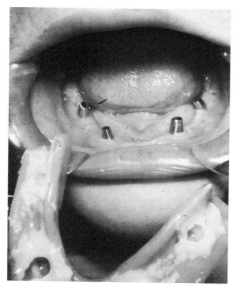

Fig. 11-143. The patient's old denture, relined with soft tissue conditioner, was placed temporarily over the implants. To make the posts parallel prior to final impressions, they were ground directly in the mouth.

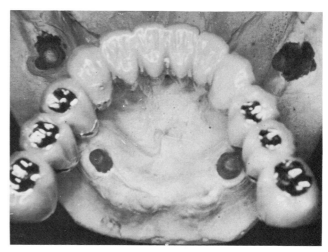

Fig. 11-144. An acrylic-over-gold full arch fixed denture with six gold occlusal stops is seen on the stone model.

case were cobalt-chrome castings, which made it impossible to bend the necks in order to parallel the posts. Because of this hardness it was also difficult to prepare the posts in the mouth with grinding stones and burs to be parallel with each other. However,

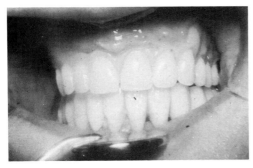

Fig. 11-145. The final prosthesis in place. Note open anterior flange in maxillary denture.

before the bridge was cemented, the posts were prepared parallel with each other.

Today titanium blades* are manufactured that allow the operator to easily bend the necks or the blade itself to fit into a curved groove. It also becomes quite simple to grind away portions of the posts for parallelism. Fig. 11-146, *B*, shows the parallelism that is readily attained with titanium blades in another edentulous mandible.

Case 12
A removable denture for an edentulous mandible using retromolar blade implants in combination with other blade type implants

In some cases where there is extreme alveolar resorption in the molar region of the mandible, ac-

*Park Dental Research Corp., New York, N. Y.

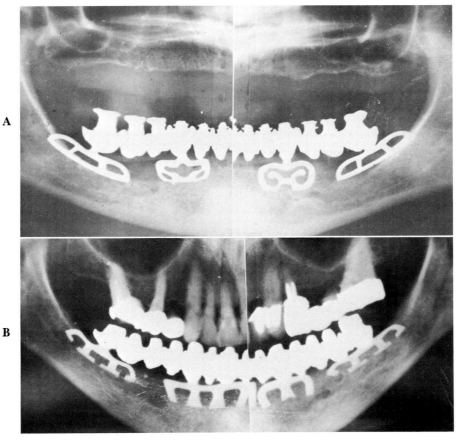

Fig. 11-146. A, The final Panorex. (From Linkow, L. I., and Weiss, J. L.: The endosseous blade: a progress report, Prom. Dent., No. 5, 1969.) **B,** Another case using blade implants as the only supports for a fixed full arch denture in the completely edentulous mandible opposing a natural upper dentition.

cording to Dr. Harold Roberts, there still remains serviceable bone in the retromolar area and in the ramus. Thus Roberts developed the retromolar blade implant (Fig. 11-147).

The retromolar blade implant is placed into the bone by first making a long incision along the fibromucosal tissue covering the alveolar crest. The mesial limit of the incision is approximately 28 mm. distal to the mental foramen and extends distally approximately 18 mm. A groove is cut with a No. 560 bur immediately below the incision into the cortical bone, extending distally approximately 14 to 18 mm. to the entire depth of the bur (5.5 mm.). The distal end of the sickle-shaped implant is then inserted into the slot in the bone below the cortical plate and is tapped distally into the medullary portion of the ramus between the buccal and lingual cortical plates until the mesial lip of the blade portion of the implant clears the anterior margin of the bony slot. Since the inferior surface of the implant is rounded, it slips gently into place posteriorly into the ascending ramus. A grooved chisel and plastic-headed mallet are all that is necessary for this procedure. With a crown and bridge remover locked behind the distal proximal surface of the protruding post, the implant is gently tapped mesially so that the mesial spur of the implant locks under the cortical plate that forms the anterior limit of the bony slot. The flaps of the soft tissue are repositioned and sutured around the protruding post. The sutures are removed in 5 to 7 days.

An impression is taken of all the protruding posts for a one-piece gold coping–dolder bar framework that is cemented into position. A removable prosthesis is then fabricated to fit over the gold framework, with or without the addition of retentive type attachments.

THE EDENTULOUS MAXILLA

Fixed restorations for the edentulous maxilla have posed a major problem in the field of implantology. Because the maxillary alveolar bone usually resorbs in a buccopalatal direction, ultimately leaving a knife-edge ridge, post and triplant implants are often unsuitable or inadequate. Perforation is common, and the danger of destroying a good portion of the alveolar crest is a real threat. In addition, because extremely thick fibromucosal tissue often camouflages a thin ridge, it is usually almost impossible to enter the bone directly at the crest to insert a post type implant. As for tripod pins, there is frequently no room to diverge them, and the thick soft tissue promotes a trifurcation involvement. Obviously, an implant had to be designed specifically for knife-edge ridge conditions. This implant is the blade.

The endosseous blade implants, although functioning in the mouths of patients for approximately 3 years, seem to be extremely encouraging for the edentulous maxillary patient. The following cases illustrate their use.

Case 13
A full arch palateless fixed restoration for a completely edentulous maxilla

Impressions were taken of the edentulous maxilla (Fig. 11-148), including an elastic impression, a bite rim and tray, a lower alginate impression, and a wax bite. At the next visit, the tray was lined with Opotow paste and placed in the patient's mouth. When it hardened, it was trimmed and the wax rim care-

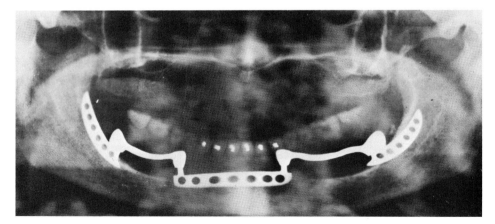

Fig. 11-147. Retromolar blade implant abutments in combination with an anterior blade acting as abutments for a removable prosthesis. (Courtesy Dr. Harold Roberts.)

fully heated. The tray was then replaced in the mouth and centric occlusion established.

A palateless denture with deep channels prepared through the tissue-bearing surface corresponding to the alveolar crest was fabricated. Appropriate implants were selected from radiographic studies (Fig. 11-149).

On the following visit the operation was begun by making a single incision from retromolar pad area to retromolar pad area with a sharp scalpel. The incised tissues were reflected with a periosteal elevator to expose the underlying bone. It is much more difficult to reflect maxillary tissue than mandibular tissue. In the mandible the cortical plate of bone is extremely compact, with a smooth surface. In the maxilla, on the other hand, the bone forming the

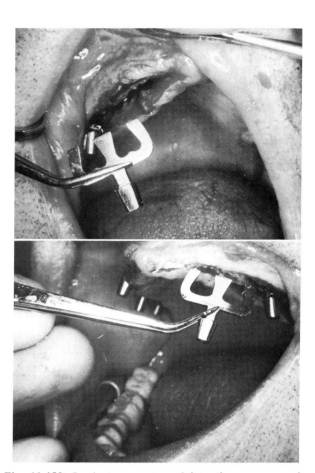

Fig. 11-150. Implants were tapped into the grooves made in the knife-edge ridge.

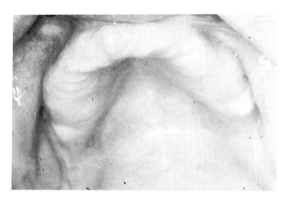

Fig. 11-148. The edentulous maxilla. Again note that the fibromucosa camouflages the underlying bone.

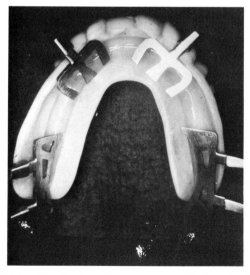

Fig. 11-149. A palateless denture was prefabricated with a continuous deep channel to accept the protruding implant posts.

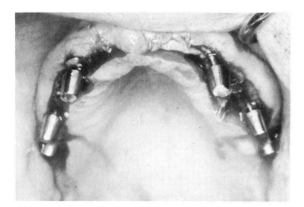

Fig. 11-151. The implants in place. Posteriorly, the double-posted implants were used for added retention of the prosthesis.

ridge is uneven and extremely porous, with the tissue tenaciously bound to it. Thus extreme care is needed to avoid tearing the tissue while separating it in order to reduce postoperative complications. As a note of interest, Linkow has never found a cortical plate of bone covering the alveolar crest in the posterior edentulous area of the maxillae from the bicuspid to tuberosity regions, no matter how long a time the area was edentulous.

Grooves the same mesiodistal length as their corresponding blades were made in the desired areas of the ridge about 6 mm. deep. The blades were set in their grooves (Fig. 11-150) and tapped in until their shoulders were below the bony ridge (Fig. 11-151). The tissue was then completely closed with surgical ties (Fig. 11-152). The palateless temporary denture was adjusted, lined with Hydrocast,* and fitted over

*Manufactured by Kay-See Dental Co., Kansas City, Mo.

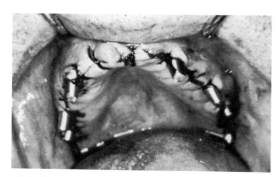

Fig. 11-152. Tissues were sutured over the implants.

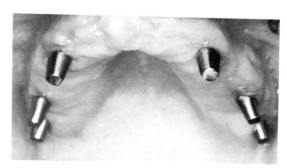

Fig. 11-153. The healed tissues 2 weeks postoperatively.

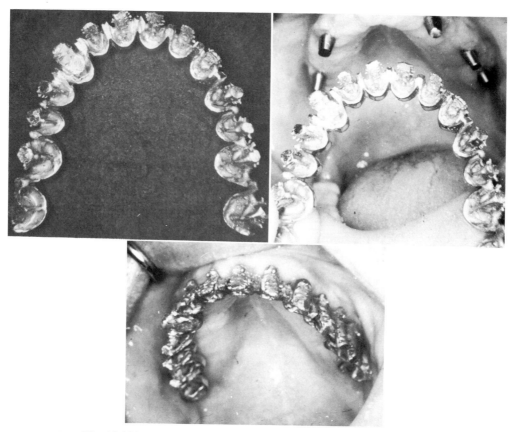

Fig. 11-154. A one-piece gold casting for an acrylic prosthesis is used.

the implant posts. It was then carefully occluded with the lower jaw.

When complete healing had taken place (Fig. 11-153), interchangeable prefabricated gold copings were placed over the implant posts. A bite registration and a full mouth plaster index were taken, picking up the copings.

At the next visit, the soldered full arch splint was tried in the mouth (Fig. 11-154). A final wax interocclusal record of centric relation was then taken for completing the bridge.

By the time the bridge was ready for final insertion, the tissues around the posts were completely healed and closely adapted (Fig. 11-155). The full arch fixed denture, made of acrylic-over-gold, was cemented over the metal posts with hard cement (Fig. 11-156). The occlusion was then carefully spot-ground for any other prematurities caused by the addition of the cement (Fig. 11-157).

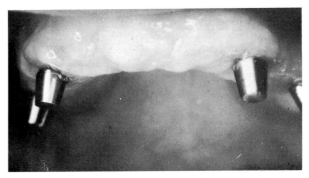

Fig. 11-155. A close-up view of the healed tissues before the final prosthesis was inserted.

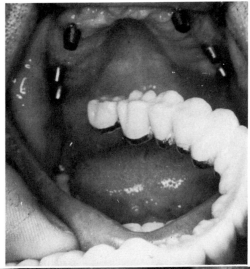

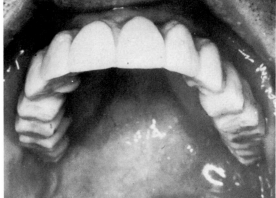

Fig. 11-156. The final prosthesis in place.

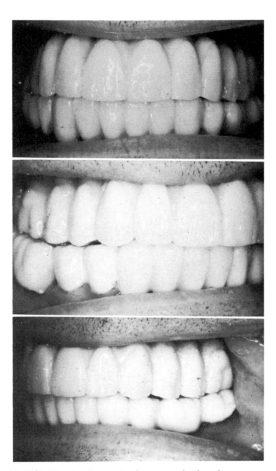

Fig. 11-157. The final prosthesis was articulated.

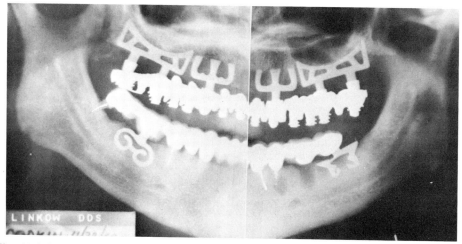

Fig. 11-158. The final Panorex. An apicoectomy had been done at the apex of the lower left first bicuspid tooth, and a tooth extraction was done 1 week before the radiograph was taken. (From Linkow, L. I.: Status of oral implants, 1969, Inform. Odontostomat., Vol. 1, 1969.)

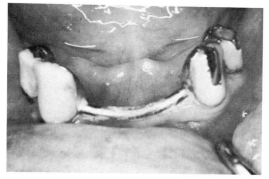

Fig. 11-159. Preoperative view of patient's existing teeth and prosthesis.

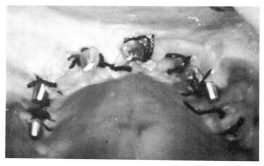

Fig. 11-160. Blade implants were placed in the edentulous maxilla and sutured.

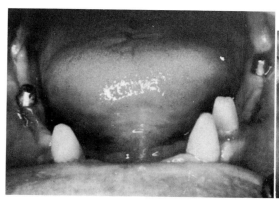

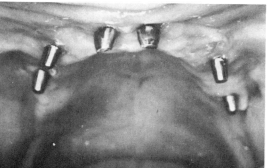

Fig. 11-161. When the tissues had healed, impressions were taken for the prostheses.

A final Panorex not only shows the full arch splint stabilized in the maxilla with four implants but also lower implants (Fig. 11-158). The two dark areas on the left side represent a recent apicoectomy at the apex of the lower first left bicuspid and a hemisection removing the mesial root of the lower right molar.

Case 14
A full arch restoration for an edentulous maxilla combined with a full arch restoration for a bilaterally posterior edentulous mandible

The patient, a 51-year-old male in good health, was wearing a full upper denture and a removable partial denture supported by four veneer crowns splinted together with a dolder bar (Fig. 11-159). Because his first lower right bicuspid lacked support-

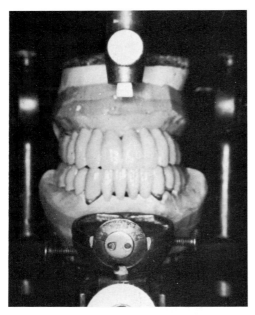

Fig. 11-162. The case was articulated on a Hanau articulator.

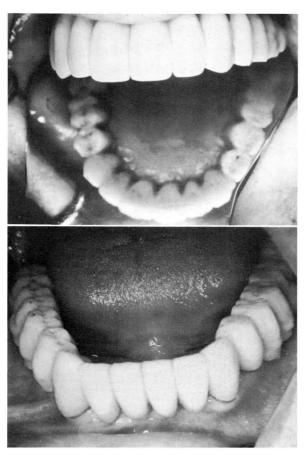

Fig. 11-163. The finished acrylic-over-gold prostheses.

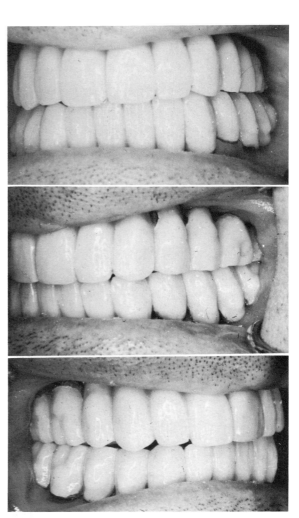

Fig. 11-164. The prostheses were articulated.

ing bone, it was extracted. The remaining three teeth were prepared for new full crown restorations.

Blade implants were set into the bone in both right and left posterior quadrants of the mandible and into the completely edentulous maxilla (Fig. 11-160). Temporary acrylic splints were processed

for the patient to carry him over until all the tissue had healed.

When the tissues had healed (Fig. 11-161), all necessary impressions were taken for upper and lower full arch fixed dentures. These were made in acrylic over gold, because the materials are lighter

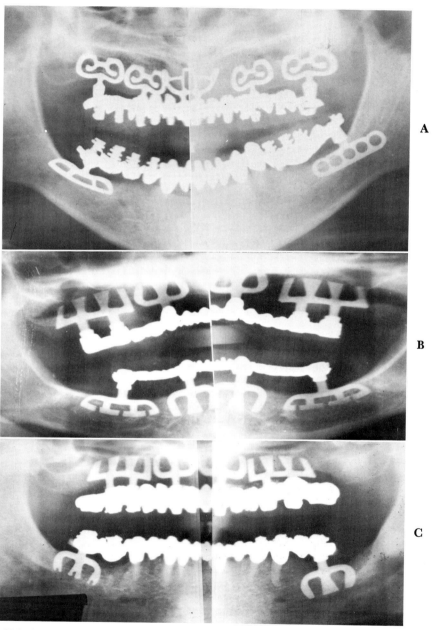

A

B

C

Fig. 11-165. **A,** A Panorex of the finished case. (From Linkow, L. I.: Status of oral implants, 1969, Inform. Odontostomat., Vol. 1, 1969.) **B and C,** Two other examples of completely edentulous maxillae restored with full arch fixed prostheses. In **B** both jaws were completely edentulous. They were restored with porcelain-baked-to-palladium-and-gold. In **C** they were made of acrylic processed to gold.

than porcelain and were articulated on a Hanau articulator (Fig. 11-162).

Today, however, Linkow often uses palladium and gold rather than platinum and gold for porcelain-baked-to-metal restorations for the edentulous maxillary cases. This creates a prosthesis even lighter in weight than acrylic processed on gold.

Both final prostheses were set over the implants in both jaws, using one of the temporary cements mixed with Vaseline or Calendula* (Fig. 11-163). The patient wore them for a few days to test for comfort and freedom from soft tissue impingements. When he returned, the bridges were removed and their tissue-bearing surfaces relieved. With oxyphosphate of zinc cement, both bridges were then cemented into their respective positions (Fig. 11-164). They were then once more carefully spot-ground for any prematurities.

A final Panorex shows both bridges in position (Fig. 11-165, A). Fig. 11-165, B, illustrates another edentulous maxilla and edentulous mandible restored with blades. Fig. 11-165, C, represents another case of a completely edentulous maxilla and partially edentulous mandible.

Case 15
A continuous blade implant for an edentulous maxilla

There are times when, because of extremely low-flaring sinuses with numerous areas of bone porosity, individual blades cannot provide adequate support in an edentulous maxilla. Therefore a continuous implant was designed by Linkow and Norman Mulnick. This implant was shaped to the contour of the crest, hopefully creating more retention by acting as a self-splinting device. It was also hoped that the relative instability of those portions of the blade set in porous bone would be compensated for by the fact that there was enough of the rest of the blade in denser bone. A few cases were tried, such as that on the edentulous maxilla detailed here (Fig. 11-166).

The soft tissue covering the edentulous maxilla was pierced from tuberosity to tuberosity along the crest of the ridge with a sharp scalpel (Fig. 11-167). The tissue was retracted with a periosteal elevator to expose the buccal and labial aspects of the ridge and part of the palatal portion. A groove was created along the center of the ridge from one side of the arch to the other with a No. 700L fissure bur. Its depth was never more than 3 mm. (Fig. 11-168).

*Homeopathic healing salve, Boericke & Tofel, Philadelphia.

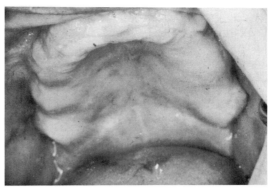

Fig. 11-166. An edentulous maxilla with very little bone below the maxillary sinus.

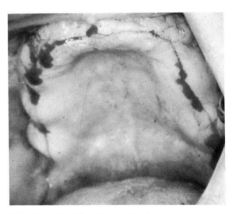

Fig. 11-167. The incision is made from retromolar area to retromolar area.

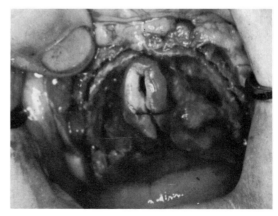

Fig. 11-168. Underlying alveolar crest was exposed and a 2- to 3-mm. continuous groove was made. (From Linkow, L. I., and Weiss, J. L.: The endosseous blade: a progress report, Prom. Dent., No. 5, 1969.)

A specially prepared tray was made and an elastic impression taken of the ridge area with the continuous groove (Fig. 11-169). The master stone model was poured into the impression. The shallow groove in the separated hardened stone model was deepened to the various depths indicated by Panorex studies of the entire jaw (Fig. 11-170). A cobalt-chrome casting was made. Like individual blades, it was wedge-shaped.

During the following visit, the tissue was once again incised and reflected, and the continuous blade

was placed inside the original groove (Fig. 11-171). It was then tapped deeper with a plastic-headed mallet and inserting instrument until its shoulder was buried (Fig. 11-172). The site was closed with interrupted sutures (Fig. 11-173), and a prefabricated

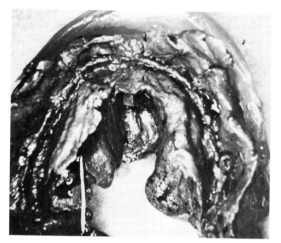

Fig. 11-169. To obtain an accurate impression, the elastic material was forced into the groove.

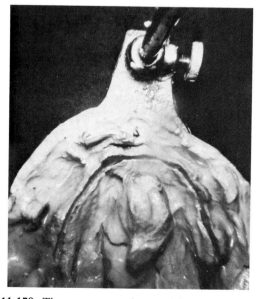

Fig. 11-170. The groove was deepened in the master stone model to comply with the x-ray interpretation.

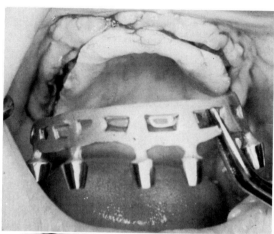

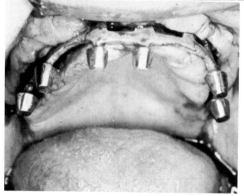

Fig. 11-171. A one-piece continuous blade was inserted into the groove. (From Linkow, L. I., and Weiss, J. L.: The endosseous blade: a progress report, Prom. Dent., No. 5, 1969.)

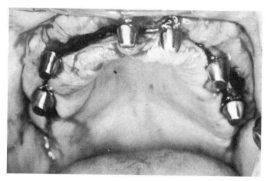

Fig. 11-172. The blade was tapped deeper until its shoulder was slightly below the alveolar crest.

temporary splint was placed over the posts to protect the site.

After the site had healed (Fig. 11-174), impressions were taken for the fabrication and completion of an acrylic-over-gold full arch splint. This was permanently seated with hard cement (Fig. 11-175).

A Panorex shows the continuous blade in place (Fig. 11-176). The patient had been successfully wearing the lower blade prosthesis nearly a year prior to the upper restoration. Since the lower restoration was one of the earlier types that was prefabricated prior to the insertion of the blades, acrylic

saddles had to be fabricated. These saddles cannot be viewed on radiographs, and thus on radiographs it appeared as though the margins of the crowns covering the implant posts were inadequate. Upon clinical observation this misconception is clearly revealed.

Case 16
A continuous palatal horseshoe blade for a fixed full arch denture

Although the early type of continuous blade seemed very promising, problems occurred. The main

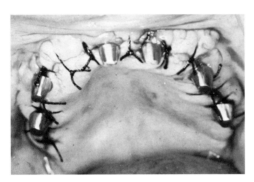

Fig. 11-173. The tissues were closed. (From Linkow, L. I., and Weiss, J. L.: The endosseous blade: a progress report, Prom. Dent., No. 5, 1969.)

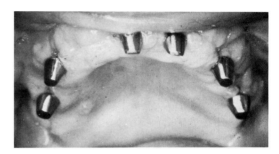

Fig. 11-174. The healed site.

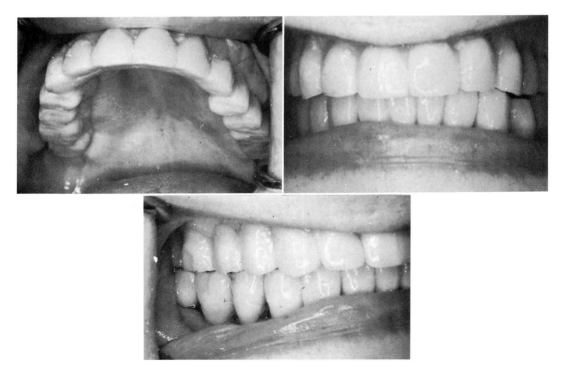

Fig. 11-175. The completed acrylic prosthesis cemented in place.

drawback was that if there was not enough dense bone, then there could not be sufficient support for a continuous blade implant. Therefore a support was added across the palate to more closely adapt the implant to its site. The implant is called the palatal bar horseshoe blade.

This patient had had recent extractions (Fig. 11-177). The fibromucosal tissue was incised and separated from the bone. Because of the palatal ex-

tensions needed in this new implant design, most of the hard palate was also exposed, including the posterior nasal spine and greater and lesser palatine foramina. The palatal tissue was then retracted in a posterior direction from the incision. Grooves were planned only for those areas where the alveolar crest was wide. In this particular case they were made in the left posterior alveolar ridge, ending anteriorly just distal to the recent open

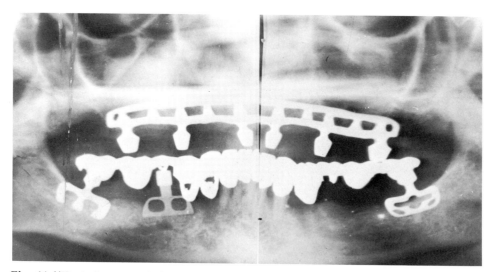

Fig. 11-176. A Panorex of the completed maxillary restoration. The mandibular restoration had been successfully functioning for over a year. Since it was one of the earlier cases the prosthesis was prefabricated before the implants were set into the bone. Large holes were made inside the pontics corresponding to the implants and then they were locked to the protruding posts with acrylic resin, which cannot be seen on a radiograph. This method is no longer done since the blades can remain unsupported for many weeks after their initial insertion. (From Linkow, L. I.: Status of oral implants, 1969, Inform. Odontostomat., Vol. 1, 1969.)

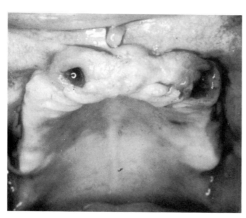

Fig. 11-177. The edentulous maxilla with recent extractions. Note the density and irregularity of the fibromucosa.

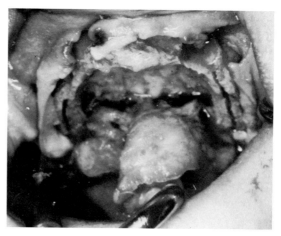

Fig. 11-178. The knife-edge ridge was only grooved laterally because the anterior portion flared.

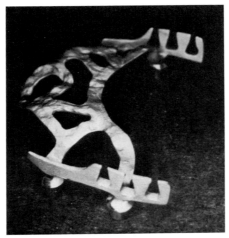

Fig. 11-179. The completed cobalt-chrome one-piece casting of the palatal horseshoe type blade.

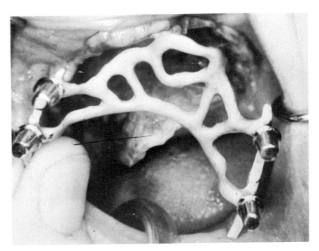

Fig. 11-180. The implant being inserted.

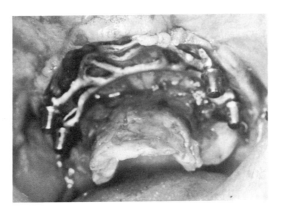

Fig. 11-181. The implant tapped into position.

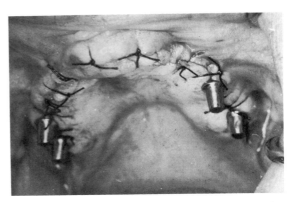

Fig. 11-182. The tissues are carefully sutured together.

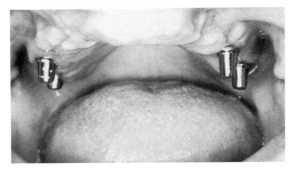

Fig. 11-183. Healing after 2 weeks.

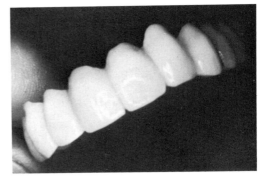

Fig. 11-184. The acrylic full arch splint.

socket, and on the right side, extending as far anteriorly as the buccolingual thickness of the bone permitted (Fig. 11-178). Anteriorly it was impossible to make a groove. Not only was the bone knife-edged, but the entire maxillary process flared out, making it impossible to parallel an anterior groove with the two posterior ones.

The elastic impression included a good portion of the palate as well as the alveolar grooves. From this impression a stone cast was poured. The design and depth of the blades were once again determined by x-rays, and the grooves were made directly in the stone model to coincide with the x-ray findings. A duplicate model on which the horseshoe palatal blade

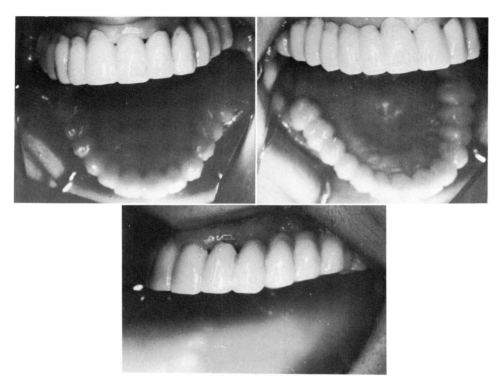

Fig. 11-185. The splint cemented in position.

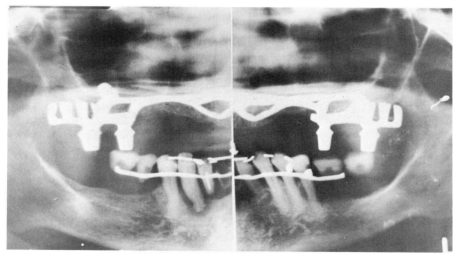

Fig. 11-186. The final Panorex. The mandibular arch was later restored.

was waxed, invested, and then cast was made from this modified stone model (Fig. 11-179).

On the next visit, the tissues were once more incised and reflected to expose the underlying bone. The palatal bar horseshoe blade was then carefully placed into the grooves (Fig. 11-180) and tapped into position (Fig. 11-181). While tapping the implant, extreme care was taken to guide its insertion so that the palatal portion became flush with the hard palate as the shoulders of the blades became level with the cortical plates of bone.

The tissues were brought snugly together over the shoulders of the implant and around the necks of the abutment posts with surgical ties (Fig. 11-182). About 10 days later the wound had healed (Fig. 11-183), and the various impression techniques were employed to complete the prosthesis which, in this case, was an all-acrylic splint (Fig. 11-184). It was cemented over the abutment posts with hard cement (Fig. 11-185). A final Panorex shows the extension of the blade across the palate (Fig. 11-186).

The palatal horseshoe type of implant can be considered to be a combined subperiosteal-endosseous implant because of its palatal extension.

Case 17
A palatal horseshoe blade implant for a removable palateless partial denture

The procedures for stabilizing a removable palateless denture with a horseshoe blade implant are basically similar to those for a fixed denture, except for the final impressions for the prosthesis itself. A removable denture rather than a fixed prosthesis becomes apparent when a sufficient amount of labial bone resorption has taken place to prevent proper esthetics to be attained with a fixed appliance.

The incision was made from maxillary tuberosity to maxillary tuberosity (Fig. 11-187). The tissues were retracted with a periosteal elevator to expose the entire hard palate. Grooves were then made in the bone and a rubber base impression taken with a specially designed tray. Some impression material was first loaded on the tray while still in a sticky form, while the rest was continously spatulated until it became putty-like. This portion was taken in the hands, forced into the shallow grooves, and molded over the ridges and palatal portion; the loaded tray was immediately placed over it and held in position for about 10 minutes. When it hardened, it was removed (Fig. 11-188), and a bone bite was then taken with wax.

Before the tissues were sutured closed, the thickness of the mucoperiosteum in all areas intended for posts was measured. This was done so that the necks of the implant would not be made too long or too short. The tissues were then sutured together.

The master stone model was poured and articulated with the lower case. The original shallow grooves made in the bone and transferred to the stone model were then deepened according to the radiographic interpretations (Fig. 11-189). The thickness or degree of taper of these grooves in the master stone cast did not matter, since it was intended that the implant be trimmed and tapered to form the characteristic wedge after casting (Fig. 11-190).

At the next visit the tissues were again incised and reflected to insert the implant (Fig. 11-191). The tissues were sutured over the implant (Fig. 11-192). When the tissues had nearly healed (Fig. 11-193),

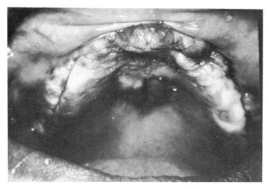

Fig. 11-187. The incision was made along the fibromucosal tissue covering the edentulous maxillary ridge.

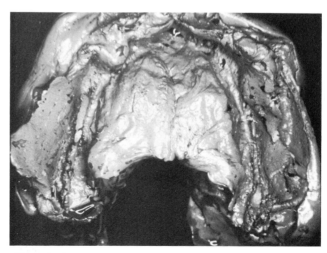

Fig. 11-188. An elastic impression was made including exposed palate and the posterior grooves.

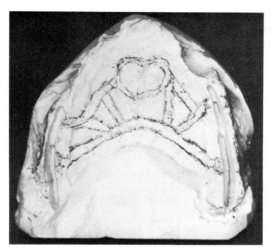

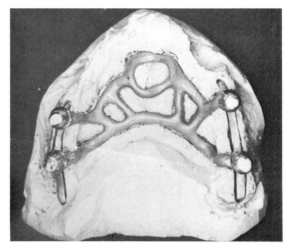

Fig. 11-189. An implant was designed on the master stone model and the grooves deepened according to the x-ray findings.

Fig. 11-190. The completed casting.

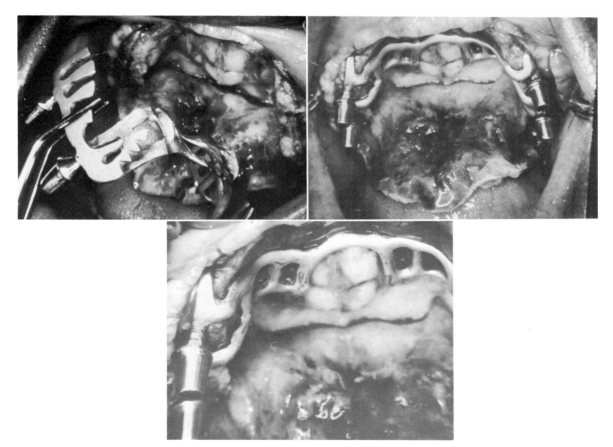

Fig. 11-191. The implant being inserted. Note its close adaptation to the palate and grooves.

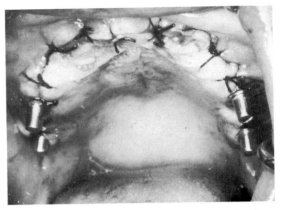

Fig. 11-192. The tissues were closed over the implant.

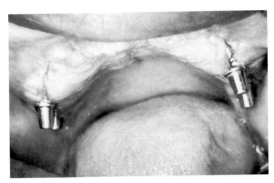

Fig. 11-193. The almost completely healed tissue 10 days postoperatively.

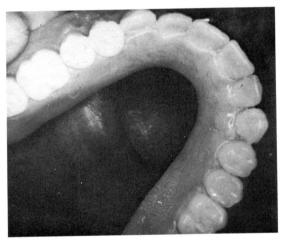

Fig. 11-194. Because so much anterior bone had been resorbed, a palateless denture with an anterior acrylic flange was fabricated.

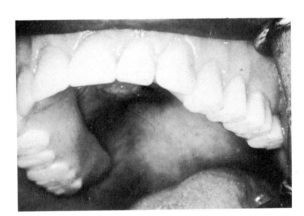

Fig. 11-195. The denture in position.

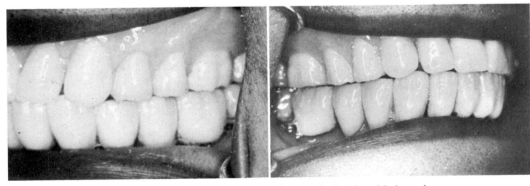

Fig. 11-196. The denture was carefully articulated and balanced.

impressions were taken for the fabrication of a palate-less removable denture (Fig. 11-194).

In such cases, the retention of a denture over protruding posts can be secured several ways:

1. Using only a functional grip of acrylic
2. Processing 360-degree clasps joined together with a connecting bar directly inside the denture (The metal superstructure is fabricated at the same time that the implant casting is made and in the same manner and form that superstructures are made for subperiosteal implants.)
3. Fabricating metal copings of gold or Vitallium

to fit snugly to the protruding posts and fastening them directly inside the denture
4. Including Gerber, Ceka, or internal clip bars for retentive purposes

Here, a frictional grip of acrylic was used (Fig. 11-195). The palateless denture was carefully articulated and balanced (Fig. 11-196). The Panorex x-ray of the completed case shows not only the maxillary palatal bar horseshoe blade implant but also a full arch mandibular splint supported by three posterior blade implants functioning successfully over 18 months previously to the upper restoration (Fig. 11-197).

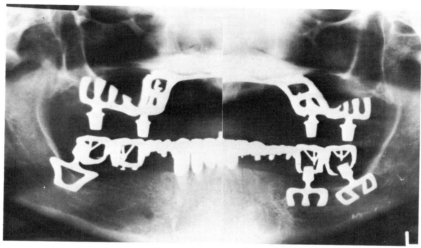

Fig. 11-197. Note how the maxillary blade circumvents the sinuses. The mandibular restoration was done 18 months previously and was of the earlier prefabricated type. (From Linkow, L. I.: Status of oral implants, 1969, Inform. Odontostomat., Vol. 1, 1969.)

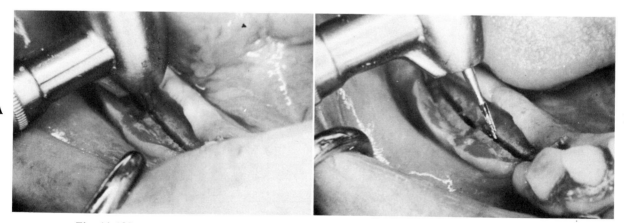

Fig. 11-198. Making a proper groove for a blade implant. A, The groove must be deep enough to accept the entire body of the blade. To do this, it is often necessary to drive the No. 700L fissure bur down to midshank. B, Note that although the groove may be deep, its bucco-lingual width is kept narrow to ensure firmly wedging the blade.

A BRIEF REVIEW
Guidelines for success

There are certain standard rules for using a blade implant. These are simple, yet essential to the long-term success of the implant intervention. They are basic, and the implantologist should rarely deviate from them. Briefly, the rules are these:

1. The fibromucosal tissues must be incised and reflected with clean, rapid surgery. The periosteum must be carefully separated from the underlying bone without mutilating or tearing it. Enough bone should be exposed to clearly view the alveolar crest, labiolingual thickness, and topography.

2. The groove in which the implant will be inserted is made with a No. 700L fissure bur. A sharp bur with water is essential to avoid overheating the bone. The bur is channeled through the center of the alveolar crest deeply enough to bury the entire blade portion of the implant. Making the groove deeper is not deleterious as long as the buccolingual width of the blade is wider than that of the groove (Fig. 11-198). The groove should be thin bucco-

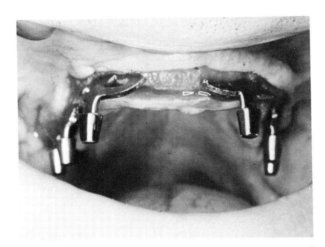

Fig. 11-199. Nearly perfect parallelism can be achieved easily with the blade. The necks are bent outside the mouth, then the blades are replaced in their grooves.

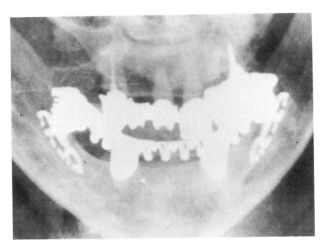

Fig. 11-200. A posteroanterior roentgenogram shows the shoulders of the blade correctly buried 2 mm. below the alveolar crest.

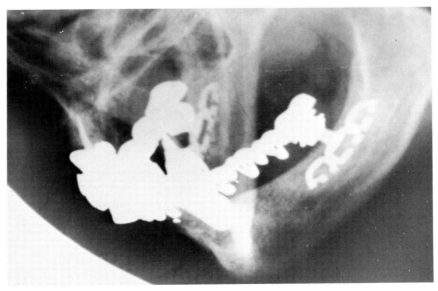

Fig. 11-201. A lateral oblique roentgenogram shows the alveolar crest covering the shoulders of the blade with at least 2 mm. of bone.

lingually to take advantage of the blade's wedging action.

3. The blade should fit passively into the groove. If the groove is curved, the blade must be bent using two flat-nosed (cone-socket) pliers until a passive fit is achieved.

4. The protruding post of the blade must be checked for buccolingual or labiolingual parallelism with the remaining abutment teeth or abutment implants. This should be done prior to tapping the implants into position. The implant is merely placed into the groove, checked, and—if adjustment is necessary—removed. With two cone-socket pliers, one holding the post and the other holding the blade, the neck is bent until parallelism is attained (Fig. 11-199).

5. The implant should be tapped gently into the groove without heavy malleting. However, if it was necessary to bend the neck of the implant, the taps should be confined to the shoulders, rather than the post. If the implant does not sink to its proper depth after a few firm taps, it must be immediately removed and the groove deepened. Concentrated heavy or prolonged malleting will result in excessive trauma to the underlying osseous structures and, consequently, a rather rapid failure.

6. The superior surface of the blade's shoulder must be buried 1 to 2 mm. below the alveolar crest. This is imperative for success (Figs. 11-200 and 11-201).

7. Mesiodistal parallelism of a protruding post can be accomplished by grinding directly in the mouth, without fear of loosening the implant.

8. The implant must be extremely tight from the very onset. A loose blade, just as a loose post type implant or triplant, can cause pain and may eventually lead to failure.

9. Once the blade has been correctly seated, the incised tissues should be carefully placed back over the bone in their respective positions. Simple interruptured sutures are sufficient to close them.

10. A blade implant need not be immediately stabilized with a temporary splint, as is always necessary with post type implants. A blade will not loosen if correctly inserted.

11. The sutures can be removed in 5 to 7 days.

12. Impressions are taken whenever the dentist believes that the soft tissues have healed sufficiently. However, the finished prosthesis should be in place no more than 4 to 5 weeks after implant insertion.

Selecting the proper implant design

There is a blade implant for almost every site and every implant problem (Figs. 11-202 and 11-203). Blades come long, short, shallow, deep, straight, or curved (Fig. 11-204). They may be set along the curve of the dental arch or at any angle to it (Fig.

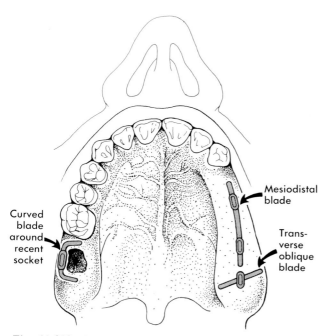

Fig. 11-202. An occlusal view of the maxillae, showing a few of the many blade designs appropriate here. Note that although the body of a blade may be set in any direction, its post follows the arch pattern.

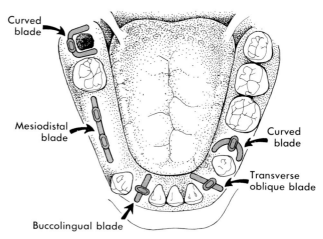

Fig. 11-203. An occlusal view of the mandible, showing several types of blade design. Note the variety of shapes, sizes, and directions in which the body can be set in the arch.

11-205). Their posts may be parallel with the broad face of the wedge-shaped body or be manufactured to follow the harmony of both arches. The operator thus has a wide range of designs from which to choose (Figs. 11-206 to 11-208).

A major problem for many operators, particularly beginners in implantology, is correctly evaluating the implant situation and choosing the most suitable design for that particular situation. Let us set up a sample problem—a full arch fixed prosthesis for an upper jaw with only two cuspid teeth remaining. Let us also assume, for purposes of simplification, that the morphology of each maxilla is the same; that is, that the right maxillary arch is a mirror image of the left.

The location and size of the maxillary sinus, as revealed radiographically, is the prime determinant in initially selecting an implant (or implants). Of

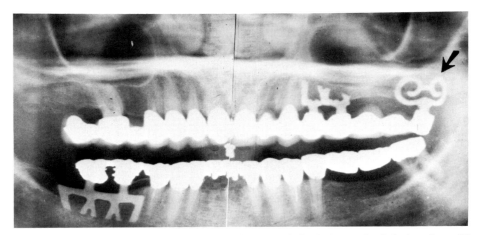

Fig. 11-204. This Panorex shows how three different blade designs suit their locations. The left maxillary tuberosity contains a curved blade *(arrow)* to obtain maximum metal-to-bone contact in a minimum amount of bone.

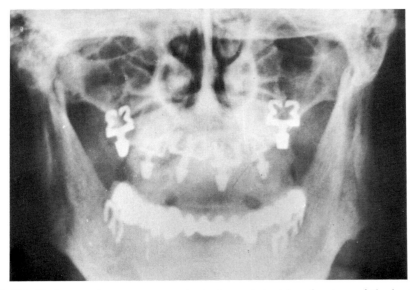

Fig. 11-205. Blades may be set at any angle in the arch to take advantage of the bony landscape. The posterior blades in the maxillae were set buccopalatally in the tuberosities. The remaining blades in both arches were inserted mesiodistally, with their broad faces lying in line with the curvature of the arch.

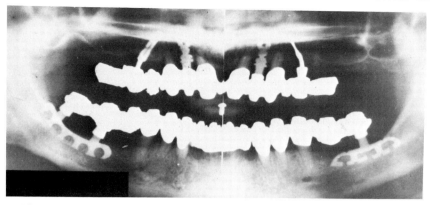

Fig. 11-206. The single tooth blades in the maxillae help stabilize anterior periodontally involved teeth. Some of these blades are obliquely set to avoid the maxillary sinus. In the mandible mesiodistal blades act as posterior abutments.

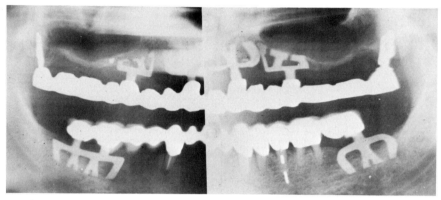

Fig. 11-207. These asymmetrical blades were specially designed to avoid penetrating the sinuses yet give maximum contact with bone.

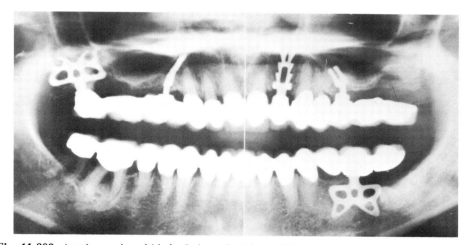

Fig. 11-208. Another series of blade designs. In this maxilla there is a mesiodistal blade in the right tuberosity, an obliquely placed buccopalatal blade in the right bicuspid area avoiding the sinus, a single tooth blade in the left central incisor region, and a transverse oblique, mesially directed blade in the left second bicuspid area avoiding the anterior extent of the antrum. The mandible contains a mesiodistal blade.

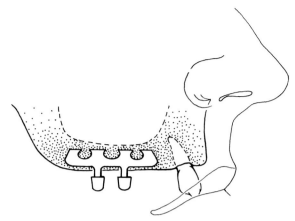

Fig. 11-209. A double-posted, mesiodistal blade lies below the sinus floor.

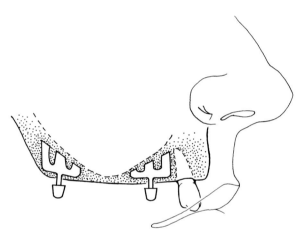

Fig. 11-210. To avoid the sinus, specially designed blades can be used anterior and posterior to it.

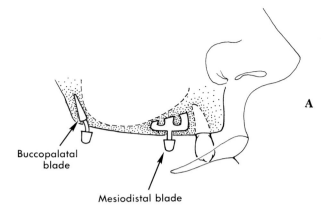

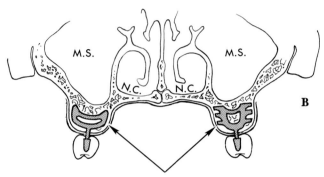

Buccopalatal blades in tuberosities

Fig. 11-211. When there is very little bone distal to the sinus, a buccopalatal blade may be used. **A,** The buccopalatal blade is angled into what little bone remains, its post bent parallel to the other implant abutment and the natural tooth. **B,** The exact location of the buccopalatal blade is clear in this cross section through the maxillary tuberosities. The blade is wedged against the cortical plates. *M.S.,* Maxillary sinus; *N.C.,* nasal cavity.

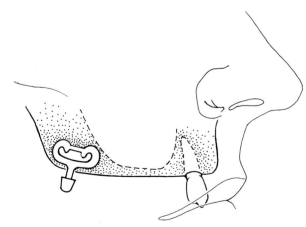

Fig. 11-212. One method of setting a blade in the maxillary tuberosity is mesiodistally.

course, conclusions drawn from radiographs must be confirmed by exposing the bone to reveal its true landscape.

When there is a good amount of alveolar bone between the floor of the sinus and the crest of the ridge, a single double-posted blade may be used in each maxilla (Fig. 11-209). This is actually an ideal situation. Surgery is needed in only one place on each side of the jaw, since it is the number and placement of the abutment posts—not necessarily the number of implants—that determines the amount of support for the bridge.

Several alternatives exist if there is little or no bone below the maxillary sinus. There may be a good deal of bone just anterior and posterior to the extensions of the sinus. Specially designed blades in

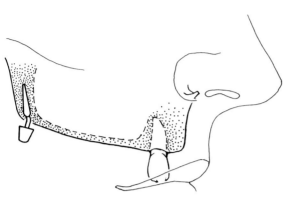

Fig. 11-213. This blade has been placed in the maxillary tuberosity in a buccopalatal direction. In some cases such an angle provides a greater mechanical advantage against lateral forces.

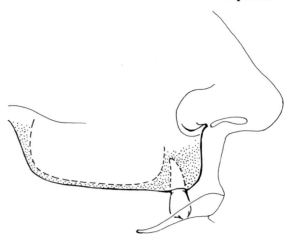

Fig. 11-214. There is not enough bone below, in front of, or behind the sinus for an endosseous implant of any kind.

these regions would provide ample support (Fig. 11-210). Or perhaps there is bone only anterior to the sinus, with very little or none distally. In this situation, another type of blade can be placed into the tuberosity in a buccopalatal direction, providing the tuberosity is wide enough (Fig. 11-211). There may indeed be a certain mechanical advantage in resisting lateral forces by setting one blade mesiodistally and the other buccopalatally.

Adequate amounts of bone may exist only in the maxillary tuberosity. If so, it must be determined whether or not the distance between the remaining cuspid and the tuberosity is too great to support a prosthesis. There is an even possibility of success if the distance is not exceptionally long (Fig. 11-212). Also, it might be more mechanically advantageous to set the blade into the tuberosity in a buccopalatal direction rather than in the usual mesiodistal direction (Fig. 11-213).

With the wide range of blade designs and possible insertion sites, it is rare when some type of blade cannot be used. One of the few remaining situations to be contraindicated for an endosseous implant intervention is one in which there is little or no bone mesial or distal to a low-flaring sinus (Fig. 11-214).

THE FAILING BLADE

A correctly inserted blade should not fail. However, occasionally one will. Failure of a blade type implant usually becomes evident from 2 to 4 weeks after its insertion, but a borderline case may take up to 6 months.

Leading causes of failure

If a blade implant fails, it is usually a result of specific mistakes made by the operator. Most of these mistakes are made during implant insertion. The basic errors are listed here for emphasis; other causes of failure are extensively discussed in Chapter 13.

1. The groove may not be deep enough to allow rapid, easy insertion of the implant so that the shoulder can be buried 1 to 2 mm. below the alveolar crest. If the groove is correct, no more than ten lightly tapped blows from the mallet should be required to properly bury the implant.

2. The groove may be too wide buccolingually. This means that the wedging action of the blade cannot be utilized. If the implant is not tight it should be removed. The mesiodistal length of the groove can be longer than the corresponding mesiodistal length of the blade because a tightly wedged blade will not slip or sink into the bone.

3. The shoulder may not have been adequately buried below the alveolar crest and wedged against the cortical plates of bone. This allows the epithelial tissue to invaginate and creep below the inferior border of the shoulder into the large openings in the body of the blade. Such invagination prevents the formation in that space of the desired fibrous tissue or bone.

Characteristics of a failing blade

Two main symptoms appear when a blade is failing: the patient complains of pain when chewing, and the implant becomes loose. At first the loosen-

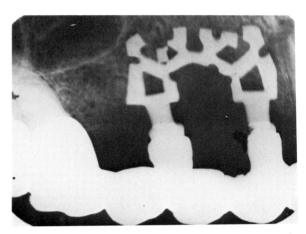

Fig. 11-215. The recessed shoulder of the "open socket" implant is buried close to the socket floor.

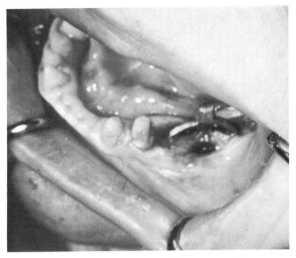

Fig. 11-216. A curved blade avoiding encroachment upon the open socket. If such an insertion is possible the patient need not wait several months until the socket heals for a fixed prosthesis.

ing may not be detected if the fixed prosthesis has already been cemented over it. However, upon severing the crown covering the implant post and separating it from the rest of the bridge, the looseness becomes apparent.

Although a failing blade, just as a failing tooth, can cause considerable bone destruction, this may not be evident in radiographs. The buccal and lingual cortical plates of bone can camouflage the true condition of the medullary bone. Also, comparing immediate postoperative and current x-rays for evidence of a blade's sinking is useless because even a failing blade does not sink into bone.

Treatment

A failing blade implant must be removed. Patchwork efforts to stabilize a loose blade are not advised; the site must be cleared of all granulation tissue and invaginated epithelial tissue.

To remove the implant three incisions are made: one directly through the fibromucosal tissues covering the superior surface of the shoulder, another along the buccal or labial surface of the blade to its entire depth, and a third along the lingual or palatal surface of the blade to its depth. The tissues are then carefully and cleanly retracted. The protruding post of the implant is firmly gripped with a wide-nosed

pliers or extraction forceps, and the implant is worked out of the bone in a mesiodistal and occlusal direction. A crown and bridge remover may sometimes be used.

Curettes and burs are then used to remove all granulation and epithelial tissue from the groove. Only after this is done can the amount of bone destruction be accurately estimated.

Whether or not immediate reimplantation is possible depends on several factors: the width of the cleaned groove, the amount of alveolar bone remaining below the floor of the cleaned groove, and the amount of bone anterior and posterior to that groove. The occlusal level of the buccal and lingual cortical plates of bone flanking the groove should also be relatively undamaged.

Basically, immediate reimplantation is possible if another blade implant, regardless of its shape, can be set in the cleaned groove deeply enough to bury its shoulder below the floor of the original groove (Fig. 11-215). Or, a curved groove may be made around the socket to carry an appropriately bent, passively fitting blade implant (Fig. 11-216).

If too much bone and surrounding cortical plates have been destroyed, at least 4 to 5 months should elapse before attempting another implant in the same site.

CHAPTER 12 Subperiosteal implants

Although this volume is primarily devoted to endosseous implants, there are certain situations in which a subperiosteal implant is preferable. The two groups of implants are not competitive; one type of implant cannot possibly be utilized successfully where the other one is indicated.

There are two schools of thought about the appropriateness of a subperiosteal implant. Both agree that the subperiosteal implant should be used only when the alveolar bone has almost completely resorbed. However, the American school, which includes such men as Gershkoff, Goldberg, Lew, Jermyn, Bodine, Cranin, Weber, Linkow, and members of the American Academy of Implant Dentistry, advise that a subperiosteal implant is successful over a prolonged period of time only when set over basal bone. Adequate amounts of this type of bone exist only in the mandibular arch, not in the maxillary arch. Maxillary bone is primarily of a cancellous, more porous structure. Therefore, with few exceptions, the edentulous maxilla is inappropriate for subperiosteal restorations.

A subperiosteal implant should be utilized for the atrophied mandible only. It should not be attempted on a mandible where much alveolar bone exists, since over a relatively short period of time— within 2 to 3 years—the alveolar bone will resorb. Subsequently the implant will probably have to be removed. In situations where teeth still exist, there is usually too much alveolar bone.

Certain Europeans, including the Spaniards Salagaray and Sol and the Frenchman Audoire, do use subperiosteal implants in the maxilla. However, these are uniquely designed to include a good portion of the hard palate, zygomatic arch, canine eminence, nasal spine, and even the pterygoid process. These men report gratifying results with their strongly braced implants. American operators, however, prefer to limit subperiosteal restorations to the mandible,

where the anatomy is more favorable for prolonged success.

The subperiosteal implant is usually cast in Vitallium* (a chrome-cobalt alloy) and consists of two major parts: a substructure and a superstructure (Fig. 12-1). The substructure, the implanted part, rests on the bone directly underneath the periosteum. It is held in position by its accurate fit and the fibromucosal tissue that tenaciously binds to it. The superstructure snaps over the protruding posts of the substructure and fits over, but does not touch, the healed soft tissues. The superstructure is incorporated into the prosthesis.

The substructure of the subperiosteal implant consists of several parts (Fig. 12-2):

1. The struts, of which there are three types:
   a. Primary struts, which bear the abutment posts. These struts should be the only ones traversing the crest of the ridge to minimize long-range problems associated with bone resorption.
   b. Secondary struts, which connect the labial and buccal peripheral strut with the lingual strut.
   c. Peripheral struts, which outline the peripheral shape of the implant.
2. The abutment posts. There should be four abutment posts, evenly spaced around the arch, for a full arch restoration. These have narrow necks around which the tissues will be sutured. Their heads will fit into the superstructure.

The substructure framework must extend to the external oblique ridges, circumvent the bundle of nerves exiting the mental foramina, extend down deep to the symphysis on the labial surface, extend deep to the genial tubercles lingually, and not go below the mylohyoid ridges posteriorly on the lingual side.

The superstructure of the implant is horseshoe-shaped and consists of four atypically clasped copings

*Howmedica, Inc., New York, N. Y.

531

joined together with a connecting bar. The super-structure becomes an integral part of the implant denture (Fig. 12-3) and "floats" it above the jaw. No portion of the tissue side of the denture should be tissue-bearing.

The implant denture should have acrylic teeth. If the patient has an existing upper denture with porcelain teeth, either make a new denture or change the teeth for acrylic ones. Sometimes a patient may

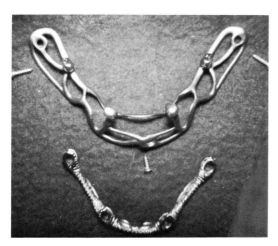

Fig. 12-1. The substructure of the subperiosteal implant is seen on top with three small set screws for primary fixation of the implant to the bone, if desired. On the bottom is seen the superstructure onto which the implant denture is processed.

complain that his implant teeth are too flat, making it difficult for him to chew. The complaint may be alleviated by the use of Hardy Mo-posteriors, specially designed posterior teeth with sharp metal occlusals (Fig. 12-4).

EVALUATING THE CANDIDATE

A mandibular subperiosteal implant should be attempted only when a conventional lower denture has repeatedly proved unsuccessful. If the failure of the conventional denture cannot be overcome by another conventional denture of a better design and fit, the implantologist should carefully evaluate the situation, checking the patient's ridge with its muscle attachments, tissue tonus, height, and thickness, as well as what exists in the opposite arch, whether it be a denture or a full complement of natural teeth. As a routine procedure a full mandibular subperi-osteal implant should never be used in the mouth of a patient who has his own full complement of teeth in the opposing jaw. Although such a case may succeed occasionally (Fig. 12-5), the trauma usually caused by natural teeth could lead to implant failure. Patients with knife-edge ridges are unsuitable candidates unless the ridge is flattened surgically; then at least 6 months to 1 year should elapse before implantation.

While endosseous blade-type implants can function normally against a full complement of opposing natural teeth, a subperiosteal implant is usually con-

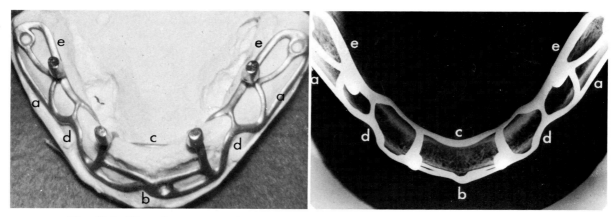

Fig. 12-2. The substructure as it appears on the master stone cast taken from a Neoplex (rubber base) impression of the exposed mandible and in an occlusal x-ray. The peripheral borders of the implant should include the external oblique ridges *(a)*, the symphysis *(b)*, and the genial tubercles *(c)*. The implant should circumvent the neurovascular bundles exiting the mental foramina *(d)* and extend to, but not below, the mylohyoid ridges *(e)*. (From Linkow, L. I.: Re-evaluation of mandibular unilateral subperiosteal implants: a 12 year report, J. Prosth. Dent. **17:**509-514, 1967.)

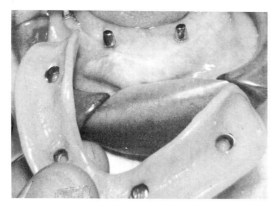

Fig. 12-3. The superstructure framework processed inside the implant denture. The tissue-bearing surface of the denture must never touch the soft tissue. In this case it is supported by the four protruding posts extending above the fibromucosal tissue. (From Linkow, L. I.: Re-evaluation of mandibular unilateral subperiosteal implants: a 12 year report, J. Prosth. Dent. **17:**509-514, 1967.)

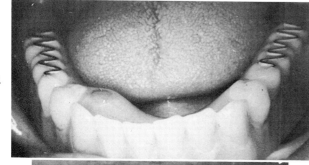

A

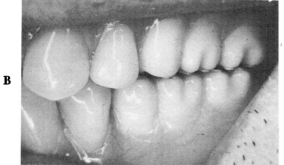

B

Fig. 12-4. A, Specially designed M.O. (metal occlusal) (Hardy) posterior teeth that consist of metal "rails" embedded inside the acrylic teeth for easier cutting of food for those patients who have trouble chewing. **B,** The superstructure implant denture in the mouth and occluded with the upper denture.

traindicated. It must be realized that since the subperiosteal implant only rests on the bone, it cannot stimulate osteogenesis. Therefore, resorption underneath it could occur if the implant were placed in a mouth with opposing natural teeth.

A thorough medical history must be taken. The history should include all those considerations extensively discussed in Chapter 6. Particularly important for a subperiosteal candidate are blood tests to determine coagulation time and any condition, such as diabetes mellitus, that might hinder healing. Alcoholics are also a poor risk as they seem to have a very slow healing potential. Unless a diabetic patient has a well-controlled condition and must have the implant in order to chew better, avoid the case. It is always a good policy for the dentist to talk directly to the patient's physician prior to implant intervention.

The site should be evaluated before surgery with radiographs. Intraoral radiographs alone should not be the determining factor for exposing any existing pathology. Lateral plate, lateral head, profile, crosssectionals, topographics, posteroanterior, and cephalometeric and pantographic roentgenograms must very often be used for proper diagnosis.

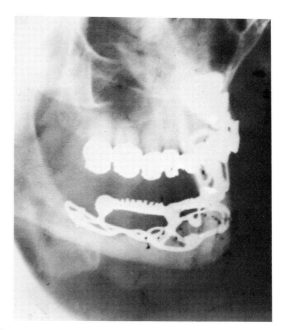

Fig. 12-5. Although this lower subperiosteal implant has been successfully functioning in the mouth opposing a full complement of upper teeth for more than 5 years, such an implant is usually contraindicated in these situations.

Any and all local pathologic conditions must first be alleviated before proceeding with the bone impression for the subperiosteal implant. Any remaining root tips, residual cysts, amalgam fillings trapped in a healed open socket, knife-edge or spiculed ridges, or hypertrophied tissue covering the mandibular bone should all be treated at least 3 to 6 months prior to implant intervention. In situations where unilateral subperiosteal implants are contemplated and some of the remaining teeth are to be utilized as natural tooth abutments, there should be no decay, abscess, or pulpitis. The mobility, periodontal condition, and occlusion of the remaining teeth should be checked.

Last, but hardly least, the operation and its prognosis should be thoroughly discussed with the patient before any work is done. The patient should

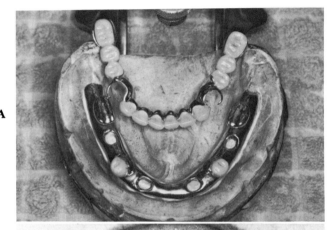

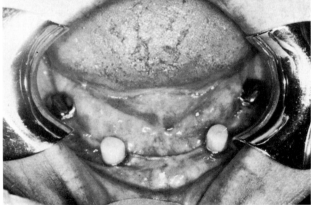

Fig. 12-6. A, A Vitallium template that was cast from a revised stone model taken from an original alginate impression of the soft tissues. The stone model is scraped to assimilate the topography of the underlying bone by the use of radiographs. (Courtesy A. Gershhoff and N. I. Goldberg.) **B,** The same case as it appears in the mouth 20 years later.

never be made to feel that his implant denture will be an overwhelming success. The entire truth about its limitations should be presented. However, many patients who were otherwise considered to be dental cripples with their routinely constructed denture have been helped greatly by the introduction of the subperiosteal implant and, in years to come, many more patients will be helped. The fact that the subperiosteal method of approach has not been used more widely has nothing to do with the degree of success. Statistical analyses of subperiosteal implants successfully functioning many years have been frequently reported and authoritatively documented (Fig. 12-6).

According to Cranin: "If the fearless practitioner who attempts to construct a conventional denture prosthesis for a totally atrophic mandibular ridge would apply the same perseverance, courage, and skill to mastering the implant technique, the problems of edentulous patients would be relegated to that small group for whom implants are contraindicated. With a greater number of doctors practicing the technique, fears would be dissipated (as they are always with the introduction of knowledge), and the implant [would] cease to be looked upon as a radical procedure to be recommended only for severely crippled patients."

Today, when some operators using modern approaches have been achieving as much as 95% success with their patients, the prognosis is optimistic.

A FULL ARCH SUBPERIOSTEAL IMPLANT

One, two, or three visits are usually required for a subperiosteal procedure. On the first, usually when the patient accepts the diagnosis and agrees to the procedure, a surgical tray to be used later for taking a bone impression is made. The following two visits are surgical, one for making the bone impression and the other for inserting the implant. Some operators prefer to hospitalize their patients for surgical visits; others prefer to have their patients ambulatory and to perform the operations in their office. The choice depends on the operator's own preferences and the patient's condition, mental as well as physical.

Obtaining the surgical tray

An acrylic surgical tray is needed to make an accurate bone impression (Fig. 12-7). Some operators make an alginate impression of the entire lower jaw over the soft tissues to make the tray. Others, including Linkow, prefer to fabricate a more accurate tray by reflecting the soft tissues to reveal the true landscape of the jaw. To do this, a bilateral inferior alveolar block and vertical block anesthesia, produced with 2% lidocaine and epinephrine 1:100,000 is first given the patient. Also injected muscularly is 2 ml. dexamethasone sodium phosphate,* an adrenocortical hormone preparation to reduce swelling. Cold cure acrylic is mixed until it is of a clay-like consistency, then it is molded to the exposed jaw, spraying cold water on it all the time to prevent burning (Fig. 12-8). The resulting tray fits quite accurately and is not overextended, as are trays fabricated in the usual manner. The tray is removed, trimmed, and punched to retain the rub-

*Merck, Sharp and Dohme, West Point, Pa.

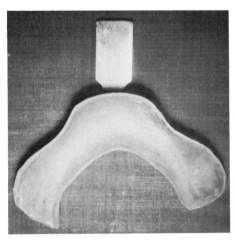

Fig. 12-7. An acrylic tray fabricated from a stone cast that has been reduced in size to assimilate the shape of the underlying bone. The stone cast had previously been poured into an alginate impression taken of the entire mandible over the soft tissue.

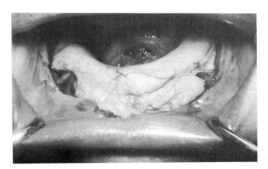

Fig. 12-8. A cold cure acrylic tray is molded directly to the exposed bone (Linkow) and removed before the heat sets in. Note the relief areas on both sides allowing for freedom of the neurovascular bundles that exit the mental foramina.

ber base material (Fig. 12-9). The only disadvantage of this technique is the possibility of the acrylic's burning the soft tissues. This can happen if most of the liquid has not evaporated before the acrylic is placed in the mouth or if the acrylic is allowed to completely set in the mouth without being cooled by water.

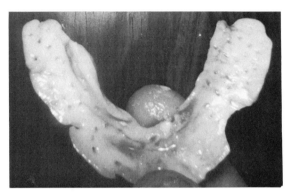

Fig. 12-9. The acrylic tray was trimmed and "punched" with many tiny holes (made with a round bur in a contra-angle) and then painted with one of the rubber adhesives, so that it could retain the rubber impression.

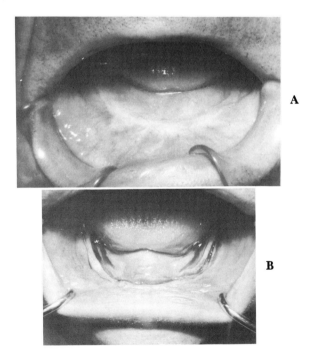

A

B

Fig. 12-10. A, The resorbed edentulous mandible just prior to the first surgical stage incision. Note how flat the ridge is when covered by the soft tissue. B, An incision was made along the crest of the soft tissue ridge directly down to the bone. It extended close to the retromolar pad areas on both sides.

However, Linkow now uses Imput,* a relatively new impression material that handles much easier than the acrylic resin. The heavy mix of Imput is used for making the tray and the light material is used for final accuracy of the bone anatomy.

Exposing the bone

To get an accurate impression of the bone, the soft tissues must be reflected. An incision is made along the crest of the edentulous ridge from one retromolar pad area to the other, making sure that the incision is clear and right down to the bone (Fig. 12-10). To help avoid stretching and tearing the tissues during reflection, a secondary bucco-lingual incision is made across the crest-line incision in the symphysis area. Secondary incisions are also made in the retromolar pad areas, but these are not single straight buccolingual cuts. A straight cut can cause a great deal of postoperative swelling and pain. Instead, a very acute V-shaped incision is made from the original incision, with the apex of the V directly in front of the retromolar pad and its legs flanking the pad area buccally and lingually (Fig. 12-11).

With a blunt instrument, such as a periosteal elevator, the soft tissues are reflected downward toward the cheeks and lips and toward the floor of the mouth, exposing the entire mandible. The lingually reflected

---

*Manufactured by Vicon Products Corp., Mamaroneck, N. Y.

tissues should be sutured so that the tongue is kept in the posterior portion of the mouth and does not interfere with the impression. This is done by simply suturing the posterior aspect of the tissue on one side with the more anterior tissue on the opposite side of the arch, and vice versa (Fig. 12-12). The

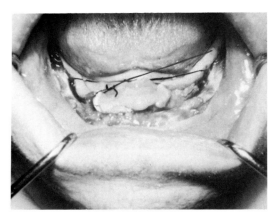

Fig. 12-12. The lingual tissue was sutured from one side to the other in a criss-cross fashion to lock the tongue away from the exposed bone so that it would not interfere with the impression, and to keep the lingual tissue away from the bone for more access of the surgical tray, so that it would fit directly over the bone for the impression.

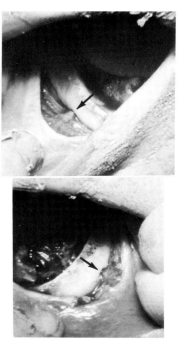

Fig. 12-13. The mental foramina on both sides of the mandible with their exiting neurovascular bundles *(arrows)* must always be exposed prior to the elastic bone impression.

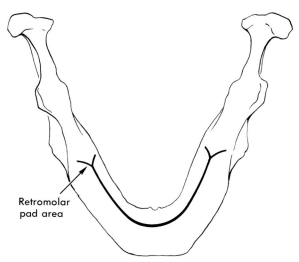

Retromolar
pad area

Fig. 12-11. A V-shaped incision was made directly in front of the retromolar pad areas. The reason for this was to prevent excessive pain, which often occurs when the incision extends beyond this area.

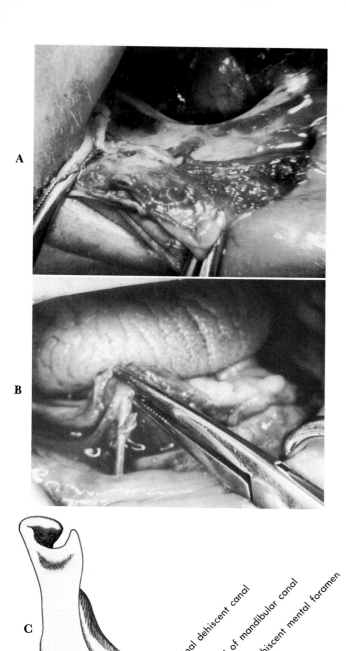

Fig. 12-14. A, The mandible has resorbed to such an extent that the mental foramen is dehiscent at the residual crest. B, Resorption of this mandible left the entire mandibular canal dehiscent. The inferior alveolar nerve is seen being held with a hemostat. C, A dehiscent mandibular canal or mental foramen can be lowered and the neurovascular bundle pushed down into it, enabling a subperiosteal implant to be placed directly over the canal with no nerve impingement.

genial tubercles should be clearly evident in the anterior lingual aspect of the jaw. The mylohyoid ridges should be seen posteriorly, because the lingual extension of the implant will end there and not go below them. Posteriorly, on both buccal aspects, the external oblique ridges should be exposed for the impression, while the entire symphysis should be exposed in the anterior inferior labial portion of the mandible.

While reflecting the tissue on both buccal aspects, the operator must be exceptionally careful not to sever or injure the neurovascular bundles of nerves and blood vessels in the areas of both mental foramina. The overlying tissue should be carefully pushed downward with a blunt instrument until a semi-crescent fan-shaped area of tissue appears. This flanks the superior wall of the mental foramen. The bundle should then be more carefully separated, exposing more of it as well as the foramen, by pushing the fan-shaped area downward (Fig. 12-13). This should be judiciously executed prior to all impression-taking. It is necessary to exactly locate these anatomic landmarks so that every available surface of bone lying above and near them can be utilized without impinging on them. Sometimes the mandible has atrophied so much that the entire mandibular canal is dehiscent (Fig. 12-14, *A* and *B*). For such conditions, Linkow has developed a technique for lifting up the exposed mandibular nerve while lowering the floor of the mandibular canal and mental foramina at the same time with a No. 6 round bur. The nerve bundle is then gently placed back into the revised canal and pushed further into it. Since a new foramen is created, there should be no impingement from the new restoration that will be fabricated for the patient (Fig. 12-14, *C*).

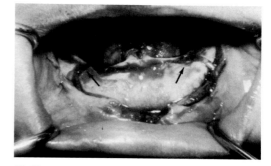

Fig. 12-15. Another case showing the neurovascular bundle of nerves exiting the mental foramina, which are both dehiscent. Arrows point to the areas of the dehiscent foramina.

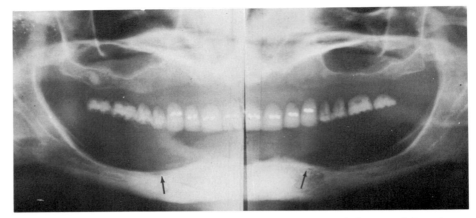

Fig. 12-16. A Panorex revealing a bilateral dehiscency *(arrows)* of the mental foramina.

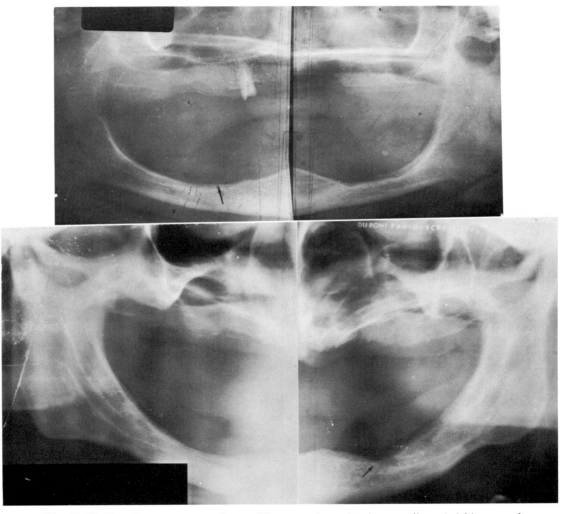

Fig. 12-17. Two Panorex x-rays of two different patients showing a unilateral dehiscency of the mental foramina on the right and left sides, respectively.

In other cases partial dehiscence results in the exposure of only the neurovascular bundle exiting from the foramina (Fig. 12-15). The mental foramina on both sides of the arch may also be unilaterally or bilaterally dehiscent. In these not too common situations, the operator must be careful to make the incision quite a bit more lingually than usual to prevent severing the exposed vessels. When the nerves in the inferior alveolar canal are exposed as a result of a dehiscency of the canal itself, the incision must be made lingual to the ridge crest to avoid the vessels. Roentgenograms help predict when these situations will occur. Fig. 12-16, a Panorex, reveals a bilateral mandibular canal dehiscence of the mental foramina on both sides. Fig. 12-17 shows two unilateral dehiscences of the mental foramina.

Making the impression

Aside from the surgery, the most important first step toward a successful subperiosteal implant is making an accurate impression including each and every imperative anatomic landmark. These landmarks are both external oblique ridges, both neurovascular bundles exiting the mental foramina, both mylohyoid ridges, the genial tubercles, and the symphysis. The importance of these landmarks cannot be stressed enough, for without the dense bone in these areas to support the metallic framework, no implant could ever be successful.

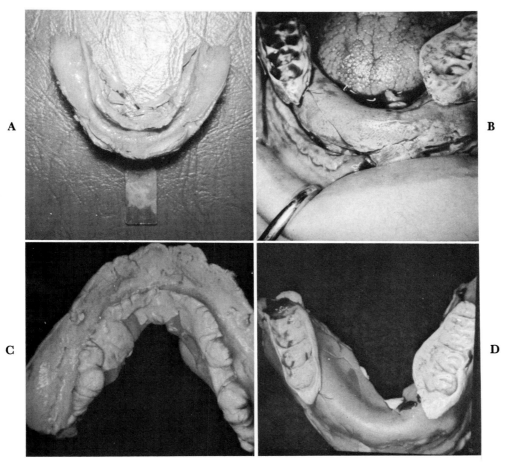

Fig. 12-18. A, The rubber impression was taken of the exposed bone that included the external oblique ridges, symphysis, genial tubercles, mylohyoid ridges, the neurovascular bundles exiting the mental foramina. **B,** The implant (silicone putty) impression is taken of the exposed mandible in heavy-bodied material. **C,** A light wash material is used for finer details. **D,** A silicone wash bite is taken directly over the heavy-bodied tray while it is still in the mouth.

The surgical tray, regardless of how it was made, should first be treated with one of the "adhesive" agents that allows the rubber to bind with it.

A rubber base material (Coe) or Neoplex (Surgident Co.) is usually the choice material for the bone impression. When using rubber, it is mixed to an even consistency and then placed into the tray and held in the mouth for at least 10 minutes to set. The advantage of using Neoplex instead of rubber, although both set at about the same time, is that the operator can mold the Neoplex in his hand like clay. He can first mold it over the exposed bone and around the landmarks before setting the tray over it. After the impression has hardened, it is removed and checked for accuracy (Fig. 12-18, *A*). Some operators take two impressions as a routine procedure. However, one lessens the danger of any impression material slipping underneath the neurovascular bundles or a dehiscent nerve. The less aggravation brought to bear on these structures, the better off the patient is.

Obtaining a bone bite

While the mandible is still exposed, a surgical bone bite using wax should be taken. The wax is merely heated and placed over the exposed bone. The patient closes in a retruded position in centric relation and meshes with the teeth of the opposite arch. This bone bite tells the technician how high to make the four abutment posts that will protrude into the oral cavity.

A more accurate wax bite may be taken with the acrylic tray containing the rubber impression still in the mouth. The resulting bite is more accurate because the rubber impression is the exact duplicate of the bony ridge. An alginate impression also must be taken of the opposing jaw.

More recent developments by Linkow include an accurate light-bodied Imput wash inside a heavier Imput body tray. While the impression is still in the mouth, another heavy-bodied Imput mix is placed against the opposing teeth and the patient is guided into centric relation. When the mix sets, it adheres to the tray; the impression of the exposed mandible and interocclusal record of centric relation are accomplished together (Fig. 12-18, *B* to *D*).

An accurate measurement of the soft tissue overlying the four areas where the abutment posts will protrude should also be taken and sent to the technician. In this manner the height of the necks can be accurately determined. The tissue in the mandible is usually no thicker than 1 to 2 mm. However, if the tissue is not measured accurately and the neck is too long, the prosthesis-bearing post may be made much too short to firmly hold the superstructure. As an example, in one case it was necessary to cast a gold coping to cover the extra long neck so that the foreshortened abutment post could gain retention (Fig. 12-19). Unnecessarily long necks may also cause tension that results in the exposure of the primary strut (Fig. 12-20). Such a situation may be

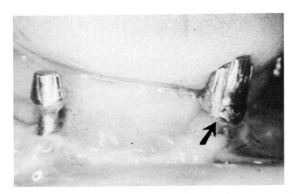

Fig. 12-19. An extended gold coping is sometimes cemented over an improperly designed implant post. In this case too much of the narrow neck below the post was exposed; the neck was made too long at the expense of the foreshortened post, greatly reducing its retentive qualities. The gold coping restores the anatomy, improving the retention required to hold the implant denture. Note also the excessively long neck and short post on the right side, which was also improperly designed.

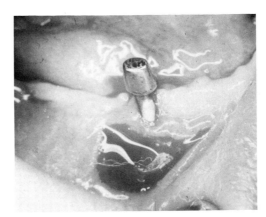

Fig. 12-20. The tissue sometimes recedes around an excessively long neck, especially if a high muscle attachment exists in the area. A relief incision is often made horizontally below the exposed strut and allowed to heal by secondary intention. This reduces the muscle pull, and sometimes the tissue readapts to its original height around the neck.

remedied by making a horizontal incision inferior to the exposed strut and severing the high muscle attachment. No sutures are made, and the tissue is treated so that healing takes place by secondary, rather than primary, intention. This relieves the pulling action of the attachment and allows the tissue to grow upward to cover the neck.

Closing the site

After the necessary impressions have been made, the site is sutured closed. This may be done with interrupted sutures, or surgical ties, which are a series of separate sutures placed about ¼ inch apart. The knots should be made to one side of the wound so that they will not press on it. Alternately, the sutures may be continuous, uniting the wound from one end to the other. Suturing in this manner is started by passing the needle through one edge of the wound and tying a simple knot. The edges of the wound are then pierced successively, making sure that the thread directly behind the needle is always under it, until the end of the wound is reached and closed with a terminal surgical knot (Fig. 12-21). Both interrupted and continuous suturing close the wound by bringing the edges together.

When the tissues are under unusual tension, as sometimes occurs between the abutment posts, surface-to-surface adaptation of the wound is preferable to edge-to-edge contact. This may be achieved with mattress sutures. Mattress sutures may be continuous or interrupted and may be buried. They do not tear the tissues as readily as surface interrupted sutures. Mattress suturing is sometimes done in combination with interrupted surgical ties.

A mattress or purse-string suture is used around each protruding post to circumvent and tightly join the tissues around the posts. Sometimes, because of the quality and thickness or thinness of the tissue, as well as its shrinkage caused by excessive time spent in making the surgical impression, tension sutures may have to be applied. This type of suturing is usually used in large open wounds to distribute the pull on the sutures over as large a surface area as possible. The needle is passed through the tissue about 1 inch away from the wound on one side and is brought out and passed through near the end of the wound on the other side. The needle is then passed back near the edge of the tissue on the first side and swept through the tissue on the opposite side about 1 inch away from the incision.

When the wound has been closed, an intraoral bandage* may be set over it to speed healing (Fig. 12-22). In addition to protecting the wound, the bandage provides medication. To make the bandage, a portion is cut to fit over the entire wound area. The paper covering the adhesive is removed and the bandage positioned and held for about 30 seconds. The adhesive contains hydrophilic compounds that hold the bandage in place from 6 to 12 hours. If possible, it is better to leave the bandage in place 24 hours.

Using a temporary denture

The patient will need a temporary denture both for functional use and to protect the wound while it is healing. Most of the patients requiring a full lower subperiosteal implant usually have a number

*E. R. Squibb & Sons, New York, N. Y.

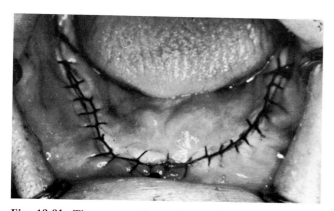

Fig. 12-21. There must always be enough sutures to completely close the wound. This case shows continuous suturing completely around the arch from retromolar pad to retromolar pad.

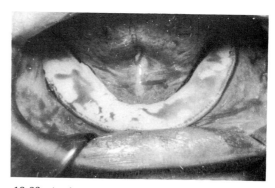

Fig. 12-22. An intraoral bandage (E. R. Squibb and Sons) is sometimes used directly over the sutured tissue.

of lower dentures on hand. As long as the teeth are acrylic, which causes less trauma, and not porcelain, the denture can easily be utilized as a temporary splint. Before any actual work is done, the dentist should choose the denture and reline it with a good soft tissue conditioner. When placed over the wound, it should be checked for proper occlusion and any high spots ground away. At this stage, if the patient does not have a denture it is usually not necessary to make one.

Postoperative treatment

The patient should be shown how to keep the wound clean and aid healing after a surgical procedure. On the first day, sterile saline packs should be changed about every 15 minutes for at least 5 or 6 hours. Icepacks should be used to reduce pain and swelling. One should be applied to the jaw for 1 or 2 hours, 15 minutes on the jaw and 15 minutes off. An analgesic, such as 30 mg. codeine phosphate, may be taken every 4 hours for pain.

On the second day, and continuing until the sutures are removed, warm saline solutions should be used to rinse the mouth. At first the solution should be swished gently around the mouth; later this should be more vigorous.

Following-up the first surgical visit

Approximately 7 days later the sutures may be removed. A 3- to 6-week waiting period is then necessary to ensure complete healing. This healing period is essential if the subperiosteal implant cannot be fabricated the very same day the impression is taken. If an attempt is made to insert the implant before the tissues have completely healed, the case could fail because the sutures probably would not hold and the implant substructure will be exposed. This point cannot be emphasized strongly enough; it is exceedingly difficult to make the tissues grow again over an exposed implant.

The Americans Cranin, Weber, and Lew and the Frenchman Audoire claim to have excellent results with a one-stage intervention procedure, which, of course, means two surgical stages within a few hours. Their approach takes about 8 hours. Early in the morning, the first surgical procedure for making an impression is accomplished, the impression is rushed to the laboratory for waxing, casting, and polishing, and then rushed back to the dentist for insertion. The wound is not sutured closed but has barely had time to begin healing. As a result the tissues are easy to reflect. There are two disadvantages to this

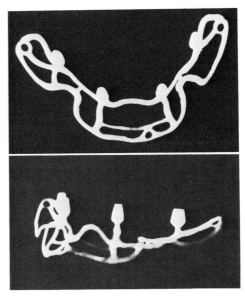

Fig. 12-23. The subperiosteal implants should always be radiographed with special x-ray equipment to be certain that no flaws exist, as they do here.

method: the lengthy day and delay that must be endured by both patient and dentist, and the fact that there isn't enough time to x-ray the substructure for flaws in the metal framework (Fig. 12-23). This is a simple and essential step to avoid using a weak implant that will probably cause trouble later.

Inserting the implant

Another bilateral inferior alveolar nerve block is given, and the original incision line is carefully duplicated with a scalpel. This line is still evident after a 6-week lapse. When reflecting the tissue away from the incision, much less resistance is encountered because the periosteum, which was separated from the bone during the first surgical visit, has not had adequate time to tenaciously rebind to the bone.

The implant is taken directly out of the autoclave and placed into the cold sterilizing solution. The sterilized implant, with the superstructure fitted over the substructure, is then inserted over the exposed bone just cleansed with warm saline solution. The accuracy of the implant's fit can be determined by the close adaptation of the substructure to the important anatomic landmarks (Fig. 12-24). When the implant has been properly seated, the superstructure is removed. If the implant is very tight, the overlying tissues can be sutured over it. However, if the fit is slightly loose because of the flat anatomy of the bone, one to three small Vitallium screws 5 to 7 mm. long can be used to hold down the implant. These screws

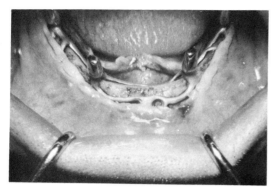

Fig. 12-24. The implant must fit over the bone with 100% accuracy.

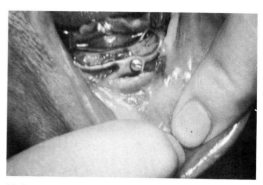

Fig. 12-25. Sometimes one to three small set screws are used to stabilize the implant to the bone.

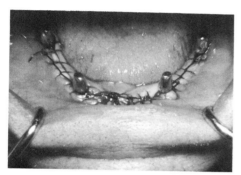

Fig. 12-26. The suturing must adequately close the entire tissue wound and closely adapt the tissue to the four protruding posts.

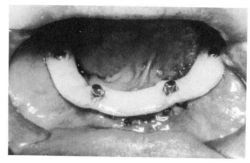

Fig. 12-27. An intraoral bandage is festooned and placed over the four protruding posts and over the sutures.

only establish primary retention; the real security develops as fibromucosal tissue binds itself in and around the meshwork of the substructure.

The holes for the screws are located in the parts of the implant that will cover the densest bone: both external oblique ridges posteriorly and the symphysis anteriorly (Fig. 12-25). Before each screw is set, a small hole is made with a No. 556 fissure bur at right angles to the surface of the bone. While inserting the screws the operator must make sure that they are going in exactly the same direction as the walls surrounding them. Otherwise the screws can create a degree of torque that will either distort the implant itself or interfere with its accurate fit and cause rapid bone resorption. Once the tissues overlying the implant have healed, the screws can be removed, if desired, but this is not necessary. A special Vitallium screwdriver is sometimes used for this procedure.

Suturing the tissues over the implant

One of the most critical steps is the suturing of the tissues to cover the entire substructure of the implant. Various thicknesses of silk ligatures are available. Wound closure with atraumatic 000 silk sutures has been the most popular.

Suturing is a time-consuming procedure, and experience has shown that the more sutures, the better (Fig. 12-26). Purse-string sutures are first placed closely around each protruding neck, making sure that the tissue closely adapts to the necks. Second, at least fifteen to twenty interrupted surgical ties should be placed through the approximating edges of the tissue between the posts or necks. Third, any tissue that seems to resist closure should be augmented with a few mattress sutures. An intraoral bandage is again fabricated to cover the sutures and soft tissues (Fig. 12-27), and the patient is dismissed with a head bandage of ice (Fig. 12-28). It is not imperative to include the intraoral bandage as a routine procedure.

Healing

There is often a considerable difference in the rate of wound healing between the first and second surgical stages. The primary surgery is on mucosal

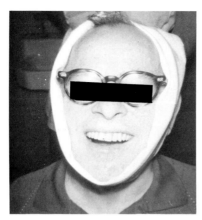

Fig. 12-28. Icepacks are placed inside a towel in the neck and chin area and tied around the top of the patient's head.

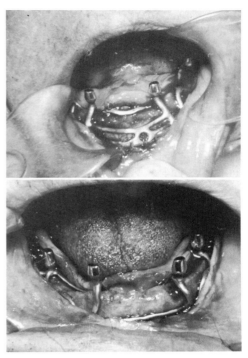

Fig. 12-29. The incision and reflection of the mucoperiosteal tissue, such as is seen in these two different cases, should expose enough of the bone so that the implant can be easily placed into position without pulling and stretching the tissue in those cases where not enough of the bone was exposed.

tissue that has either never been operated upon or not operated upon for many years. There is a fairly good blood supply, which allows for rapid healing of the wound. Another important factor at the first surgical stage is that the tissues are merely joined together and do not have to be stretched over an implant, as is done during the second stage. Also, during the first stage the fibromucosal tissue is very widely reflected in order to expose enough of the bone for a bone impression. This makes this tissue more mobile for suturing.

Healing after the second surgical stage is more complicated. Scar tissue has developed all along the original incision site and in the approximating tissues. Scar tissue has a greatly reduced blood supply, and its fibrous tissue content is greatly increased. It is into this avascular bed of scar tissue that the second surgical incision is made. Because of this lack of an adequate blood supply, the healing over the implant is retarded and could take place by secondary intention, or healing by granulation tissue. This is less desirable because granulation tissue cannot be controlled, and the tissue never adheres as closely to the protruding posts as it does with healing by primary intention.

Several techniques have been tried to compensate for or alleviate the problems associated with the second surgical stage. The amount of time between the first and second stages has been increased to as much as 2 months to allow for complete cicatrization across the original incision. Some operators restrict the amount of tissue reflected, thinking that this helps reduce postoperative swelling, pain, and edema and speeds healing. Just enough tissue is in-

cised and reflected to allow the implant to be slipped into position. However, postoperative results in this manner are not as good as when larger incisions and reflections are made (Fig. 12-29).

Without generous reflection, the tissue flaps are less mobile and the approximation of their edges is often obtained at the expense of stretching the tissues. Complicating this situation is the fact that the tissues also have to be stretched over the substructure of the implant. By limiting the amount of tissue freed from the bone, less is available for stretching over the implant.

An extremely effective method of dealing with delayed healing by secondary intention has been devised by Metz. He advocates a modified advancement flap technique that avoids many of the problems of reincising the original site. The second surgical phase is performed from 6 weeks to 2 months after the first surgery. At this time the incision begins at the point where the distal post will be located. This is easily determined by placing the framework in the mouth before the surgery and marking

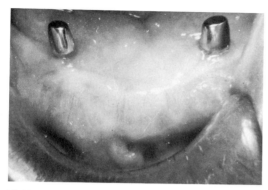

Fig. 12-30. With clean and proper sugery, healing takes place uneventfully. Notice the tissue around the implant posts as they appeared 12 years postoperatively.

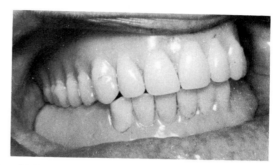

Fig. 12-31. A temporary acrylic stent obtained from a surgical bone bite is fabricated.

the soft tissue with an explorer. To ensure room for the small 7-mm. set screws that might be needed to hold the implant in place, the incision can be extended about 5 mm. posteriorly across the retromolar pads to give sufficient access. The entire incision, however, is made in the buccal and labial mucosa and carried deep enough to assure adequate blood supply. It is not made along the crest of the ridge, as was done during the first surgical phase. Since the incision involves cutting a portion of the buccinator and mentalis muscles, care must be taken not to carry the incision too deeply or the proximal portion of the muscles will have a reduced blood supply.

After careful separation of the mucoperiosteal tissue from the bone and flapping it lingually to expose the ridge, two very small holes are made in the mucosa to allow for the protrusion of the anterior abutments. By this method Metz avoids the entire avascular area resulting from the first operation. As a result healing of the previously intact, highly vascularized buccal and labial mucosa is rapid, occurring in about 3 days. The sutures should not be removed for at least 6 days to ensure adequate fibroblastic proliferation to hold the wound closed.

The flexibility of this outer tissue flap reduces problems in wound closure. However, the main complication in this technique is incising too deeply. This may result in cutting away some of the blood supply to the mentalis or buccinator muscles, causing sloughing of some portions of these muscles.

Although Metz's approach and those of some other operators are useful, Linkow believes that clean, aseptic, and intelligent surgery over the original in-cision causes a minimum amount of trauma and healing is quite good (Fig. 12-30).

Setting the temporary denture over the implant

Immediately after the tissue has been sutured, the original or a new prefabricated temporary denture should be fitted over the four abutments. If an old denture is used, its tissue side should be completely hollowed out with a heatless stone or a vulcanite bur so that it can fit directly over the four protruding implant abutment posts without interfering with occlusion.

If a new denture is made, it need only have six anterior acrylic teeth and two posterior acrylic occlusal tables (Fig. 12-31). No matter which denture is used, it should be tried in the mouth and balanced. The denture should not be in premature occlusion; the bite should not be beyond the original vertical dimension. Fast-setting acrylic should be mixed and placed inside the denture, which is then placed into its proper position over the four implant abutments, and the patient is asked to bite into centric occlusion.

It is imperative to remove the denture long before the acrylic sets, because excess acrylic can slip underneath the abutments to the narrower undercut necks and prevent removal of the denture. Therefore a good procedure is to take the denture on and off every 20 seconds or so as the acrylic sets. As soon as the acrylic starts to get hard, the denture should be left outside the mouth. All excess acrylic inside the post areas of the denture should then be removed so that no undercuts exist. Sometimes, too, a soft denture reliner is used if the operator deems it necessary. It is advisable to slightly hollow out the post holes with a tapered diamond stone so that the denture easily fits over the posts. Also, the denture must not contact the underlying tissues, so it becomes necessary to reduce the tissue-bearing surface of the denture between the four holes.

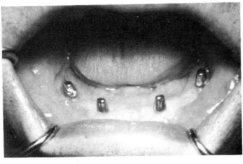

Fig. 12-32. Healing of the soft tissues covering the implant usually is completed 3 to 6 weeks after its insertion.

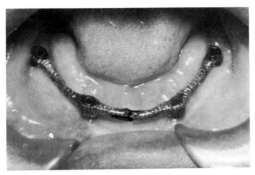

Fig. 12-33. The superstructure framework is placed over the protruding implant posts.

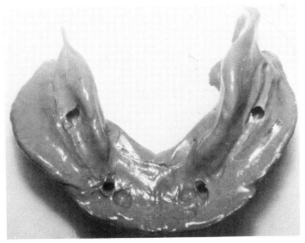

Fig. 12-35. The superstructure framework is then "picked up" with an elastic impression.

Making the impression for the final implant denture

After about 3 to 6 weeks, the implant should have completely set and the surrounding tissues should be sufficiently healed to take the final "pick-up" impression for the final implant prosthesis (Fig. 12-32). The superstructure framework is first placed over the four implant abutments (Fig. 12-33), and an accurate wax or stone occlusal record of centric relation is taken and the vertical dimension established (Fig. 12-34). The superstructure is then picked up with one of the elastic impression materials (Fig. 12-35) or with one of the alginate materials (Fig. 12-36). All the soft tissue underneath the superstructure should be included in this impression. Instead of processing the denture, a wax-up of acrylic teeth fitted to the metallic superstructure should be tried during the next visit so that the bite, articulation, vertical dimension, and balancing of the case can be corrected (Fig. 12-37). Finally, the com-

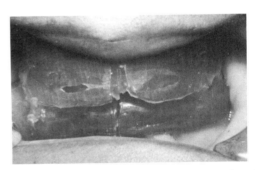

Fig. 12-34. A wax interocclusal record of centric relation is taken.

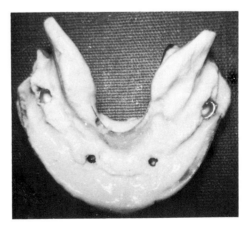

Fig. 12-36. Sometimes an alginate impression is used to "pick up" the superstructure.

pleted, processed denture is fitted and rearticulated for high spots, prematurities, and impingements (Fig. 12-38). The teeth should be acrylic and the upper denture, if present, should also be fabricated at the same time with acrylic teeth. The differences in size between the old denture used as a temporary bridge and the implant denture can be seen in Fig. 12-39. Because the implant denture obtains its retention from the implant posts, it is never as large or as long as a conventional denture.

Follow-up

The patient should be recalled at least every 3 months for periodic check-ups regarding the fit, proper balance, and articulation of the case, if at all possible. Periodic roentgenograms of the osseous structures in relation to the implant should be taken

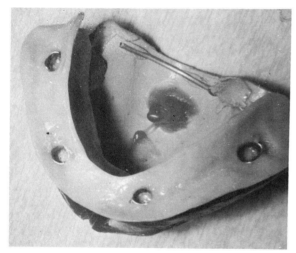

Fig. 12-37. The lower subperiosteal implant is fabricated to the metal superstructure. The upper denture is also completed.

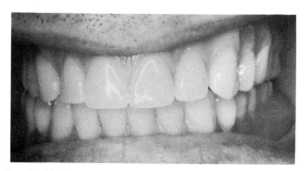

Fig. 12-38. The completed case must be carefully balanced. No portion of the tissue surface of the implant denture must touch the fibromucosal tissue. The denture is implant-borne only.

at least once each year to check for bone resorption (Fig. 12-40).

MARZIANI'S FULL ARCH RESTORATION

A popular European method for subperiosteal implantations is that of the Italian, Marziani. Unlike the American method of designing and fitting a cast Vitallium implant over the bone, Marziani utilizes a tantalum mesh that he molds over the site in one stage. Tantalum is well tolerated by the tissues and is easily cold-worked to fit the exposed bone.

Marziani claims that his technique has two distinct advantages. First, using tantalum eliminates the inconvenient risks that exist when casting Vitallium. The tantalum is supplied in a flat sheet that is a meshwork with standardized holes (Fig. 12-41). The abutments, also standardized, can be inserted in any desired hole. Each abutment consists of three parts: a fixation screw, a tubic pin, and a vent.

Second, only one operative procedure, rather than two, is necessary. The problems that may arise from reincising the site do not exist.

Preliminary procedures

The first steps in inserting a full lower tantalum subperiosteal implant involves taking an alginate impression of the entire lower jaw over the soft tissue. An upper impression and a wax bite are also made. A full lower denture is waxed up on the articulated model and tried in the mouth.

The tantalum meshwork is cut with metal shears

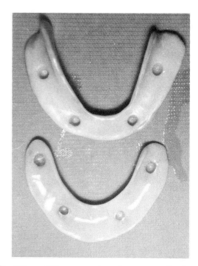

Fig. 12-39. The difference in the size of the completed implant denture (bottom) is much smaller than the temporary denture (top) that was originally the patient's standard type denture.

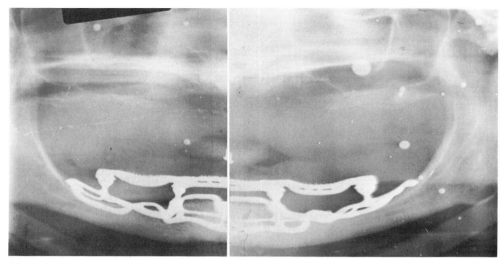

Fig. 12-40. A Panorex showing the close adaptation of the implant denture to the bone of a resorbed mandible.

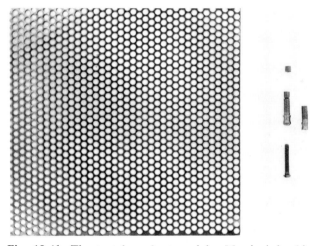

Fig. 12-41. The tantalum sheet used by Marziani for his specially designed subperiosteal implant.

to form the dental implant. The size and shape of the "cutout" are determined by evaluating radiographs and study models.

Four holes—parallel to one another and corresponding to the position of the abutments—are drilled perpendicularly into the stone model with the aid of a parallelometer. Steel pins are then inserted into these holes. The tantalum "cutout" is placed on the stone model, where it is fixated by means of the four protruding steel pins. The first shaping of the "cutout" is done by molding it to the previously prepared stone model. The heights of the abutment posts are established on the articulator according to the amount of occlusal clearance desired when the jaws are in centric occlusion. The molded tantalum "cutout" is cleansed thoroughly with carbon tetrachloride and a 5% nitric acid solution and then sterilized.

A prefabricated tray of acrylic, in either one or two sections, is then prepared prior to incising the site for the bone impression.

Operative procedures

An incision is made along the crest of the ridge and the tissues are retracted, exposing the bone. Any bone leveling that might have to be accomplished is done at this time.

The molded tantalum "cutout" is then tried over the bone without the four abutments. Some modifications in its shape and size can be done at this time. The operator must be sure to relieve the implant in the area of both mental foramina. While the tantalum is in place over the bone, four notches 1 mm. deep are drilled in the bone to receive the screw heads. The meshwork is then removed.

With the prefabricated tray, a rubber base bone impression of the entire exposed mandible is taken. It is allowed to set in the mouth and is then removed. A model is poured into the impression with quick-setting stone.

When the stone has set, four parallel holes are drilled into the model using a parallelometer. These holes correspond to the notches made in the bone. Four steel pins with collars are then set into the

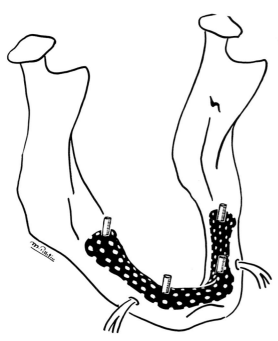

Fig. 12-42. The Marziani-designed tantalum subperiosteal implant.

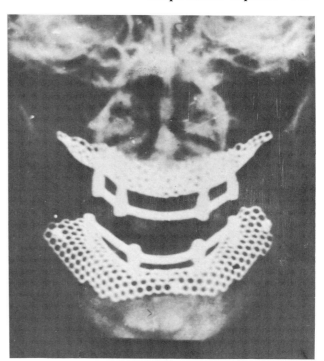

Fig. 12-43. A posteroanterior roentgenogram showing a maxillary and mandibular tantalum subperiosteal implant.

holes in the model. These pins secure the "cutout" during the pressing procedure and maintain the surfaces around the holes through which the abutments will be inserted.

The meshwork is carefully molded to the stone model, and the abutment posts are affixed parallel to one another either by welding or by screws. The implant is once more cleansed with carbon tetrachloride and a 5% nitric acid solution and then sterilized.

Finally, the implant is positioned over the exposed mandibular bone (Fig. 12-42). For immediate fixation, a few screws are passed through the implant and into the bone in the areas of the external oblique ridges and symphysis.

The tissues are sutured over the implant and the prefabricated lower denture is hollowed out and fitted to the four abutments with the use of fast-setting acrylic. The case is occluded and balanced out. Roentgenograms are taken periodically to analyze the situation (Fig. 12-43).

Unilateral implantations following slightly modified procedures are shown in Fig. 12-44.

UNILATERAL SUBPERIOSTEAL IMPLANTS

Each unilateral implant of American design inserted by Linkow prior to 1955 had to be removed.

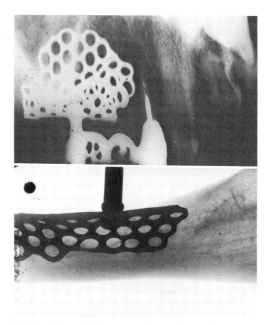

Fig. 12-44. Two different unilateral tantalum type subperiosteal implants.

These partial subperiosteal implants were designed to utilize the same anatomic landmarks as did the full subperiosteal implant. Most other operators also found these implants unsatisfactory because they were unsuitable both in design and method of implantation.

There are basic differences between utilizing a limited site and utilizing the full lower jaw. The lingual tissue covering the mylohyoid ridges is usually much thinner than that in the buccal and occlusal areas. Thus, with the old designs the tissue became extremely taut as it was stretched over the implant. This eventually caused a breakthrough of the lingual border of the implant, with the formation of granulation tissue between the border and the bone, and the implant failed. In those implant designs where the lingual peripheral border was not extended below the mylohyoid ridge, there was very little resistance against lateral forces. Eventual dislodgment of the implant occurred, with granulation tissue growing underneath the implant and dislodging it even more.

After considering these difficulties, Linkow introduced his open lingual finger unilateral design in 1955. To reduce or eliminate lateral displacement, the lingual surface of the implant was extended some distance below the mylohyoid ridge, following the contour of the bone (Fig. 12-45). To reduce or eliminate the stretching of the thin lingual tissue over these extensions, notches about 1 mm. deep were made with diamond stones in the bone to accept the fingers (Fig. 12-46). The seated lingual fingers

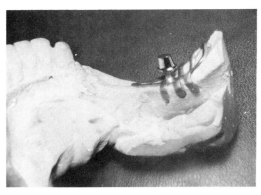

Fig. 12-45. Lingual fingers (Linkow) extend below the mylohyoid ridge into previously prepared notches to give the unilateral subperiosteal implant added retention and stability. (From Linkow, L. I.: Re-evaluation of mandibular unilateral subperiosteal implants: a 12 year report, J. Prosth. Dent. 17:509-514, 1967.)

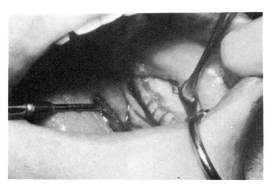

Fig. 12-46. The basal bone is exposed, showing the lingual notches below the mylohyoid ridge. The exposed external oblique ridge is seen on the buccal aspect.

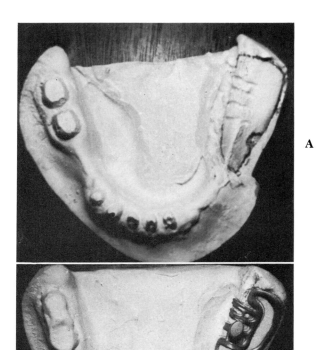

A

B

Fig. 12-47. A, The master stone cast illustrating the depth and angulation of the lingual notches as well as the external oblique ridge and part of the mental foramen. B, The implant fits flush onto the stone model and the lingual fingers fit flush into the prepared grooves.

thus fit flush with the bone, thereby eliminating stretching the tissue (Fig. 12-47).

Some operators criticize notching the bone for a subperiosteal implant because their experiences in making grooves in other regions of the jaw have led to bone resorption and, consequently, loose-fitting implants. From a great deal of clinical experience, Linkow has found that notching the lingual cortical plate below the mylohyoid ridge has led to little or no resorption in most cases. Three to six weeks after the notches have been made, the lingual fingers fit snugly into the grooves.

Because the lingual peripheral border of the older implant designs was a continuous strut that extended over the mylohyoid ridge, more exposure would rapidly take place once a part of the strut became denuded. Therefore the inferior peripheral border was discontinued. The fingers were left open at their ends so that they were completely inde-

pendent of each other. In this manner, if any portion becomes exposed, it can be quickly cut off from the rest of the implant and not affect the remaining portions. Fibromucosal tissue quickly fills in the vacated space and covers the bone.

Unlike implantations done with the older type unilateral designs, cases using the open lingual finger implant have proved successful over many years.

The technique used for inserting a unilateral open lingual finger implant differs slightly from that used for seating a full arch implant for a completely edentulous mandible. All teeth that are to be included in the implant bridge are prepared and impressions of them are taken. These include compound tube impressions, a wax bite, an alginate impression of the opposing jaw, and an alginate impression of the prepared teeth and the edentulous area that is to house the implant. From this latter impression, an all-acrylic temporary splint is fabricated to fit over the prepared natural tooth abutments and the implant abutment, to stabilize it immediately after it is placed in position (Fig. 12-48).

A bone impression must be taken to fabricate the implant itself. To do this, an incision is made from the retromolar pad area, across the crest of the ridge, and anteriorly toward the last two remaining abutments. Here the incision should extend from the crest to the distoproximal surface of the last abutment

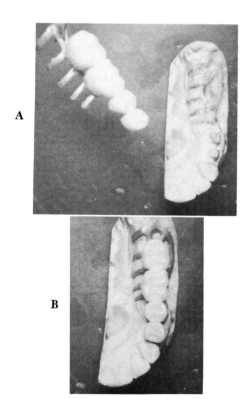

Fig. 12-48. **A,** A temporary acrylic splint is prefabricated and adjusted to fit over the protruding post of the implant posteriorly and over the anterior tooth abutments anteriorly. **B,** The accurately fitting temporary acrylic splint positioned over the tooth and implant abutment. It is used for immediate immobilization of the implant. (From Linkow, L. I.: Evaluation of the unilateral subperiosteal implant; eight year report, Dent. Dig. 68:213-217, 1962.)

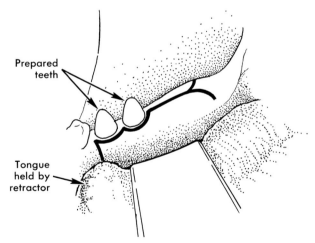

Fig. 12-49. An incision is made from the retromolar pad area to the distoproximal surface of the prepared second bicuspid tooth and is continued along the gingival sulcus to the mesial aspect of the prepared first bicuspid tooth. From this point a vertical downward incision is made so that the tissue can easily be retracted.

tooth, where it should continue buccally along the gingival sulci of the abutment teeth. When it reaches the mesial aspect of the most anterior abutment tooth, the incision is angled downward toward the inferior buccal border of the mandible (Fig. 12-49).

The bone exposure should include the external oblique ridge from the retromolar pad area to the area of the nearest natural tooth abutment. The mylohyoid ridge and the lingual surface of the mandible should be exposed, especially in the area where the lingual grooves will be made.

The tissue is peeled away, making sure that all the periosteal tissue against the bone is completely reflected. It is not usually necessary to suture the lingual tissue away from the bone to expose it, as is done during the completely edentulous impression technique. It is relatively easy to obtain a bone impression in the small unilateral edentulous area.

Before the impression is taken, the lingual grooves are made. The length of these grooves is determined by the contour of the bone's lingual surface. If there is a severe undercut from the crest of the ridge extending downward to the lingual surface, the grooves must start near the crest of the ridge and proceed downward to the point where the ridge turns sharply inward. Usually when these severe undercuts exist, the lingual grooves are much shorter. The grooves are made with a narrow tapering diamond point bur and are usually ½ to 1 mm. deep and 1½ mm. wide—the depth and width of the implant fingers. The grooves should have no sharp line angles (Fig. 12-50).

A quick-setting acrylic mix is then manipulated and molded in the operator's hands until it turns to a dry, clay-like consistency. It is then immediately molded over the exposed bone to form the neces-sary accurate tray. Cold water should be constantly sprayed on it while in the mouth, and it should be removed before it becomes too heated. It is hollowed out slightly, small holes are drilled through it for retention, and it is coated with a good adhesive agent.

Rubber base or Neoplex impression material is then mixed and placed inside the tray, and the tray is positioned over the site and held for 10 minutes. The tray may be removed, so that the impression may be checked for accuracy, and then replaced, but this is not necessary. A full lower alginate impression of all the prepared abutments as well as of the entire acrylic tray with the rubber base impression is taken. After the alginate has set, the entire mass is removed intact (Fig. 12-51) and the tissues sutured

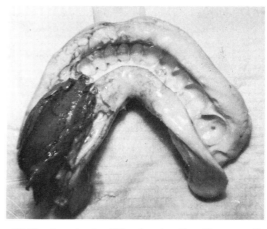

Fig. 12-51. An elastic (Neoplex by Surgident or Coeflex rubber base by Coe) impression of the bone is taken and "picked up" with a full mouth alginate impression that also includes the prepared abutment teeth.

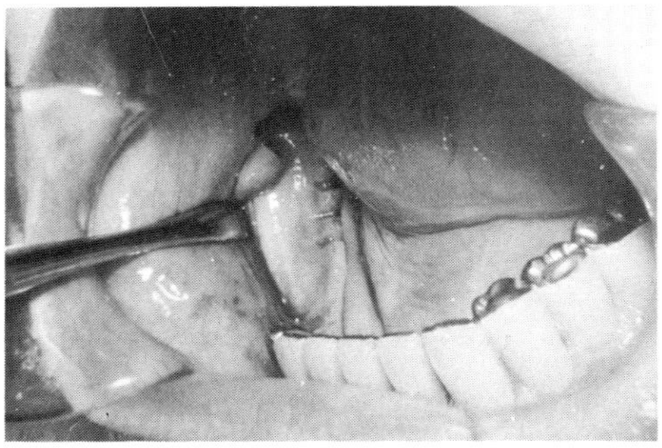

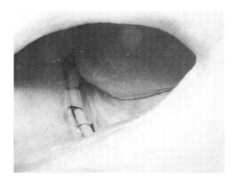

Fig. 12-50. The lingual notches are usually ½ to 1 mm. deep and 1½ mm. wide, and all line angles are rounded out.

Fig. 12-52. The tissue wound is sutured.

closed (Fig. 12-52). Linkow now prefers using Imput for the fabrication of the tray and impression.

Suturing is done in the same manner as for the completely edentulous implant patient. Sometimes an intraoral bandage is used over the sutured tissues to protect them from movements of the tongue, cheeks, and lips.

A surgical wax bite of the exposed mandible in relation to the opposing complement of teeth is also taken.

The master stone model is poured. From this model both the metallic implant and the temporary acrylic splint, if one is to be used, are fabricated (Fig. 12-53). The temporary splint fits over both

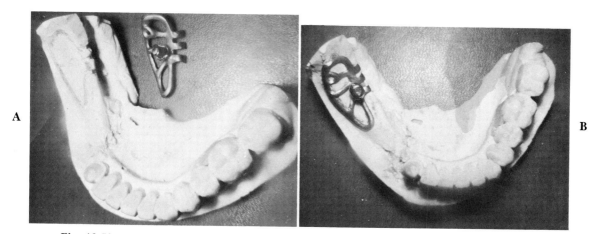

Fig. 12-53. A, The unilateral subperiosteal implant is seen next to the stone cast showing the duplicate bone area with the lingual notches. **B,** The implant fitted snugly over the model.

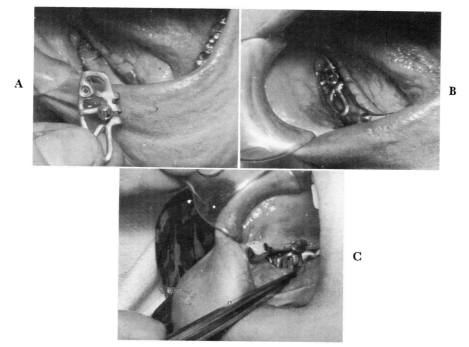

Fig. 12-54. A, The implant just prior to its insertion over the exposed bone during the second surgical stage procedure. **B,** The implant should accurately fit over the exposed bone. **C,** Lingually, the fingers fit snugly into the previously prepared grooves.

the tooth abutments and the implant abutment to immediately stabilize the implant. If a fixation screw is to be used to stabilize the implant, then the acrylic splint is not necessary.

The sutures are removed in about 5 to 7 days. The tissue is usually ready for the final setting of the unilateral implant approximately 3 weeks after the initial bone impression was taken.

To insert the implant, the tissue is incised along the exact line of previous incision, and the soft tissues are gently retracted, exposing the bone. The sterilized implant is then placed into its exact position (Fig. 12-54).

The accuracy of its insertion may be tested by placing the temporary acrylic splint over the implant and natural tooth abutments. If the splint has been fabricated properly and the fit of the implant is accurate, there should be no difficulty in positioning the splint. The splint, after being ground into proper occlusion, is then removed from the mouth so that the wound may be closed.

The lips of the wound are closely adapted to the protruding implant post by first making either a mattress or a purse-string suture around it and using surgical ties to approximate the remaining tissues.

With a temporary cement, the acrylic splint is set into position to protect the prepared tooth abutments and to immobilize the implant. The splint also places the implant into immediate functional occlusion.

The sutures should be removed anywhere from 7 to 10 days later. If any of the implant framework has become exposed, and if this situation was not corrected within 48 hours, there is little sense in resuturing the site. It simply will not heal correctly. The only proper procedure is to remove the implant, allow the tissue to heal for at least 2 months, and then reincise the tissue and reset and resuture it over the implant a second time. Sometimes in these situations it may be necessary to make new lingual grooves. This, of course, will necessitate taking new impressions for another implant.

After the tissue has completely healed, the final procedures for completing the fixed partial denture are begun. The previously fitted castings are placed over all the tooth abutments. A gold coping, which was fabricated at the same time as the implant, is fitted over the implant abutment. A wax interocclusal record of centric relation and a plaster index are taken, as well as an alginate impression of the teeth in the opposing jaw for the fabrication of the fixed partial denture. The fixed denture is cemented over the posts using the same procedures as for any ordinary type of fixed partial denture (Fig. 12-55). The x-ray of the completed case is shown in Fig. 12-56.

BILATERAL SUBPERIOSTEAL IMPLANTS

Basically, the surgical procedures for restoring bilaterally edentulous mandibles with partial subperiosteal implants are the same as for unilateral restorations. The remaining teeth are prepared for crown restorations before implant surgery. The first surgical stage for the bilateral bone impression is then done (Fig. 12-57). A wax bite, plaster index, and opposing upper alginate impression are taken.

If desired—as shown in another very similar case—all of the castings covering the natural tooth abutments and any pontics existing between may be soldered together and the facings processed. However, the casting covering the tooth abutment nearest the implant should be fabricated as a thimble instead of a veneer casting (Figs. 12-58 to 12-60). A veneer

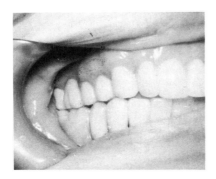

Fig. 12-55. The partial fixed bridge is cemented with hard cement over the implant and tooth abutments.

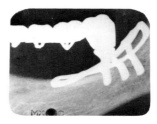

Fig. 12-56. A periapical postoperative film of the completed case. (From Linkow, L. I.: Re-evaluation of mandibular unilateral subperiosteal implants: a 12 year report, J. Prosth. Dent. 17:509-514, 1967.)

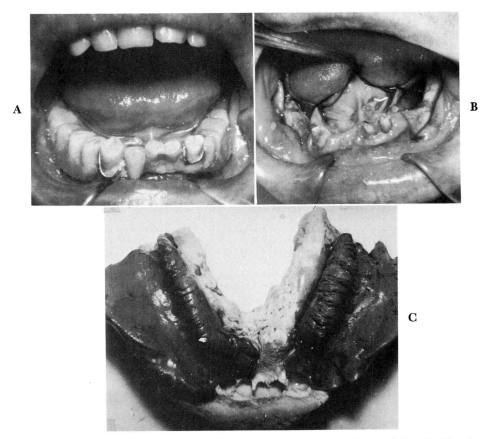

Fig. 12-57. A, A preoperative patient with only three anterior teeth remaining. B, The three teeth had been previously prepared for full crown coverage. The fibromucosal tissues are retracted posteriorly and bilaterally to expose the underlying bone. C, Bilateral rubber base (Neoplex) impressions are taken and picked up, if desired, with either a full arch plaster or an alginate impression, which includes the anterior tooth preparation.

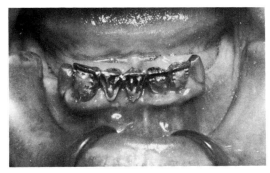

Fig. 12-58. During the healing of the soft tissues after the first surgical stage, the castings are fitted over the remaining abutment teeth with the pontics soldered to the rest of the framework.

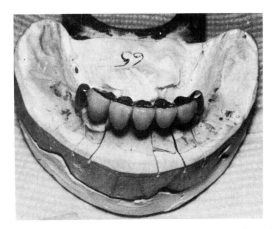

Fig. 12-59. The anterior fixed partial denture is fabricated with gold occlusals and acrylic facings.

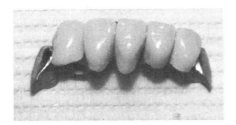

Fig. 12-60. Cantilevered off each of the last abutment teeth on each side is a gold thimble that acts as the anterior abutments for the two posterior fixed partial dentures that will be supported by the implants posteriorly.

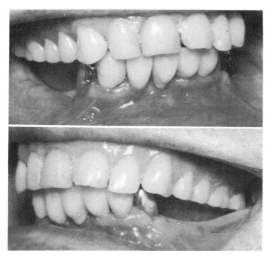

Fig. 12-61. The anterior prosthesis is fitted into position.

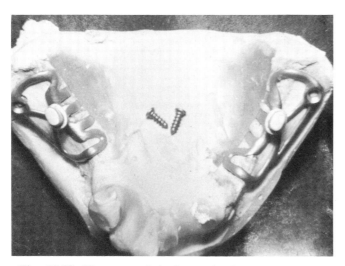

Fig. 12-62. The cast cobalt-chrome implants are seen on the model. Two small cobalt-chrome set screws are sometimes used for securing the implants to the bone. They are screwed through the two openings seen on the distobuccal aspects of the implants.

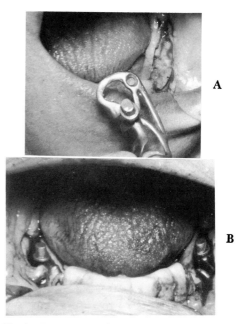

Fig. 12-63. A, The implant is ready to be placed over the exposed bone. B, Both implants are seen fitting accurately to the bone.

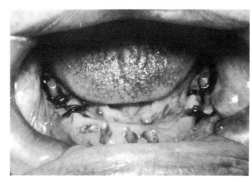

Fig. 12-64. The tissues are closely adapted to close the wounds and to closely cover the necks of the implants.

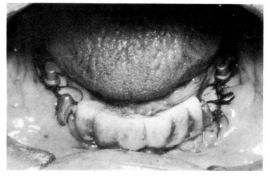

Fig. 12-65. A temporary acrylic splint is sometimes fabricated if the fixed partial denture is not fabricated prior to the implant insertions.

casting may also be fabricated to fit over each thimble. In this manner, the entire processed bridge, including the two cantilevered thimbles, can be immediately cemented into position (Fig. 12-61).

The second surgical stage takes place anywhere from 3 to 4 weeks after the initial surgery. Before inserting the implants the castings are checked for their fit on the master stone model (Fig. 12-62). Some castings, such as the ones used in this case, may contain a small hole in the region of the external oblique ridge. This is for the insertion of a small Vitallium set screw. A hole is made in the bone with a No. 556 fissure bur, and the screw is inserted

through the implant and into the bone. Usually the screw is not needed because the lingual finger design provides enough retention.

The implants are placed on the exposed bone (Fig. 12-63), and the tissue is sutured (Fig. 12-64). At this time the anterior processed fixed partial denture can be cemented into position, or—as in this case—the temporary anterior acrylic splint is used (Fig. 12-65).

After healing, the temporary splint is removed. The anterior prosthesis is seated, the veneer castings (if done this way) are positioned over the thimbles, and the prefabricated gold copings are placed over the implant abutments. A wax interocclusal record of centric relation and a plaster index to complete the bridges are taken. The bridges are then cemented into position.

There is a simpler method for making the final impression for the two posterior bridges. An elastic impression of the two cantilevered thimbles and the implant post abutments is taken and a one-piece casting for each bridge made (Figs. 12-66 and 12-67). This procedure makes it unnecessary to first cast veneer crowns to fit over the cantilevered copings and to fabricate gold copings to fit over the implant

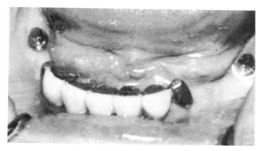

Fig. 12-66. Healing around the protruding posts is usually uneventful if the operator follows good surgical and prosthetic principles. (From Linkow, L. I.: Re-evaluation of mandibular unilateral subperiosteal implants: a 12 year report, J. Prosth. Dent. **17:**509-514, 1967).

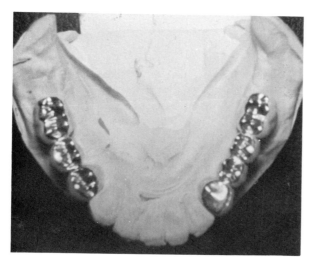

Fig. 12-67. Two bilateral fixed partial dentures are fabricated from the impressions taken of the implants and anterior gold thimbles.

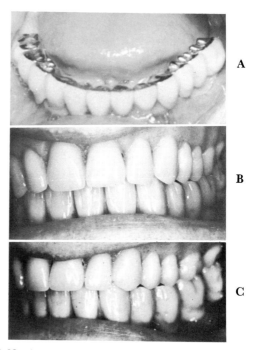

Fig. 12-68. **A,** The bridges are cemented into their positions with oxyphosphate of zinc. **B and C,** Anterior and lateral views. A new maxillary denture with acrylic teeth was made in conjunction with the lower prosthesis.

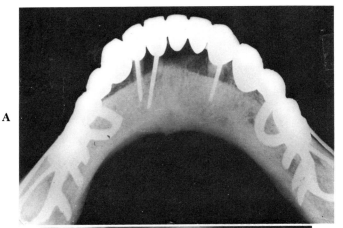

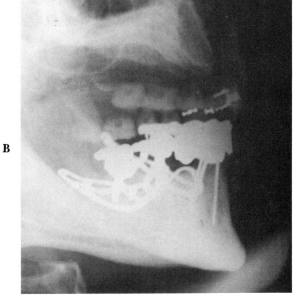

Fig. 12-69. A, A cross-sectional occlusal x-ray showing both subperiosteal implants in close position over the bone. Three endodontic root stabilizers were used to stabilize the three remaining anterior teeth. **B,** A lateral plate showing the subperiosteal implants and endodontic stabilizers in position.

posts. Also, no solder joints are needed. The bridges are then cemented (Fig. 12-68).

Radiographs of the finished case are seen in Fig. 12-69.

MAXILLARY SUBPERIOSTEAL IMPLANTS

For many years American operators have avoided maxillary subperiosteal implants. A few practitioners, including Gershkoff and Goldberg, have reported some long-term maxillary implant successes functioning over 10 years, but most operators have been discouraged by the high proportion of failures. From other countries come reports of greater success. Bello from South America claimed that a maxillary subperiosteal implant that he did on his wife was functioning splendidly after 12 years. Salagaray and Sol of Spain and Audoire of France have been doing successful subperiosteal implants in the maxilla for a number of years.

Failures in the maxillary subperiosteal implants have been attributed mainly to poor design of the framework and poor surgical and impression techniques. However, the most common cause of failure may be attributed to the fact that there is little dense bone in the maxilla to bear the subperiosteal implant. Whereas the mandible usually has relatively flat dense cortical plates after alveolar bone resorption, the maxilla resorbs to thin, irregular ridges—frequently knife-edged—with a very thin layer of cortical bone, especially over the posterior ridges.

Many different designs have been created for maxillary subperiosteal implants, some of which included the hard palate while others did not. In Linkow's opinion, the following design features should be included for the maxillary superiosteal implant to enjoy long-term success. There should be a minimal amount of primary struts across the alveolar bone. Strong bony landmarks should be used as foundations. These include the base of the anterior nasal spine, the zygomatic arch, the canine eminence, and sometimes the lateral surface of the pterygoid plate (Fig. 12-70). A brace should be laid across the hard palate. The anterior and posterior palatal struts going from left to right should be as far away from one another as possible, with a few cross struts between them.

In addition to the contraindications typical to all implant candidates, a maxillary subperiosteal implant should never be done if the mandible has a full complement of natural teeth or if the patient suffers with sinusitis, postnasal drip, or similar conditions.

To take the bone impression, the site is anesthetized. Two percent lidocaine and epinephrine 1:100,000 infiltration injections are given in the buccal and labial folds, palatal tissue, and infraorbital regions. Posterior superior alveolar and anterior palatine injections also may be given, if desired.

The fibromucosal tissue is incised down to the bone around the entire crest of the ridge, from maxillary tuberosity to maxillary tuberosity (Fig. 12-71).

The tissue is retracted with a periosteal elevator, and the eggshell thin periosteum is carefully separated from the underlying bone without tearing it (Fig. 12-72). If the periosteum is badly mutilated, an increased amount of bone resorption will occur

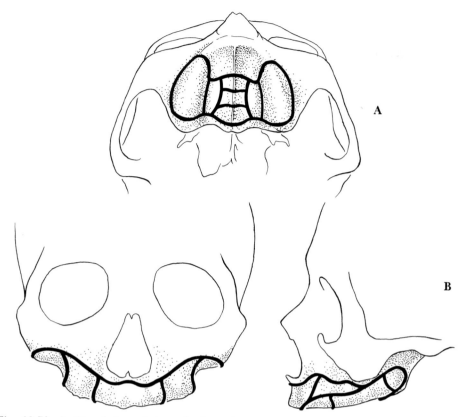

Fig. 12-70. **A,** The design of the palatal portion of the subperiosteal maxillary implant must be as broad as possible (Linkow). **B,** The peripheral borders should end close to the base of the anterior nasal spine, extend high into the canine eminence and slightly below the infraorbital canals, and extend further distally along the zygomatic arch and along the lateral wall of the pterygoid plate.

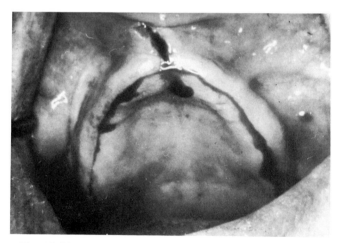

Fig. 12-71. An incision is made along the crest of the ridge from maxillary tuberosity to maxillary tuberosity. Sometimes a vertical accessory incision is made; this can be seen in the anterior region above the primary incision.

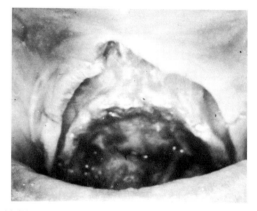

Fig. 12-72. The fibromucosal tissue on the labial and buccal aspect is retracted to expose the base of the anterior nasal spine as well as the canine eminence, zygomatic arch, and pterygoid process. The palatal tissue is retracted to expose the entire hard palate, and sometimes the posterior nasal spine and greater and lesser palatine foramina.

because of delayed healing. The soft tissue covering the palate should be reflected posteriorly until the greater and lesser palatine foramina and posterior nasal spine are almost exposed. Reflecting the nerve endings exiting from the anterior palatine foramina very rarely results in parasthesia. Labially, the tissue is retracted to expose the hard bony portion existing

in the canine eminence and the inferior border of the anterior nasal spine. The hard bone in the region of the zygoma is also exposed so that, superiorly, the extension of the implant framework will almost reach the infraorbital foramina. Posteriorly, the peripheral border should reach up to or toward the pterygoid process.

A quick cure acrylic tray is adapted to the exposed maxillary bone in much the same manner as in the mandible (Fig. 12-73). The tray is trimmed, punched, and treated with adhesive (Fig. 12-74), and the rubber base bone impression is taken. It should include the hard palate, nasal spine, canine eminence, and part of the zygomatic arch (Fig. 12-75). A surgical wax bite and elastic impression of the lower jaw are also taken. Again, Imput is now used

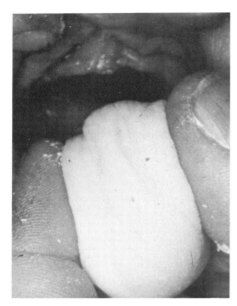

Fig. 12-73. Cold cure acrylic monomer and polymer was mixed. When it became clay-like in texture, it was manipulated over the exposed maxillary bone to reach the proper peripheral borders onto which the implant would rest.

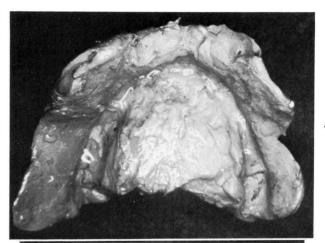

A

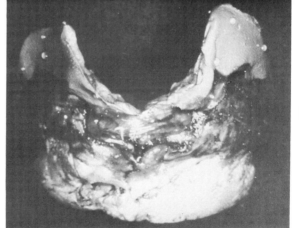

B

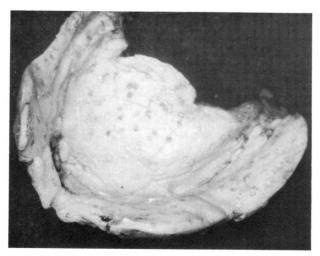

Fig. 12-74. When the acrylic tray hardened, it was trimmed and made more retentive for the rubber impression by notching its inner and outer surfaces with a round bur in a contra-angle. It was then painted with one of the rubber adhesives.

Fig. 12-75. A, The rubber base impression. B, The anterior extension of the rubber base (Neoplex by Surgident) impression. A wax interocclusal record of centric relation is seen attached to the lower portion of the acrylic tray.

more frequently by Linkow. Its advantage is that it can be molded into position, and when it sets it can be used as the tray itself since it sets harder than rubber base.

The tissue is sutured and the denture fitted (Fig. 12-76) and postoperative instructions are given to the patient, including the use of saline rinses, ice-packs, and analgesics. Because of a more adequate blood supply, the palatal tissues heal more rapidly than do the tissues covering the mandibular bone. About 6 days later the sutures are removed, and the patient's old denture is again hollowed out and relined with a soft tissue conditioning material. This prevents dropping of the palatal tissue.

The master stone cast is poured and articulated from the surgical bone impression (Fig. 12-77) and the implant cast (Fig. 12-78).

About 3 to 6 weeks after the first surgical stage,

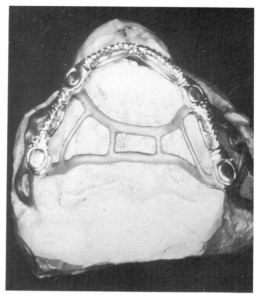

Fig. 12-78. The maxillary implant fits accurately over the duplicate bone model. The superstructure framework was fabricated the same time that the substructure was cast.

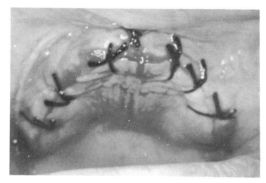

Fig. 12-76. The tissues were sutured together.

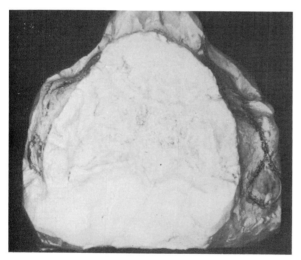

Fig. 12-77. Note the knife-like ridge of the maxilla seen on the master stone model.

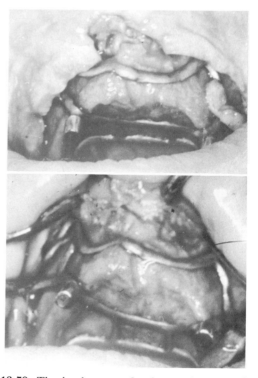

Fig. 12-79. The implant was fitted over the exposed bone. It must fit accurately.

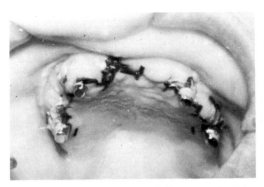

Fig. 12-80. The tissues were carefully sutured with mattress or purse-string suturing around each post, with interrupted surgical ties between them.

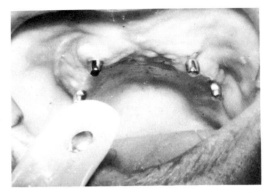

Fig. 12-82. The palateless implant denture is ready to be inserted after the healing is complete.

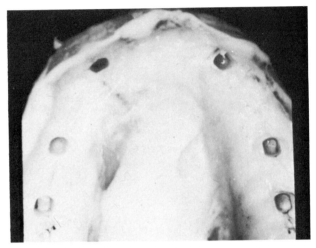

Fig. 12-81. The patient's old denture is sometimes used temporarily by first hollowing it out so it will not interfere with the four protruding posts and then relining with one of the soft reline materials, such as Hydro-Cast (Kay-See Dental Manufacturing Company) and Softtone (Bosworth Company).

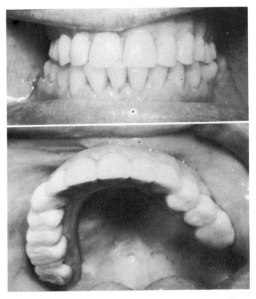

Fig. 12-83. The palateless denture is implant-borne and never touches the fibromucosal tissue.

the second surgical incision is made directly over the original incision and the implant is set over the bone (Fig. 12-79). Purse-string sutures are placed around each protruding post. As many surgical ties and mattress sutures as are needed are placed between the four abutment posts (Fig. 12-80).

The old denture in the area of the posts is hollowed out so that there is no interference (Fig. 12-81), and the denture is relined with the soft tissue conditioner. If the patient has no old denture, a new temporary denture is fabricated from the surgical bite and positioned directly over the implant framework. Postoperative instructions are once again given to the patient.

The sutures are removed about 1 week later. Any necessary adjustments with the fit and occlusion of the temporary denture are made. When all healing has taken place (Fig. 12-82), the final palateless implant denture is processed. The cast metal superstructure is placed over the implant posts, and a wax bite registration of centric relationship is taken. The superstructure is picked up with an elastic impression. The wax-up of the maxillary denture with acrylic teeth is tried in the mouth. (If the patient also has an edentulous lower jaw, the lower wax-up should be accomplished at the same time.) The completed denture is inserted and balanced (Fig. 12-83). A Panorex shows the finished case (Fig. 12-84).

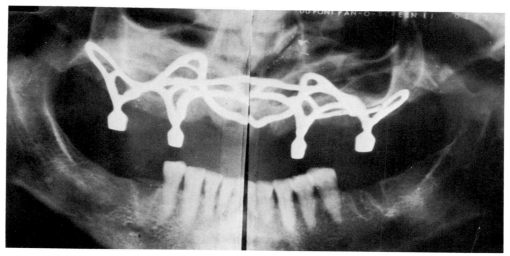

Fig. 12-84. A Panorex x-ray of the subperiosteal implant shows the topography of the bone that it covers. This implant should have been contraindicated because it opposed natural teeth.

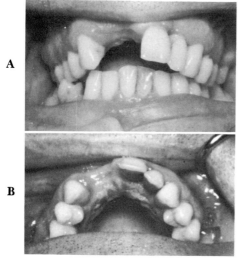

Fig. 12-85. A, A preoperative picture showing missing right central and lateral incisors. B, There were no caries or preexisting fillings in any of the teeth.

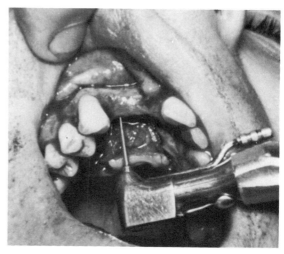

Fig. 12-87. Transfixation pins were drilled through the alveolar bone from the palatal surface to the labial surface deep in the canine eminence.

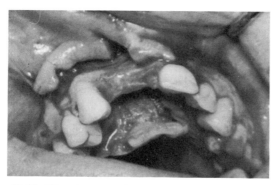

Fig. 12-86. The tissue was incised to expose the underlying bone.

PARTIAL MAXILLARY SUBPERIOSTEAL IMPLANTS WITH HORIZONTAL TRANSFIXATIONS

Horizontal pins may be used to help stabilize and support a maxillary subperiosteal implant. In this case, a 32-year-old man was missing right maxillary central and lateral teeth (Fig. 12-85). He had neither decay nor fillings in any of his maxillary teeth. His anterior quadrant flared out anteriorly so that there was an overjet of about 5 or 6 mm. over the lower teeth. In order to spare the neighboring teeth from full crown restorations, a unilateral subperiosteal implant was fabricated with two horizontally placed transfixation pins to stabilize the implant.

To make the bone impression, infiltration anesthesia was given labially and palatally. An incision was made along the edentulous ridge crest from the mesial surface of the left central incisor to the mesial surface of the right cuspid. The incision became continuous labially and lingually with the gingival tissue that was attached at the neck lines of neighboring teeth. The tissues were reflected to expose a good portion of the labial and palatal plate of bone (Fig. 12-86).

With a special twist drill the same diameter as the

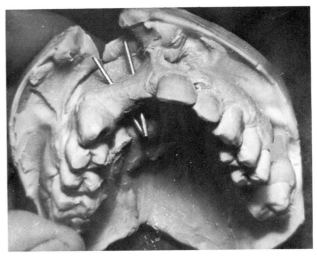

Fig. 12-90. The master stone model was poured into the impression with the pins horizontally fixed inside.

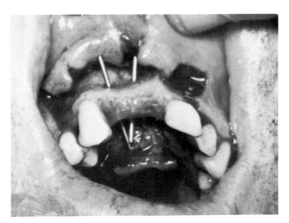

Fig. 12-88. Both pins remained transfixed through the bone prior to the elastic impression.

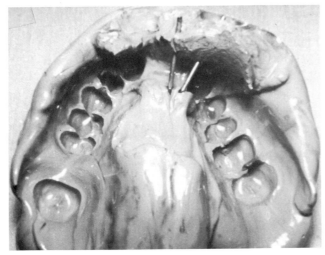

Fig. 12-89. The pins were first removed from the mouth after the elastic impression hardened and were then slipped back into the impression after it was removed.

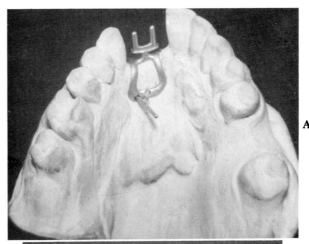

A

B

Fig. 12-91. A, The unilateral subperiosteal implant with specially cast cobalt-chrome pins is seen on the master model. B, The labial ends of the transfixation pins were fabricated with a wider head to prevent them from slipping through the holes in the substructure framework.

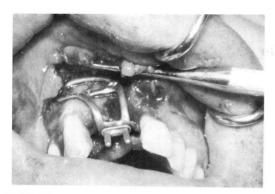

Fig. 12-92. The implant was fitted over the exposed bone.

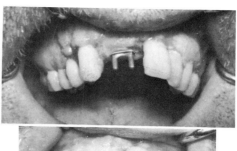

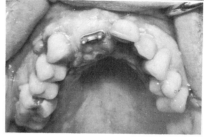

Fig. 12-95. After 3 weeks the tissue around the implant was completely healed.

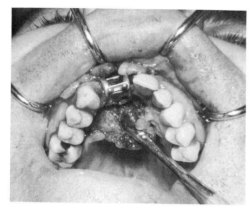

Fig. 12-93. The implant was locked tightly to the bone when the lingual extensions of the transfixation pins were "riveted" to the lingual peripheral border of the substructure by grinding them flat with a heatless stone.

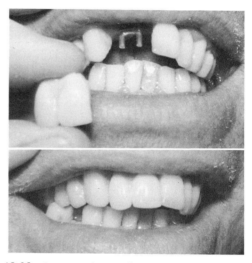

Fig. 12-96. A two-unit acrylic splint was cemented over the protruding posts.

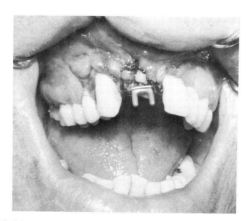

Fig. 12-94. The tissues were sutured to cover the implant and to closely adapt around the protruding post.

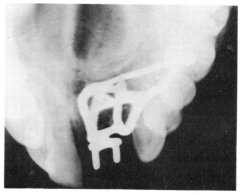

Fig. 12-97. A cross-sectional occlusal x-ray shows the subperiosteal implant with the horizontal transfixation pins.

pins, the bone was traversed palatolabially, high in the area of the canine eminence (Fig. 12-87). The bur should go completely through the bone in a slightly upward and distal direction. A second twist drill of the same diameter was then drilled through the bone in the area of the canine eminence, but mesial to the first bur and in a mesial direction. Both transfixation pins were then inserted completely through the two holes made in the bone (Fig. 12-88). Both were then backed out so that their palatal ends were flush with the palatal bone.

An impression of the exposed bone was taken with a specially prepared partial tray—fabricated by removing its labial flange—and with one of the elastic impression materials. At least one tooth on each side was also included. With the impression material still in the mouth, the pins were immediately pushed palatally before the material set.

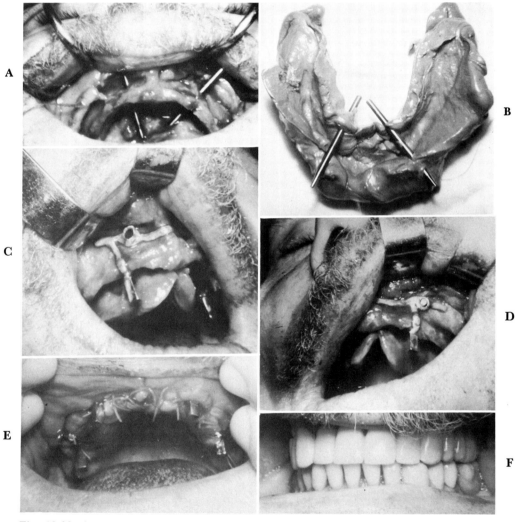

Fig. 12-98. A, Another case showing two transfixation pins of a much larger diameter than those of the previous case. B, The horizontal transfixation pins were placed back into the elastic impression. C, The subperiosteal implant was closely fitted to the bone. Note the circular hole at the superior peripheral border of the implant. D, The transfixation pin was placed through the hole on the labial border and traversed the bone horizontally to end through the other side of the hole on the palatal aspect. E, The tissues were sutured so that they closely adapted to close the incision. F, The completed case—an all-acrylic full arch splint processed over gold copings.

After the elastic set, the two pins were pulled out of the impression in a labial direction so that the impression could be removed without tearing the material. The two pins were then immediately replaced into the elastic impression (Fig. 12-89). A surgical wax interocclusal centric relation bite and an alginate impression of the lower arch of teeth were also taken.

A master investment model was poured into the elastic impression with the seated fixation pins (Fig. 12-90), and the subperiosteal framework was waxed up directly on the model. It was then cast after the fixation pins were removed (Fig. 12-91).

After the wound had healed, the tissue was once more anesthetized, incised, and reflected to expose the underlying bone. The sterilized subperiosteal frame-

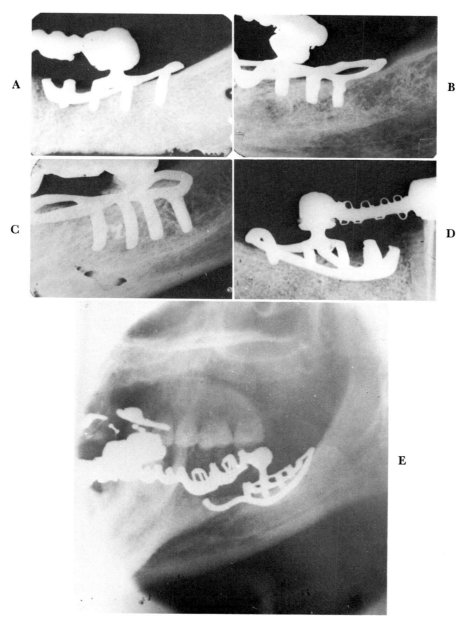

Fig. 12-99. Periapical intraoral x-rays of five different cases utilizing the unilateral subperiosteal implant as the posterior abutments. These cases with the lingual fingers have been in the mouths of these patients from 7 to 12 years. **A** shows a 12-year postoperative radiograph.

work was placed over the bone (Fig. 12-92), and one by one the transfixation pins were set horizontally through the holes previously made in the bone. These pins were held in place because one end had been flattened before insertion to prevent slipping through the holes. Once a pin had been inserted, that portion protruding from the implant was cut off and flattened against the implant by rotating a heatless stone with running water. No part of the implant or pins thus protruded excessively (Fig. 12-93).

Sutures were applied to close the wound (Fig. 12-94), and after 5 or 6 days they were removed with uneventful healing. About 3 weeks later, the tissues were completely healed (Fig. 12-95). Impressions were taken for a two-unit splint to fit over the implant (Fig. 12-96). A cross-sectional x-ray shows the implant in position (Fig. 12-97).

MISCELLANEOUS CASES

Horizontal transfixation pins may also be used to help stabilize a full arch implant for a completely edentulous maxilla (Fig. 12-98). These pins

are larger than those used for partial restorations and do give some added retention. An acrylic-over-gold thimble fixed full arch denture was fabricated for this patient.

Partial mandibular implants are shown in Fig. 12-99. Some of these implants, which are the lingual finger design, have been functioning as long as 12 years.

In some cases it is necessary to use both endosseous and subperiosteal implants (Fig. 12-100). Again the type of implant depends on the condition of the site. The endosseous implants were inserted after the subperiosteal implants had been cast from direct bone impressions. Both types of implants were inserted simultaneously and splinted together with a fixed full arch denture. Fig. 12-100, C, shows three blades and one unilateral subperiosteal implant supporting a full arch fixed prosthesis.

UNIVERSAL SUBPERIOSTEAL IMPLANTS

Sometimes, instead of making bilateral posterior subperiosteal implants when a few remaining anteri-

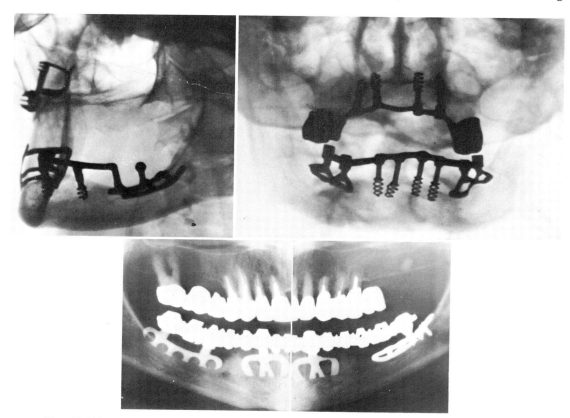

Fig. 12-100. In some cases a combination of endosseous and unilateral or bilateral subperiosteal implants is sometimes used.

or teeth exist, the utilization of a full subperiosteal (Universal-Weber) implant can be accomplished with the teeth still in place. The framework includes four posts and the substructure avoids impingement upon the anterior teeth. In this manner if the anterior teeth ever have to be extracted, a full arch implant denture can be utilized to fit over the existing posts of the subperiosteal implant.

The following case clearly illustrates the technique. Only three anterior teeth remained; these supported a five-unit splint (Fig. 12-101, *A*).

The remaining anterior teeth were prepared for full crown restorations. It was necessary to eliminate

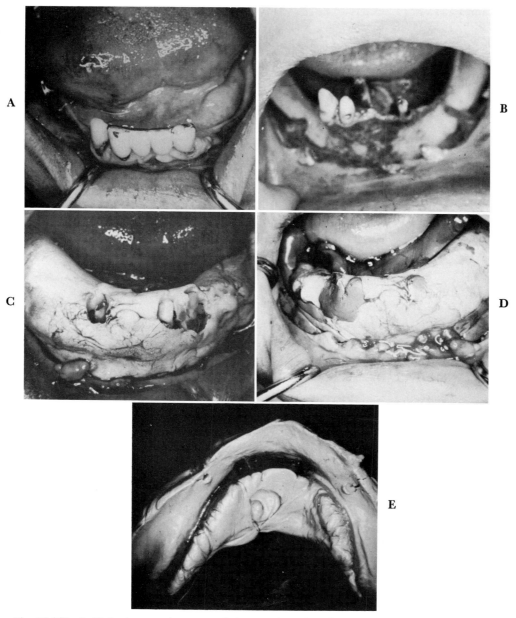

Fig. 12-101. A, Only three teeth supported the anterior splint. **B,** The abutment teeth were prepared for full crown restorations and the tissue retracted to expose the bone. **C,** A cold cure acrylic tray was molded to the exposed bony landmarks. **D,** A rubber base impression was taken. **E,** The impression also included the three tooth impressions.

as much tooth structure as possible so that the teeth would not interfere with the peripheral struts of the subperiosteal implant framework that straddled them. An incision was made from the retromolar pad on one side to the pad area on the other side. The incision extended to the distoproximal surfaces of the terminal abutments on each side. The tissues were retracted in the edentulous areas and from the gingival attachments around the remaining teeth with a blunt periosteal elevator.

It was necessary to expose the same bony landmarks as is done when doing the full subperiosteal implant procedures (Fig. 12-101, *B*).

An acrylic tray was fashioned to fit over the pre-

pared teeth in the anterior quadrant and over both posterior edentulous areas (Fig. 12-101, *C*). A rubber base impression of the entire mandible was taken (Fig. 12-101, *D* and *E*). It became necessary to expose as much of the symphysis and genial tubercles as possible so that the framework of the implant could encircle the teeth without the teeth interfering

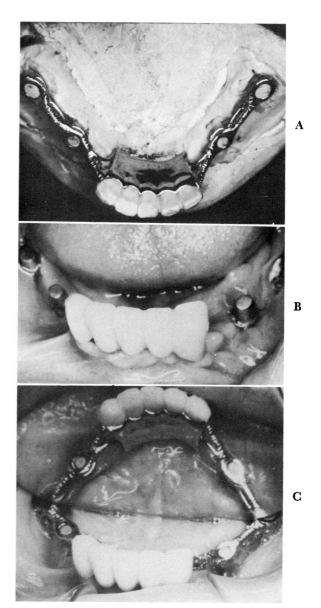

Fig. 12-103. A, The implant superstructure is processed from an impression taken after the anterior restoration is completed. It contains a lingual type Kennedy bar to further support the anterior teeth. **B and C,** The superstructure is fitted in the mouth.

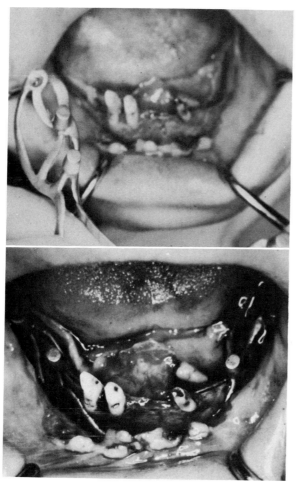

Fig. 12-102. The universal subperiosteal implant is fitted to the bone. There should be no interference from the anterior teeth.

with the insertion of the implant (Fig. 12-102). The tissues were sutured together covering the implant.

The anterior fixed partial prosthesis was processed independently of the subperiosteal implant, although the anterior framework could also have been fabricated from the original rubber base impression that was taken for the implant fabrication.

The anterior restoration must be completed prior to the final impression for the implant denture, since the superstructure framework will contain a continuous Kennedy-type lingual bar that will closely adapt to the lingual surfaces of the anterior fixed restoration (Fig. 12-103). The processed implant denture was fitted into position and properly articulated (Figs. 12-104 and 12-105).

A Panorex shows the completed case. An endodontic stabilizer was used to support one of the anterior teeth (Fig. 12-106).

The rationale for the universal subperiosteal implant opposed to two unilateral subperiosteal implants makes a good deal of sense for specific situa-

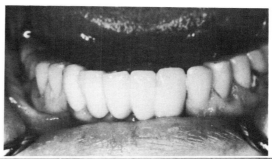

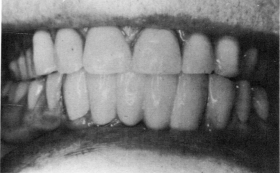

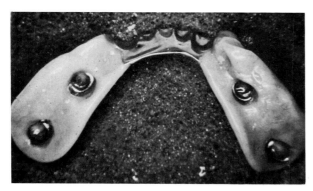

Fig. 12-104. The completed case.

Fig. 12-105. The processed universal implant denture was fitted over the protruding implant posts and the articulation carefully checked.

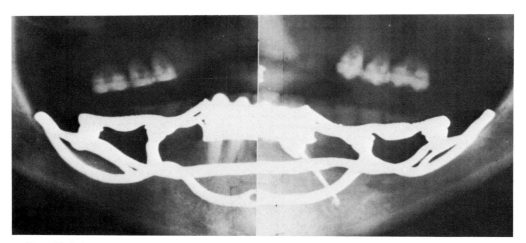

Fig. 12-106. A Panorex of the completed case. Note the endodontic endosseous stabilizer giving added support to the left cuspid.

tions. From a physical point of view alone, a full arch horseshoe type universal subperiosteal implant is more stable than unilateral types, since it utilizes the symphysis and genial tubercles and also extends to both sides of the arch, which increases stability and primary retention of the implant. An added safety gap is included in the universal implant in that if ever the anterior teeth should have to be extracted, the

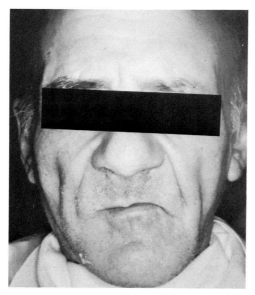

Fig. 12-107. A preoperative photograph of a disheartened patient.

patient still can retain a full arch implant denture without any further surgery.

MAXILLARY TOROPLANTS

Maxillae exhibiting very little or no bone below the maxillary sinus and nasal vestibulum along with the clinical appearance of extremely flat ridges have always presented problems in the fabrication of well-fitting dentures. Patients with this condition cannot obtain dentures that are stable and retentive enough to satisfy them.

The introduction of mucosal inserts is certainly not advisable, for they might be pushed into the superficially located maxillary sinus. Subperiosteal maxillary implants would also fail in such situations, since the metal struts of the substructure crossing over the atrophied alveolar crest would eventually sink into the antrum and nasal cavities.

Since the hard palate is the only area in the maxilla that is of a permanent type bone, while all the rest of the maxillary osseous structures are of a transient type, Linkow decided to utilize only the hard palate—and he thus created the toroplant.

A preoperative photograph of the patient as well as a preoperative Panorex of his edentulous jaws are seen (Figs. 12-107 and 12-108).

Clinically, the soft tissues covering the atrophied maxillary alveolar ridge created a very flat appearance, making it extremely difficult for an adequately fitting conventional denture (Fig. 12-109). A sub-

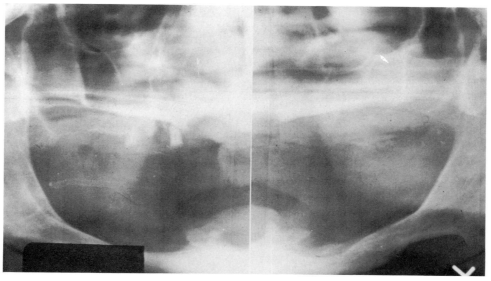

Fig. 12-108. A preoperative Panorex radiograph of both arches.

periosteal implant was made for the atrophied lower jaw (Fig. 12-110).

Technique

An incision was made along the soft tissue covering the residual bony crest from tuberosity to tuberosity (Fig. 12-111, *A*). The tissue covering the hard palate was carefully retracted, exposing the posterior nasal spine and a portion of the greater and lesser palatine foramina (Fig. 12-111, *B*). An acrylic tray was fabricated directly over the hard palate (Fig. 12-111, *C*).

A rubber base impression was taken of the exposed palate using the acrylic tray for support (Fig. 12-111, *D*), and the tissues were sutured (Fig. 12-111, *E*). A wax interocclusal record of centric relation was then taken.

The implant was cast in cobalt-chrome. It contained two holes to accommodate two Vitallium screws to fix the implant to the hard palate. The casting also included three parallel posts 12 mm. long (Fig. 12-112, *A*). The implant was radiographed commercially to check for any porosities (Fig. 12-112, *B*).

Two weeks later the tissue was again incised and retracted and the toroplant was screwed directly to the hard palate (Fig. 12-113). The tissues were then sutured. The three posts can be seen protruding through the central area of the soft tissues covering the hard palate (Fig. 12-114, *A*).

A hole was made in the bite registration to accommodate the protruding implant posts (Fig. 12-114, *B* and *C*). The palatal portion of the tray was then relined with quick cure acrylic resin in order to obtain an accurate seat over the three posts (Fig. 12-114, *D*). A wax interocclusal record of centric relation was taken.

The tissue healed uneventfully around the protruding implant posts in less than 10 days (Fig. 12-115, *A*). The tissue-bearing surface of the bite registration trays was lined with silicone material, and a final wax interocclusal record of centric relation was accomplished (Fig. 12-115, *B*).

A specially designed template was cast in gold. It contained two resilient anchorage attachments* that were only 1 mm. in height (Fig. 12-116). The circumferential attachments become an integral part of the denture.

*Rothermann's Resilience Anchorage-Eccentric 747, Cendres & Metaux, S. A. 2501, Biel-Biemme, Switzerland.

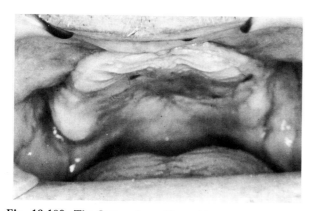

Fig. 12-109. The flattened maxillary ridge.

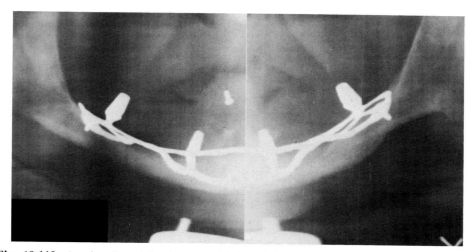

Fig. 12-110. A subperiosteal implant was fabricated for the mandible. Note the absence of bone below the sinus in the maxilla.

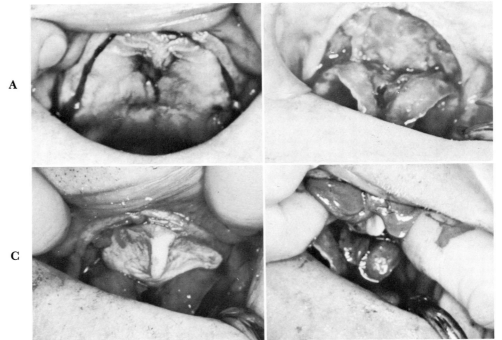

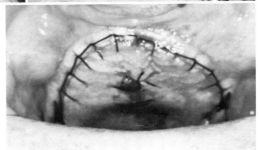

Fig. 12-111. A, The incision was made. B, The palatal tissue was retracted. C, An acrylic tray was cold cured. D, A rubber base impression of the hard palate was taken inside the acrylic tray. E, The tissues were sutured together.

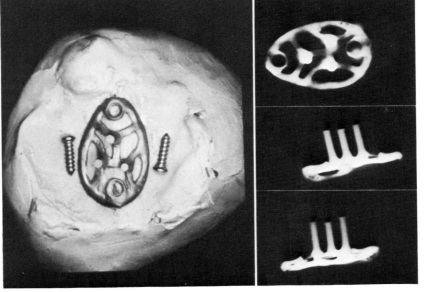

Fig. 12-112. A, The subperiosteal toroplant contains three parallel posts and two holes for fixative screws. B, The casting was commercially radiographed for porosities.

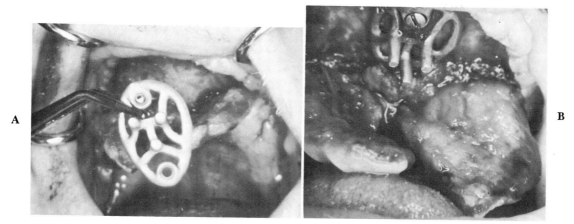

Fig. 12-113. A, The implant was fitted to the hard palate and, B, secured to it with fixation screws.

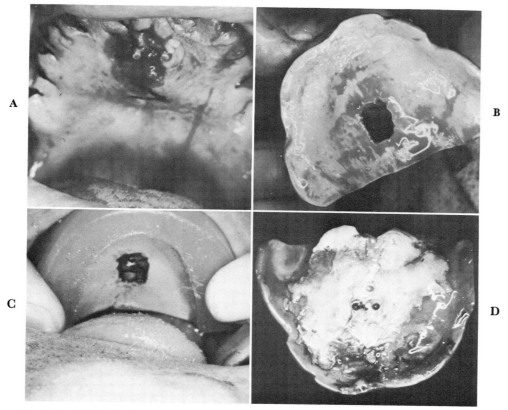

Fig. 12-114. A, The tissues were sutured along the alveolar crest. The three protruding posts were "punched through" the palatal tissue, so no sutures were required. B and C, A hole was cut out through the palatal portion of the bite registration block so that it would not interfere with the three protruding posts. D, An acrylic liner was placed inside the bite block to obtain an accurate seat over the implant posts.

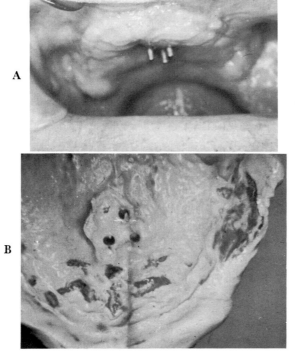

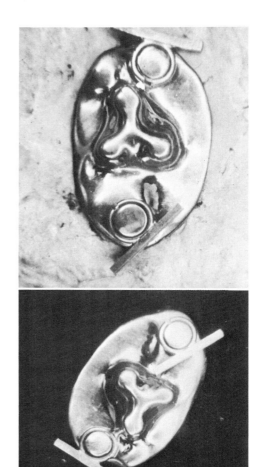

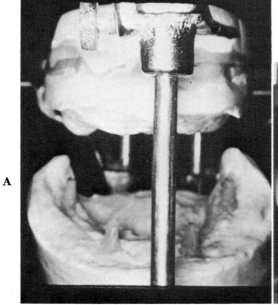

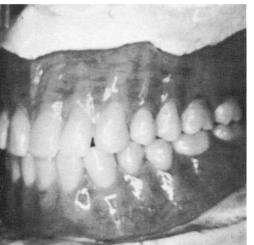

Fig. 12-115. **A,** Healing around the posts was uneventful. **B,** The inside of the bite registration block was relined with silicone and a final wax interocclusal record of centric relation was taken.

Fig. 12-116. A specially designed template with unique ring lock–resilient type attachments was fabricated.

Fig. 12-117. **A,** An excessive amount of intermaxillary space existed between both atrophied arches. **B,** The implant dentures mounted on the articulator.

The upper and lower master casts were articulated (Fig. 12-117, *A*). In the completed dentures (Fig. 12-117, *B*) the maxillary denture snapped over the palatal attachments, and the mandibular denture fit over the mandibular subperiosteal implant that was needed.

The undersurfaces of both dentures reveal the special attachments (Fig. 12-118, *A*).

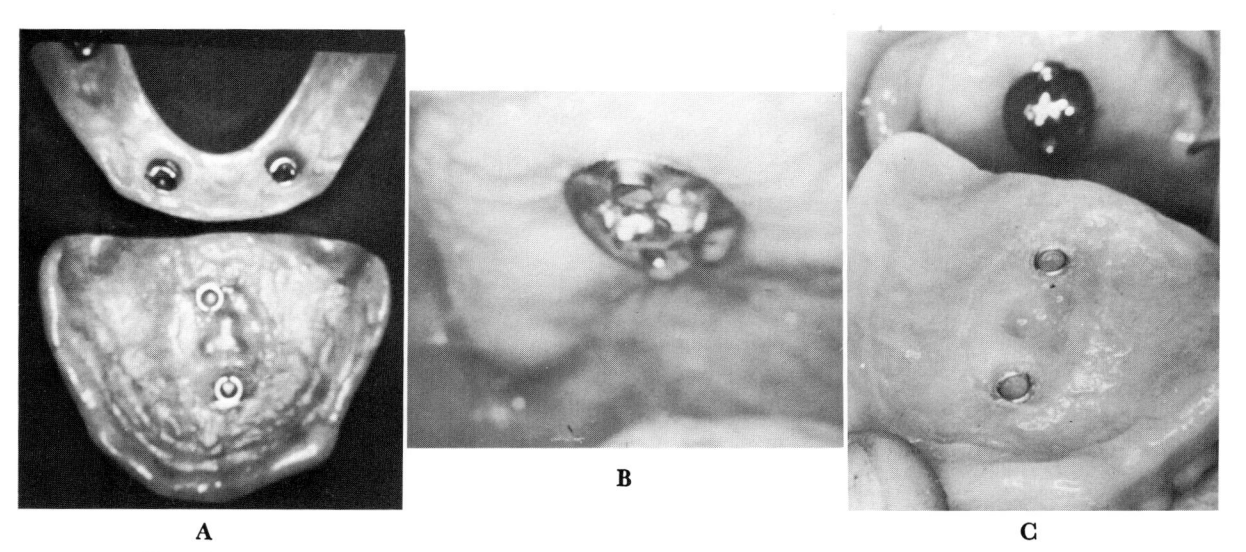

Fig. 12-118. **A**, The undersurface of both dentures. **B**, The template cemented over the implant posts. **C**, The maxillary implant denture was snapped over the male attachments connected to the template.

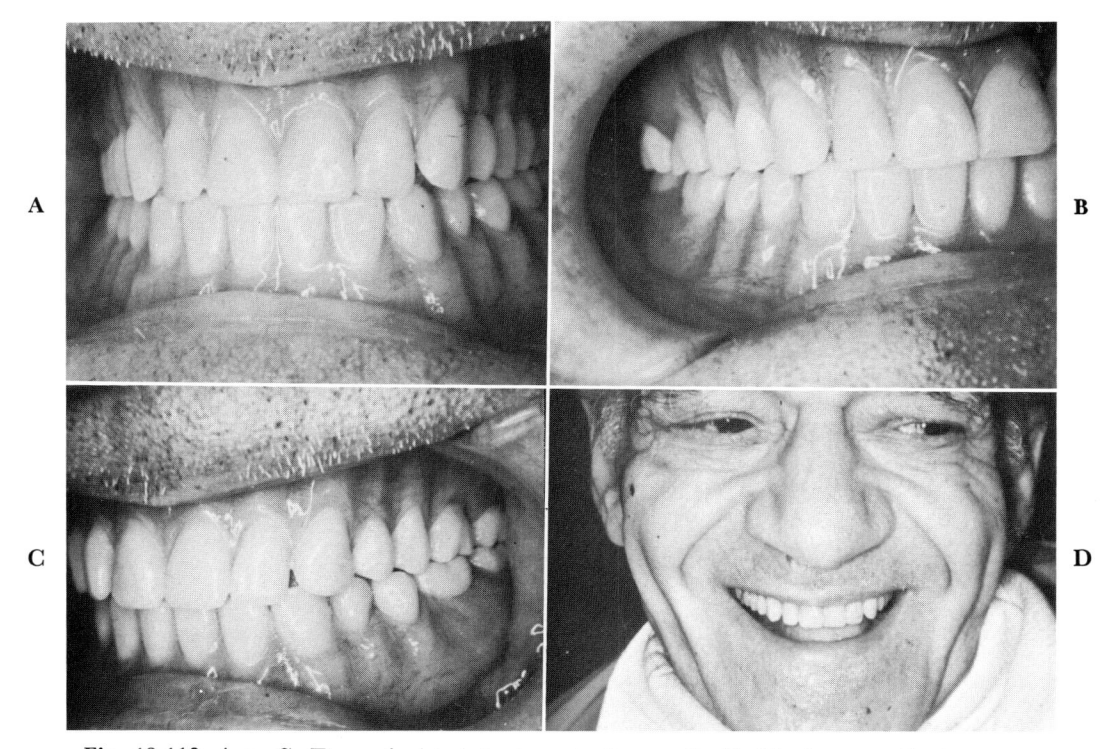

Fig. 12-119. **A** to **C**, The articulated dentures in the mouth. **D**, The happy patient.

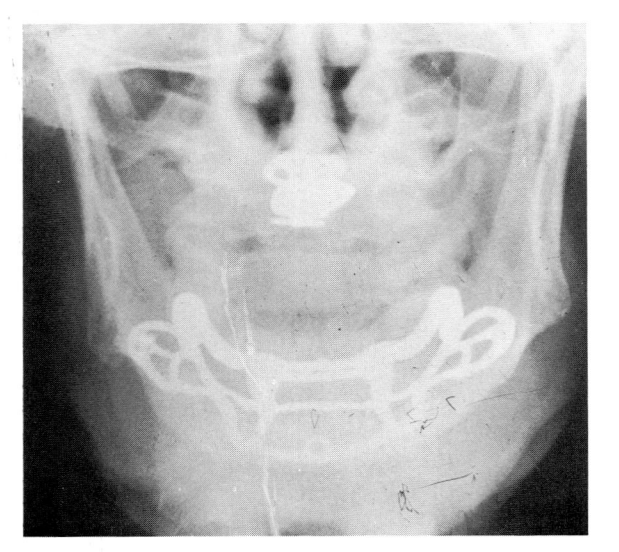

Fig. 12-120. A posteroanterior roentgenogram of the maxillary toroplant and mandibular subperiosteal implant.

The template was cemented over three protruding implant posts with hard cement. The excess cement squeezed through tiny vents along the lateral walls of the gold covering the implant posts (Fig. 12-118, B). The implant denture was then seated into position by snapping the female attachments over the male attachments, which were soldered to the palatal template (Fig. 12-118, C). The dentures were carefully articulated and balanced (Fig. 12-119).

The completed case is seen in the patient's mouth (Fig. 12-119, D), and a final posteroanterior roentgenogram shows the lower subperiosteal implant and the maxillary toroplant (Fig. 12-120).

Because the resilient type of attachments were fixed to a rigid palatal template supported by the toroplant, the maxillary denture was able to move from side to side, using the soft tissues to take away some of the load from the hard palate.

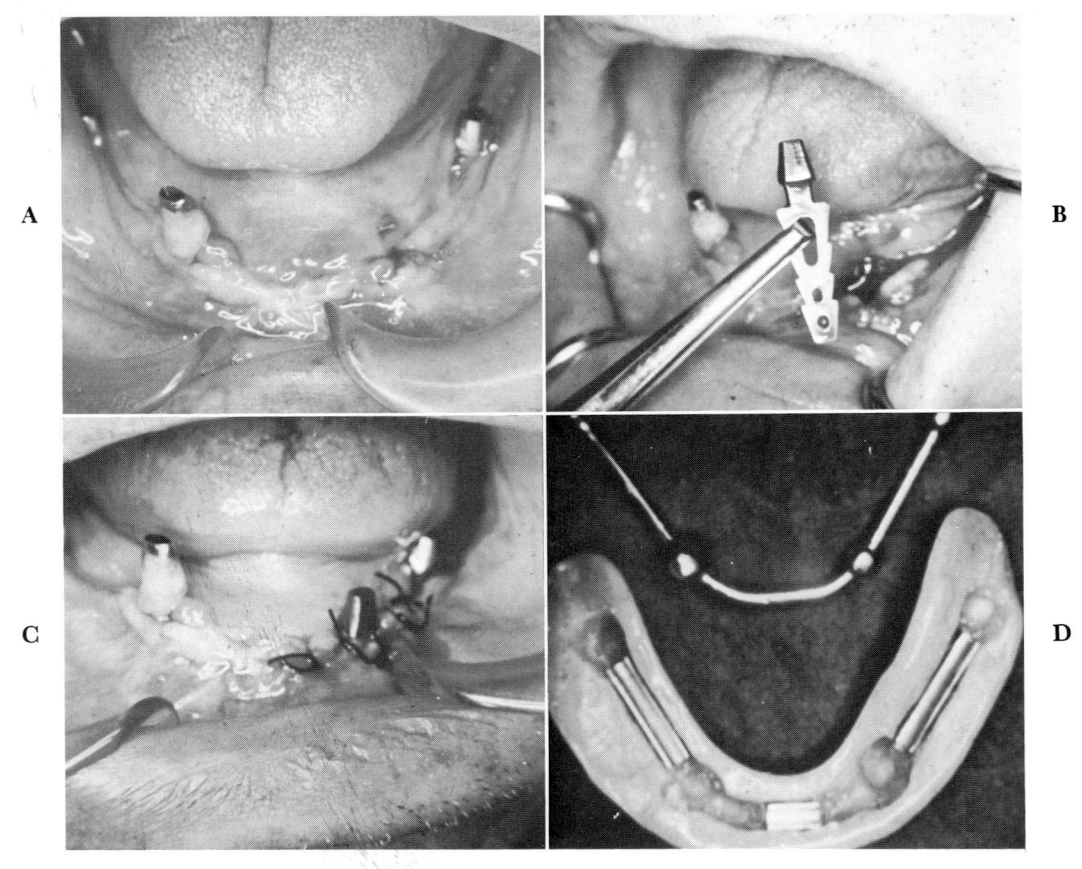

Fig. 12-121. A, The left anterior post was broken off from the substructure framework. B, A single tooth endosseous blade implant was tapped into the bone between the buccal and lingual peripheral struts of the subperiosteal implant. C, The tissues were sutured around the neck of the blade. D, A gold mesostructure and denture containing internal clip bars were fabricated.

ATYPICAL SITUATIONS

Because of improper instructions given to the laboratory technician, a subperiosteal implant can sometimes be cast with an extremely long neck at the expense of a shorter post. This creates not only a looser fit of the superstructure but also causes a weak link in the implant framework in the area of the lengthened neck.

Such a case occurred with one of Linkow's patients. The unique ingenuity in step-by-step procedures for restoring the arch is shown in the following illustrations.

The neck of the left anterior post broke, leaving only three posts connected to the substructure (Fig. 12-121, *A*). Notice that acrylic resin was added around the long neck of the right anterior post, which aided in retention for the superstructure as well as strengthened the extra long neck. A single tooth blade implant was then tapped into a groove previously prepared in the bone in the same area where the neck had broken. The blade was set into the bone between the buccal and lingual peripheral struts (Fig. 12-121, *B*). The tissues were sutured close to the neck of the blade (Fig. 12-121, *C*).

After 5 or 6 days the sutures were removed. When healing had been completed, a hydrocolloid impression was taken of the four posts and a wax interocclusal record of centric relation was obtained. An alginate impression of the upper denture was also taken.

The casts were articulated and a mesostructure containing four gold copings soldered to one another with a dolder bar was fabricated. A new implant

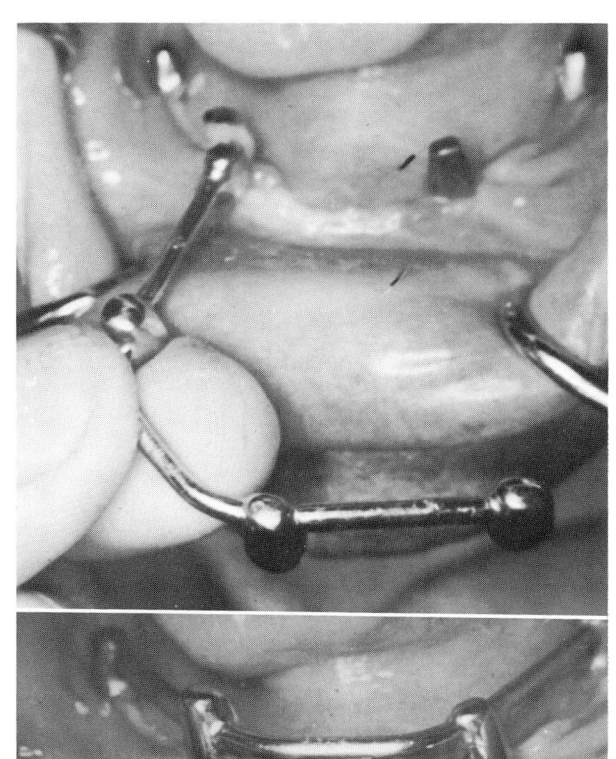

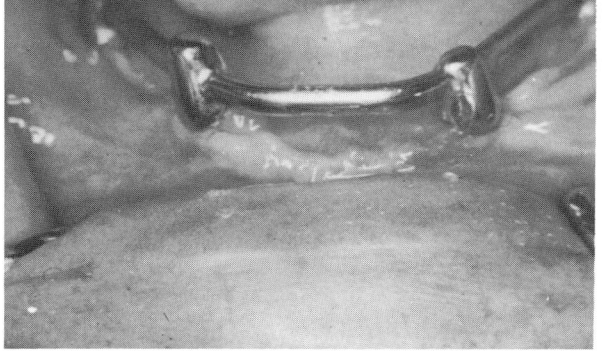

Fig. 12-122. The mesostructure was cemented over the four implant posts.

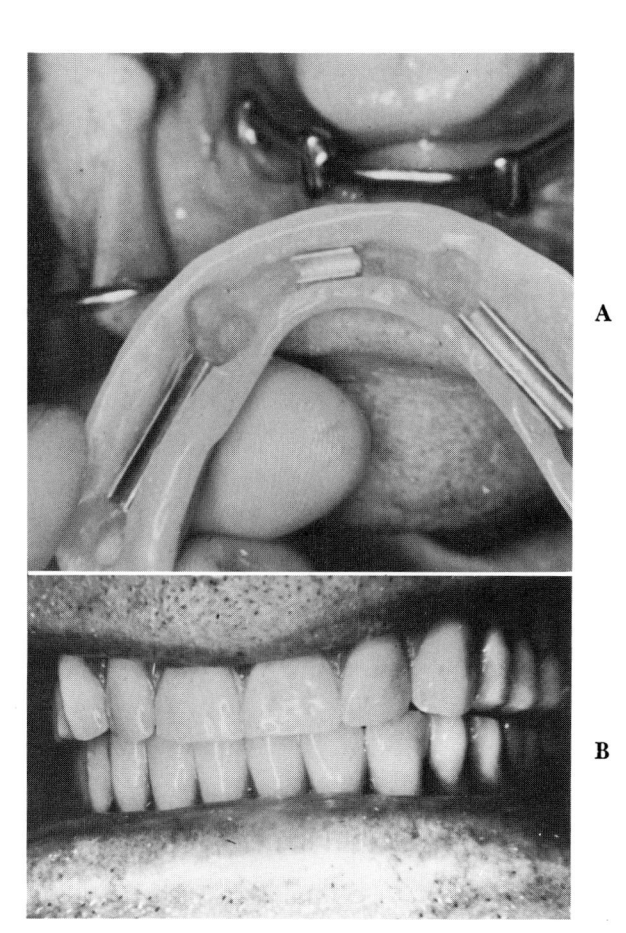

Fig. 12-123. The lower implant denture with its internal clip bar attachments was placed over the mesostructure and articulated with the maxillary denture.

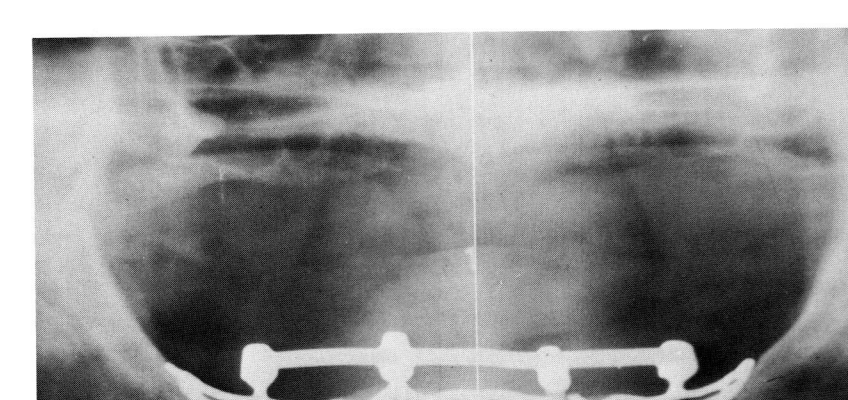

Fig. 12-124. The endosseous blade implant *(arrow)* is seen splinted to the three remaining subperiosteal implant posts with the gold mesostructure.

denture containing internal clip bars was also fabricated (Fig. 12-121, *D*). The mesostructure was cemented over the implant posts (Fig. 12-122). The implant denture was fitted over the mesostructure and articulated (Fig. 12-123).

A Panorex (Fig. 12-124) shows the completed case. Note the single blade implant in the left cuspid region splinted to the remaining three subperiosteal implant posts with the fixed mesostructure (arrow points to the endosseous blade implant).

CHAPTER 13 Endodontic implants

Endodontic implants are similar to prosthodontic implants in many respects. However, they serve another purpose—the stabilization and preservation of remaining natural teeth, not the replacement of lost teeth. For this reason, their uses, techniques of insertion, and potential problems are quite different.

The classic method for stabilizing loose teeth is to bridge them by external splints to existing natural teeth. This is usually temporarily adequate in cases involving a single loose tooth. However, when several loose teeth are involved or when no firm natural teeth remain for splinting, problems arise.

In addition to external bridging to stabilize loose teeth, several other methods have been tried. Cross, in 1957, experimented with raising the periodontal crest by bone grafting. Reattachment operations with or without bony or cartilagenous implants have also been tried. The most fertile avenue of exploration was initiated in 1943 by the Strock brothers. They reported a method of reinforcing anterior teeth whose roots were abnormally short as a result of incomplete formation or amputation necessitated by disease. The Strock technique consisted of thoroughly removing the pulp tissue in the canal, amputating part of the root apex, and removing all the granulation tissue. A tantalum or Vitallium wire rod implant was then inserted through a root canal filling material. This implant extended into the area where the original root existed. It was found that normal reorganization and regeneration of bone into the cavity and around the apical end of the rod took place, resulting in increased stability of the tooth.

Other operators utilized or varied this idea. The Italian, Luigi Marziani, using tantalum rods, verified the Strocks' observations. Sonza and Bruno (Uruguay, 1954), Raphael Cherchève (France, 1955), Hans Orlay (England, 1960), Staegemen (1961), and Held, Spirgi, Pfifer, and Cumasoni (1958) all experimented with stabilizing loose teeth by splinting them with combined endodontic and implant techniques.

The value of the endodontic implant was firmly established by the discovery of the effectiveness of inserting the implant past the level normally occupied by the root and as deep into dense cortical bone as possible. The mechanical principle is simple: by pushing a rigid post through the tooth deep into the bone and cementing the intradental part to the root canal walls, the fulcrum of the movement of a loose tooth is moved deeper into the jaw, the support in the bone is increased, and the mobility of the tooth is lessened. This means that the vicious spiral of excessive mobility causing destruction of the periodontium, which in turn causes even more mobility, is stopped, and immediately healthier conditions prevail.

With the tooth stabilized, the periodontal membrane can regrow if prior damage has not been too extensive. Bone condenses around the apex of the tooth and the implanted pin. This, plus general reconditioning, leads to even further security of the tooth.

Because the endodontic implant is completely embedded in the tissues and does not protrude into the mouth, there is no danger of infection via open communication with the mouth or of irritation caused by chemical reactions aggravated by saliva or substances put into the mouth.

There is substantial radiographic evidence that endodontic implants are well tolerated by the tissues and that bone does regrow up to the implanted pin. As for histologic evidence, few studies have been done on the healing processes and eventual tissue structure around a successful implant. However, it can be safely assumed that the histologic features characteristic of an endodontic implant do not differ

581

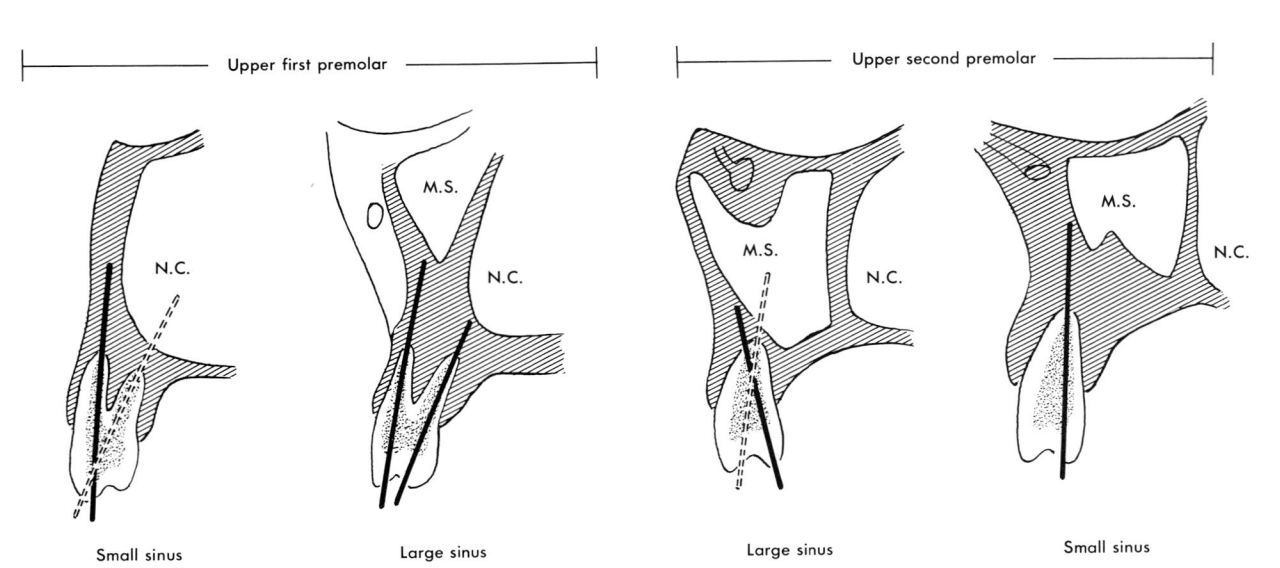

Fig. 13-1. The extended axes of the root canals in relation to the nasal cavity *(N.C.)* and the maxillary sinus *(M.S.)*. The solid axes indicate ideal placement sites for endodontic pins. The dotted lines indicate possible perforation of a sinus. Even if these axes are followed, perforation may be avoided by using shorter pins. There is usually at least 5 mm. of bone available for the intraosseous part of a stabilizer in such cases. (Redrawn from Orlay, H. G.: Splinting with endodontic implant stabilizers, Dental Pract. (Bristol) 14[2]:481-491, 1964.)

radically from those of other implants. At first the debris of the operation will be resorbed, and later a very thin layer of fibrous tissues, about 2 to 3 cell diameters thick, will surround the implant in the reorganized bone. One investigator, experimenting with dogs, reported finding layers of epithelial cells of Malassez around the deeper part of his implant. This could be theoretically possible where epithelial tissue has invaginated down to the apex of the tooth. In this situation by perforating the periodontal membrane to set the implant deep in bone, some epithelial cells might be carried down into the bone and proliferate there. However, the presence of these cells seems to be of no practical clinical importance.

EVALUATING THE CANDIDATE

The probable success or failure of any type of surgery depends upon the patient's general health, local conditions, and attitude. As has been extensively discussed previously, the patient's general health should be good. Any systemic condition, particularly involving the blood or bone, that might affect healing should contraindicate the procedure. When the implantologist is in doubt about the patient's general health, he should consult the patient's physician.

Periodontal conditions

The dentist is the best judge of local conditions. Obviously, only patients who carry out proper oral hygiene should qualify, and all should be instructed how to brush the teeth and otherwise care for the mouth after the procedure.

About 80% of all presenting patients have teeth loosened by periodontal disease. Of these, two-thirds involve the lower front teeth. Periodontal disease, except in very advanced cases, is not a contraindication. As long as at least 3.5 mm. of viable periodontal membrane is visible on a radiograph, the operation is possible.

It is difficult to advise whether periodontal treatment should precede or follow the endodontic implantation. Each case must be determined by its particular circumstances. Generally speaking, very loose teeth should be stabilized first; otherwise they may become too weak for any treatment. But whether before or after implantation, all periodontal treatment necessary must be performed for long-term success.

Anatomic considerations

Although the anatomy of the jaws differs a great deal from patient to patient, there are a few general

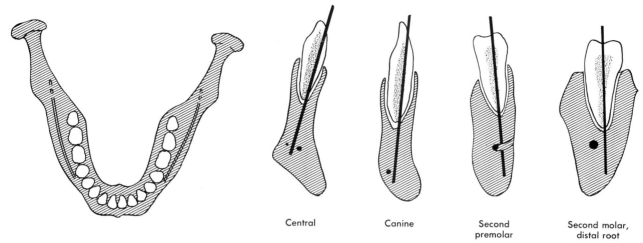

Central | Canine | Second premolar | Second molar, distal root

Fig. 13-2. In the mandible, the extension of root axes will bypass the mandibular canal in most cases. Except in the incisor region, if the canal should continue anteriorly beyond the mental foramen, the canal lies buccal to the axes. Also, in the incisor region the vertical distance, apex to canal, is usually great. However, the canal very rarely continues beyond the mental foramen. (Redrawn from Orlay, H. G.: Splinting with endodontic implant stabilizers, Dent. Pract. (Bristol) 14[2]:481-491, 1964.)

rules and consequent suggestions for varying their applications. The primary rule is that the implant should extend into the bone as deep as is anatomically possible; the denser the bone, the better the stabilization. In the maxilla, the amount of bone between the apex of the tooth and the nasal cavity or the maxillary sinus is the main factor determining the possibility of implantation and the probability of success. The more bone height present and the smaller the cavity, the greater the success rate. However, even in unfavorable cases sufficient bone usually can be found by utilizing the nasal spine, the front parts of the septum, the canine prominence, the triangular mass of bone on the palatal side of the incisors, and sometimes even the zygoma and the tuberosity (Fig. 13-1).

Perforation of the maxillary sinus by a pin implant should naturally be avoided. Although the ciliated epithelium will tolerate the emerging post in the same manner as the stratified oral epithelium will tolerate the emerging cones of prosthodontic implants, the pin will be unstable. A protruding post will irritate the nose, and crusts of dry mucus will accumulate around it.

Two areas of compact bone are visible on occlusal radiographs of the mandible. The implant posts should reach at least one of these areas, if not penetrate right into it, to give the end of the post a firm grip.

There is very little danger of injury to the mandibular nerve in endodontic implant stabilization. The mandibular canal lies lateral to the alignment of the teeth (Fig. 13-2). The small branches of the nerve are rarely harmed. Because those fibers serving the lips and gingivae leave the bone at the mental foramina, they are usually well out of the operatory site.

Although it is not necessary when inserting endosseous or subperiosteal implants, the operator wishing to insert an endodontic implant must contend with tooth anatomy. One of the most important considerations is the direction of the root canals. The axes of root canals do not coincide with the axes of the crowns of the teeth. This frequently makes it necessary to enlarge the root canal considerably to accommodate the rigid post. Sometimes parts of the incisal edges or even of the labial surface of a tooth must be sacrificed for this purpose.

Often, the direction in which the pin should be inserted for maximum support in bone does not correspond with the direction taken by the axis of the root canal. Sometimes this is easily remedied by enlarging the canal. In an upper central incisor, for example, the coronal part of the canal may be enlarged distally and the apical area mesially. This alters the ultimate direction of the post so that it becomes embedded in the nasal spine, permitting better fixation through the use of a longer implant

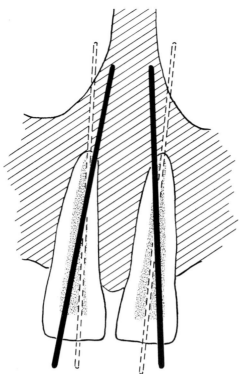

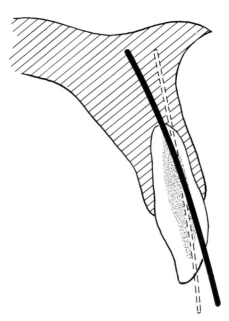

Fig. 13-3. The pins may be angled to lodge in the nasal spine and septum. This permits using longer pins than could otherwise be used if the axes of the root canals were followed (dotted lines). To angle a stabilizer toward the nasal spine, the root canal must be enlarged distally at its crown and mesially at its apex. (Redrawn from Orlay, H. G:. Splinting with endodontic implant stabilizers, Dent. Pract. (Bristol) **14**[2]:481-491, 1964.)

Fig. 13-4. Angling the pin along the axis of the alveolar bone (solid line), rather than along the axis of the root canal (dotted line), often gives greater stability. (Redrawn from Orlay, H. G.: Splinting with endodontic implant stabilizers, Dent. Pract. (Bristol) **14**[2]:481-491, 1964.)

(Fig. 13-3). Another method of gaining more support in bone is to widen the canal lingually so that the axis of the alveolar process may be followed (Fig. 13-4).

In dealing with roots with bends, the operator should resort to intentional perforation. Of course, that part of the canal apical to the perforation must be previously sealed with gutta-percha. Such teeth seem to be particularly well stabilized, having been made "two-rooted" by the operation. As for multirooted teeth, they can be extremely well secured by placing an implant in two or three roots.

The problem of reconciling the optimum direction of an implant with tooth anatomy will lessen as the operator gains experience.

TOOLS AND MATERIALS

Provided that the operator has the usual endodontic and periodontic equipment, only a few new tools and materials are needed for endodontic implantations.

Stabilizer pins. Four standard endodontic implant stabilizers are suitable for most cases. They are all 60 mm. long, the thickest tapering from 2 to 1.25 mm., the thinnest from 1.25 to 0.7 mm. (**Fig. 13-5**). Assuming that threaded pins might provide a greater hold in bone, some operators have tried them (Fig. 13-6). However, the threads are too close together to allow bone to grow between them, and the only advantage of the threaded pin is that cement adheres somewhat better to it.

The metal of which the implant is made must be biologically compatible with the tissues in which it is set. Results with the chrome-cobalts Virilium and Vitallium have been very good. Certain titanium alloys, such as Plantanium* (with and without sapphire coating), have been excellent. Although tanta-

*Manufactured by Implant Research Corp., Pennsaukin, N. J.

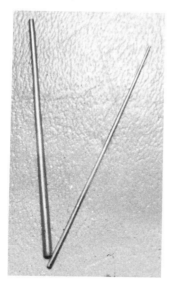

Fig. 13-5. Two of the many sized endodontic stabilizers. The rigid ones are cast in Vitallium*; the more resilient ones are tooled in titanium.†

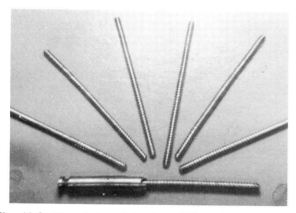

Fig. 13-6. Threaded endodontic stabilizers have also been used. The main advantage is that threading provides more retention for cementation to the inside walls of the root canal.

lum also would seem a good choice, it is considered by many operators to be too pliable.

Drilling tools. Although in ordinary endodontic work reamers more than 23 mm. long and above gauge 5 or 6 are rarely required, reamers from 31 to 36 mm. with gauges up to 15 must be available for endodontic implants (Fig. 13-7). Until recently such reamers were handmade, but now a few manufacturers are producing them.

For drilling through the hard compact bone of

*Howmedica, Inc., Chicago, Ill.
†Park Dental Research, New York, N. Y.

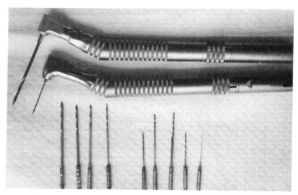

Fig. 13-7. The engine-mounted tapered and cylindrical reamers, which are different in length: 21 mm., 30 mm., and 36 mm. Note the difference in working length between a normal reamer mounted on a normal contra-angle handpiece (bottom) and a long reamer mounted on the miniature contra-angle handpiece (top). Another 2 mm. can be gained by using a pedohead contra-angle. Angle handpieces also permit easier viewing. (From Orlay, H. G.: Endodontic implants, J. Oral Implant Transplant Surg., pp. 44-53, 1965.)

the mandible, a cable dental engine is more powerful than the Doriot engine. This engine should be reinforced with a speed-reducer, which at the same time can also reduce the danger of overheating the bone. Further useful gadgets are a miniature, or lilliputian, contra-angle handpiece to drive the reamers deeper into the bone, a diamond disk to mark and cut the posts and to grind them if necessary, and some strong curved pincers to grip the implant posts firmly.

To keep the operational area free from flooding, saliva ejectors and walling the teeth with small interchangeable gauze pieces suffice. Rubber-dam cover is also helpful.

Cements and filling materials. Once the site has been created, cement is needed to bind the implant to the root canal walls. For that portion of the stabilizer flush with the root apex, any nonsoluble endodontic cement may be used. The remainder of the stabilizer coronal to the root apex will be covered with oxyphosphate of zinc cement.

Because cement can irritate bone and prevent healing, a substance is needed to prevent it from reaching and filling the periapex. For this Kri paste is used. Kri paste is a mixture of iodoform powder with methylated and camphorated parachlorophenol. It was introduced into European endodontics for root canal filling by Professor Wlakhoff of Warzburg, Germany, about 1925. It was relatively

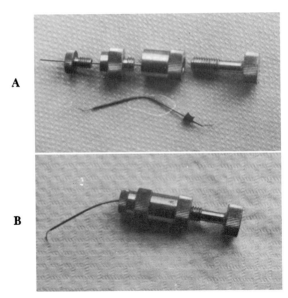

Fig. 13-8. The Morgan (Evamore) paste propelling screw. **A,** The apparatus disassembled. **B,** The apparatus assembled, with iodoform (Kri I) paste extruded.

unknown in the United States until recently. In addition to acting as a mechanical barrier to cement, Kri paste also is a good local disinfectant, is resorbable, and can arrest hemorrhage. It is also easy to deposit and, if necessary, remove.

Ledermix paste has been mixed with Kri paste to enhance its antibiotic and anti-inflammatory properties, but the results do not differ from those of using Kri paste alone. As a barrier, Kri paste alone seems best.

To insert the Kri paste to the apex of the tooth, an Evamore (Morgan) paste-propelling screw is recommended (Fig. 13-8). It is, of course, possible to position the paste by other means, such as Lentulo spirals, but the Evamore screw will greatly facilitate the work.

Anesthetics. The kind and amount of anesthetic needed depends upon the site. For front teeth, regional anesthesia is recommended to lessen irritation. For lower premolars and molars, infiltration anesthesia is advisable because it does not dull the main mandibular nerve. Although the danger of injuring this nerve is very slight, it should nevertheless be considered. If the nerve is sensitive, the patient can warn the operator of approaching danger.

Sometimes it may be expedient to instill anesthesia by pressure or to inject a few droplets of anestheticum through the foramen into the periapex of the tooth. Because the bone itself exhibits no pain,

only a few drops for the periapex and the periodontium are needed. Although this technique is deemed dangerous by some dentists, extensive experience with hundreds of cases indicates otherwise.

The usual premedication and postmedication drugs, both anodynes and antibiotics, may be given, although they will rarely be necessary.

OPERATIVE PROCEDURES

Inserting an endodontic implant for tooth stabilization is basically a two-part operation. The first part is an endodontic procedure, which consists of removing the pulp tissue in the canal, sterilizing the canal, and then packing it with the proper filling material. The second phase is the implant procedure, which consists of entering the bone beyond the apex with proper spiral rotary instruments, stopping existing hemorrhages, treating the osseous tissue with antibiotics, and, finally, inserting the endodontic implant with the proper cement.

The step-by-step techniques of creating the site and setting the implant vary slightly from operator to operator. One of the most simple and effective approaches is that of Hans Orlay. Orlay's procedures, diagrammed in Fig. 13-9, are as follows.

First, the root canal is trephined. When sufficient bone is available at the apex of the tooth to hold the pin, the implant will be inserted along the axis of the root canal. This frequently necessitates entering the tooth on the incisal edge or some visible part of the crown, as the rigid endodontic implant usually cannot be bent to follow the curved pattern of the tooth.

Second, the canal is widened following Wlakhoff's method to permit the eventual passage of root canal instruments up to gauge 15. This is done by alternating tapered and cylindrical reamers, sizes 3 or 4. At first the enlarging should stop just short of the apex, which should be protected by Kri paste in order to avoid contamination with debris. During this process the canal should be frequently cleaned and irrigated.

Third, the canal is widened to a 9 or 10 cylindrical bur without piercing the apex. Again Kri paste is used in the apical region as a mechanical barrier.

Fourth, the endodontic pin is inserted to see whether it fits properly. An x-ray is taken to determine how far it extends into the tooth. If the proper depth has been reached, just shy of the apex, the pin is marked. Because the labial and linguopalatal emergence points may differ as much as 3 or 4 mm., marks should be made circumferentially. Now the interdental length of the implant has been established and the implant is withdrawn.

Fifth, rotary burs are used to pierce the apex, which is enlarged until the pin or post can pass through. Enlarging the apical foramen removes a great deal of cementum. This cementum is particu-larly prone to infection and, by destroying it, the danger of a later infection is greatly diminished. Because this stage shortens the root about 1 mm., it is a kind of "inner apicoectomy."

The burs pass into the bone, gradually deepening the bore hole as much as anatomically possible and

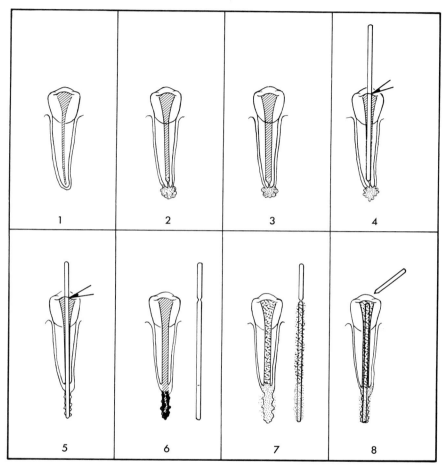

Fig. 13-9. Orlay's eight-stage endodontic pin insertion procedure.
1, The root canal is trephined and the entrance made funnel-shaped for easier access.
2, The canal is widened, stopping just short of the apex, which has been filled with Kri paste to avoid contamination with debris.
3, With Kri paste in the apex, the root canal is enlarged to the diameter of the pin. At this point, the apex is still unpierced.
4, The pin is inserted and its emergence point marked. This establishes the intradental depth of the pin.
5, The apex is pierced and enlarged. The bone is prepared for the pin gradually, deepening and enlarging the site. Roentgenographic control is essential. The post is inserted and its new emergence point marked.
6, The pin is withdrawn, and hemorrhaging is arrested. The pin is deeply notched.
7, After the canal is cleaned and dried with ether, Kri paste is applied to the apices of both the canal and the pin and cement applied to their respective superior portions. The pin is then inserted.
8, The excess length is snapped off and any remaining space treated. The implanted tooth is then immediately stabilized. (Redrawn from Orlay, H. G.: Endodontic implants, J. Oral Implant Transplant Surg., pp. 44-53, 1965.)

widening it to accept the post. Because of the various densities of the tissues to be penetrated, this stage is particularly dangerous in respect to instrument fracture. It should therefore be done with special care, starting with small diameter reamers and proceeding slowly, with frequent counterclockwise reversing, débridements, and irrigations to remove the shavings and blood clots.

Another danger encountered at this stage is the tooth's turning or even being extracted by the rotational force of the reamer. This is particularly true in cases where the periodontium is very weak or has been extensively destroyed. If the tooth does move, the borehole in bone may be drilled in a wrong direction. If the borehole is made in a wrong direction, the tooth and hole in bone will be improperly aligned. Therefore loose teeth should be temporarily stabilized by some extraneous means. Usually a firm grip between the fingers will suffice, but other methods of fixation, such as pressing onto an existing denture, wire-looping, or splinting with composition-impression material, may prove necessary.

Small mistakes are sometimes unavoidable but can usually be corrected by spot-grinding. Teeth accidentally extracted by rotational forces during reaming are not necessarily lost; they can be reimplanted. Their sockets should be artificially deepened before reimplanting and stabilizing such teeth with endodontic implants to provide a better hold in the bone.

Once the hole in bone is created, the post is inserted to its base and its depth verified by an x-ray. At this stage, it is easy either to deepen the borehole or, if necessary, to retract the post from the deep end of the borehole. After a satisfactory depth has been determined, the new emergence point is marked on the post. The post is withdrawn, and a circular notch is ground slightly below the emergence point mark just deep enough to ensure an easy break in the last stage of the operation. The reason for notching the post below the last emergence mark is so that the pin will not protrude at the incisal edge or rest right at it. In notching the post, care must be taken not to cut too deeply; the post may break prematurely, making it difficult to set the implant at the exact depth intended. On the other hand, if the notch is too shallow, too great a force will have to be used to break the post, and it may even be necessary to cut it with diamond disks. This could overheat the implant in the bone and would make proper filling of the trephined cavity impossible.

Sixth, bleeding from the borehole into the root canal must be arrested. Usually instilling 3 to 4 droplets of epinephrine solution (1:100) or Calyxl is effective, but firmly packing the foramen and the periapex with Kri paste invariably helps. After arresting the hemorrhage, the canal walls are throughly cleaned and dried with ether. Failure to do this endangers cementing the implant to the canal walls.

Seventh, the implant and canal are ready for cementing. The apex of the tooth has already been packed with Kri paste. If this has been done properly, it should prevent any cement from reaching the bone. Thin-flowing oxyphosphate of zinc cement is then pressed into the root canal with a Jiffy tube. That part of the implant to lie in bone is coated with a thin layer of Kri paste (and/or Ledermix paste), and that part to remain in the root canal is covered with a more sticky cement mix. The operator can deduce from his two sets of markings which part will lie flush with the apex of the tooth. This section is coated with a nonsoluble endodontic cement, the rest with viscous oxyphosphate of zinc cement. The coated post is then quickly pushed into the borehole until the uppermost mark is slightly below the trephine opening. Heated, softened gutta-percha is used to press the cement firmly home between the stabilizer and the canal walls.

Eighth, a few moments before the cement sets, the surplus part of the stabilizer is broken at the circular notch and discarded. Then the gutta-percha is pressed further into the cavity, and any remaining space is filled with cement. Once the cement has set and the surface has been trimmed, the implantation is completed. The tooth is immediately stabilized, and its firmness will increase as bone reforms around the endodontic post.

With the stabilizer pin in place, the tooth is usually well protected against tongue thrusts and other buccolingual movements. However, Linkow feels that splinting the affected tooth is also necessary to protect it from lateral movements. A single pin has little retentive power in bone and acts only to improve the root-to-crown ratio. As a narrow post, it can also serve as a pivot, particularly if the tooth is very loose. For this reason, splinting is advised in most cases. Naturally, a multirooted tooth with more than one pin implant has less chance of being rotated, and splinting in such cases may be superfluous.

A more simplified implantation technique is that of Edelman and Linkow. This technique, instead of

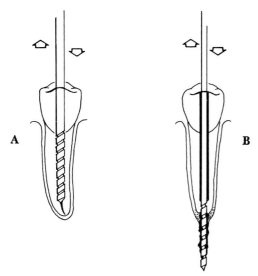

Fig. 13-10. In this simplified technique, only two drills are necessary: **A,** one to prepare the root for the pin, and **B,** a smaller one to pierce the apex and prepare the site in bone. To prevent binding and bone injury, drilling is done with an in-and-out movement and is accompanied by a coolant. The endodontic implant is made of Plantanium. (Courtesy The Implant Research Corporation.)

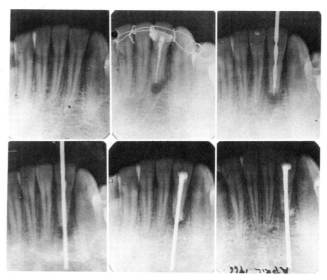

Fig. 13-11. A number of months after an apicoectomy and gutta-percha root canal filling was done on a right loose lateral incisor, the filling was removed and replaced with an endodontic root stabilizer. Within 1 year after its insertion the radiolucency completely disappeared. (Courtesy Dr. V. Bloch.)

gradually enlarging the root canal with a series of instruments, employs only two drills (Fig. 13-10). With one, an endodontic stabilizer drill whose diameter is slightly larger than the implant itself, a borehole large enough to accept the implant is created in one stage. With this drill the root canal is bored to about four-fifths of its depth. To prevent binding and bone injury, the drilling is done with an in-and-out movement, accompanied by a coolant. When the root canal has been bored to the proper depth, a smaller diameter endodontic stabilizer drill is used. It perforates the apex of the root and goes into the bone as deep as anatomically possible.

An appropriate sized Titanium endodontic root stabilizer is then fitted into the canal and x-rayed. Any adjustments as to depth and seating must be made before final cementation.

Before cementation, cortisone (Metimyd Ointment) is syringed into the trephined dry bone beyond the apex and also placed on the apical tip of the stabilizer. The cement-coated implant is placed into the canal and pushed into position. The implant is then tapped into the bone another millimeter with a mallet. The protruding part of the implant is snapped off, and the finishing stages proceed much as already described.

The two-stage endodontic pin implant process is clearly illustrated radiographically by two cases. In Fig. 13-11 a right lateral incisor had a periapical lesion and was loose as a result of an accident. The nerve was removed, an apicoectomy was performed, and the tooth immobilized with .010 ligature wire. Within a year after endodontic stabilizer insertion, the periapical radiolucency had disappeared.

Another patient fractured a right mandibular central incisor in an automobile accident, severing the nerve in the canal. Pain and looseness of the coronal half of the tooth was obvious. Removal of the damaged nerve and insertion of an endodontic root stabilizer rigidly held the coronal portion of the tooth to the root (Fig. 13-12).

No matter which technique is used to set the implant, the benefit of endodontic implant stabilization is almost immediately apparent. The patient is able to masticate a few minutes after the operation. The self-cleansing lacking in loose teeth will be improved almost automatically. In addition, the patient need no longer fear loosening his teeth further by brushing them. After stabilization proper oral hygiene is again possible. The tongue and lips, which are always loosening mobile teeth, will cease to do

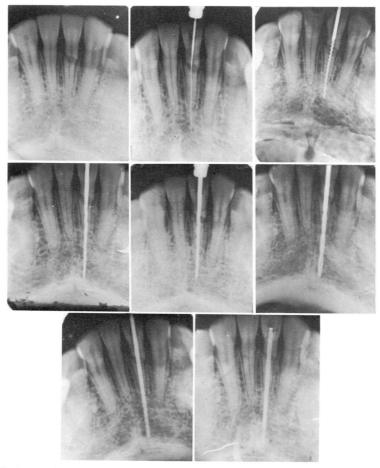

Fig. 13-12. A completely fractured right mandibular central incisor is supported by an endodontic root stabilizer.

so. Psychologically, the patient will regain confidence in his teeth.

APPLICATIONS

The main application of endodontic pin implants is the stabilization of teeth loosened by periodontal disease (Fig. 13-13). Although implantation will alleviate the problem of mobility immediately, it should not be considered a panacea for all other palliative measures, such as gum treatments, gingivectomies, and deep scaling. The periodontal problem must be treated, either before or after the implantation, at the operator's discretion.

In cases of severe periodontal disease there is little hope of periodontal membrane regeneration or bone regrowth. Even after treatment, a periapical focus may remain or appear after implantation. However, the infection never spreads along the im-

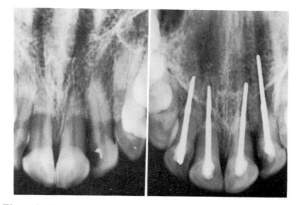

Fig. 13-13. Here endodontic stabilizers help support four loose anterior maxillary teeth.

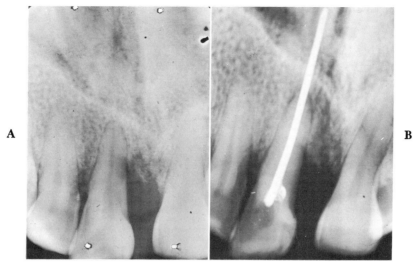

Fig. 13-14. Stabilization of the only loose tooth in the dental arch. The patient has an excellent set of natural teeth. Stabilization of the only periodontally involved tooth in the arch prolongs the eventual need for a fixed bridge or partial denture. The x-rays show, **A,** the preoperative site, and, **B,** the pin 5½ years after insertion. (From Orlay, H. G.: Endodontic implants, J. Oral Implant Transplant Surg., pp. 44-53, 1965.)

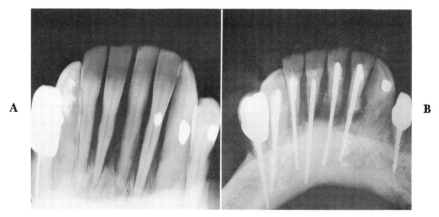

Fig. 13-15. An advanced case of periodontal disease. **A,** Bone loss and subsequent mobility are evident in the immediate preoperative x-ray. **B,** Five and one-half years later, the teeth are still functioning members of the dental arch and some bone has regrown. (From Orlay, H. G.: Endodontic implants, J. Oral Implant Transplant Surg., pp. 44-53, 1965.)

plant deeper into the bone (Fig. 13-14). In evaluating the success of the stabilization procedure, clinical soundness and adequate function should be the criteria rather than radiologic evidence (Fig. 13-15).

One of the most obvious uses of the endodontic stabilizer is to reestablish the proper crown-to-root mechanical ratio after an apicoectomy. By introducing stabilizer implants that extend beyond the bone removed at the tooth's apex into dense, undisturbed bone, the proper mechanical ratio is reestablished and the tooth is once again firm (Fig. 13-16).

Endodontic implant stabilization can be combined with post-crowning. This approach is particularly useful for stunted roots (Fig. 13-17) or roots shortened by resorption or mutilating apicoectomies, or when the taper of the root cavity is unfavorably divergent. Using a chrome-cobalt post as a sprue, a model is constructed for a stabilizer-plus-cone by direct inlay technique. The model is then cast in the usual way. After final shaping in the mouth, a jacket is made over the cone. Two or three sessions are required for this combined process, and the borehole should be kept clean between sessions by sealing a temporary post into it.

A potentially widespread use of endodontic implants is the conservation and stabilization of remaining natural teeth for use as bridge abutments (Fig. 13-18). The stabilized teeth help prevent denture shifting and its consequent problems.

The left second molar, saved as a posterior abutment for a fixed partial denture in Fig. 13-19, has been radically treated with an endodontic implant. The obliquely set stabilizer has been functioning well for 5 years. Because the tooth is so extremely tipped mesially, the implant acts as a mesial root.

Even part of a tooth may be saved to act as an abutment post, as shown in Fig. 13-20. Here only

one root of a multirooted tooth remains, the others having been removed either because of a bifurcation or trifurcation involvement or because of a periapical lesion. Complete bone healing can readily be seen.

The reimplantation of teeth may be facilitated

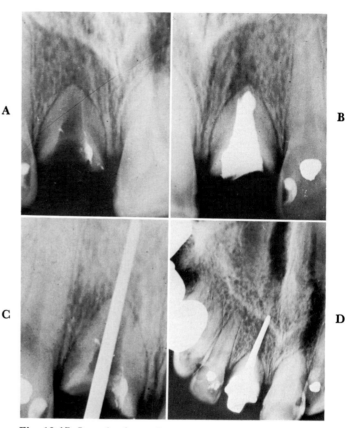

A

B

C

D

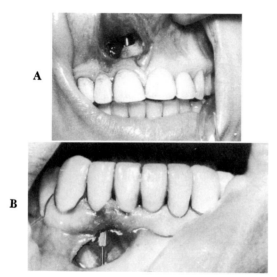

A

B

Fig. 13-16. Endodontic root stabilizers are useful in conjunction with apicoectomies to reestablish the root-to-crown ratio. A, A maxillary case; B, a mandibular case. (From Linkow, L. I.: Pin implants, Prom. Dent. 3:4-15, 1968.)

Fig. 13-17. Lengthening a short root to accept a restoration. A, An extremely short root on a central incisor prevented a retentive fitting post crown. B, The short root was first prepared and filled with Kri I paste. C, The Virilium post was fitted and cemented. D, the tooth was still functioning more than 4 years later. (Courtesy H. G. Orlay.)

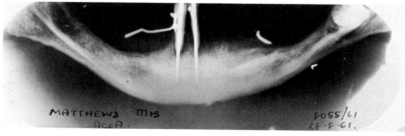

Fig. 13-18. Stabilizers are most successful in the lower anterior region. Their greatest value is in stabilizing the few remaining teeth so that they could be used as abutments for the support of a partial removable appliance instead of a full denture.

by endodontic implant procedures. In cases of intentional reimplantation, such as that of the upper impacted canine shown in Fig. 13-21, the tooth should be removed from the impacted position only after the new socket has been prepared. The tooth should be positioned in its new socket and checked for alignment and proper occlusion. Then root canal treatment and drilling of the site for the pin should take place.

Reimplantation plus endodontic implant stabilization can be very useful after accidental injuries to teeth. Fig. 13-22 shows a tooth that was accidentally knocked out and reimplanted later in the ordinary way. Two years later progressive root resorption had loosened the tooth considerably, and endodontic implant stabilization was attempted. The resorption stopped and the tooth became firm again, although little bone reconstruction occurred.

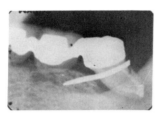

Fig. 13-19. Sometimes pins can be passed through the tooth obliquely to help support it. Here an extremely mesially tipped mandibular second molar stabilized by an endodontic stabilizer acting as another root is seen. (From Linkow, L. I.: Pin implants, Prom. Dent. 3:4-15, 1968.)

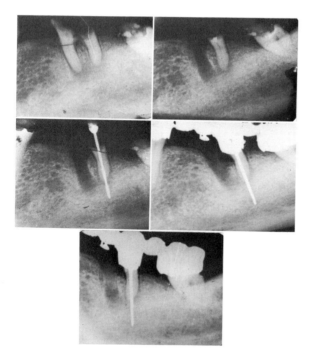

Fig. 13-20. Endodontic stabilizers are often used to stabilize a remaining root after the other roots were resected and removed.

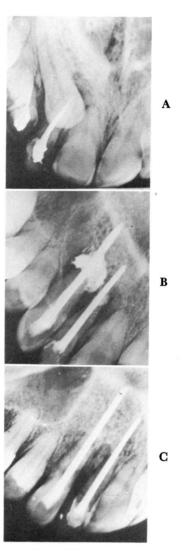

Fig. 13-21. Endodontic stabilizers are also used commonly in conjunction with reimplanted teeth. **A,** A preoperative x-ray shows a palatally impacted canine and deciduous canine. The deciduous canine was removed and the impacted canine was surgically removed and reimplanted into the socket of the deciduous tooth. At the same time the displaced lateral incisor was forcibly pushed into alignment. **B,** Both teeth were endodontically stabilized (immediate postoperative x-ray). **C,** Three years later the x-ray shows the teeth still functioning well. (From Orlay, H. G.: Endodontic implants, J. Oral Implant Transplant Surg., pp. 44-53, 1965.)

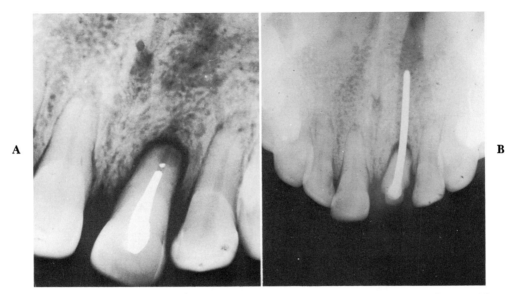

Fig. 13-22. Saving a reimplanted tooth. A few minutes after it was knocked out, this central incisor was root-treated (Wlakhoff method), reimplanted, and externally splinted for about 4 weeks. **A,** Two years later the tooth was so loose that endodontic splinting was required. **B,** Five years after splinting, the tooth—which now carries an acrylic jacket crown—is a good member of the dental arch. (From Orlay, H. G.: Endodontic implants, J. Oral Implant Transplant Surg., pp. 44-53, 1965.)

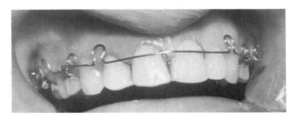

Fig. 13-23. As a result of an accident to a 16-year-old girl undergoing orthodontic treatment, her right lateral incisor was so loose that it came out of the socket with an alginate impression.

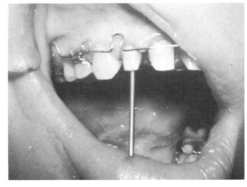

Fig. 13-24. The right lateral incisor and both central incisors were prepared for full crown restorations. The canal of the tooth was then treated and the tooth reimplanted with a stabilizer.

Accidental injury to a 16-year-old girl undergoing orthodontic treatment necessitated reimplantation (Fig. 13-23). As a result of a fall, the girl's lateral incisor was so loose that it came out of her mouth when an alginate impression was taken for fabricating a removable splint. With the tooth outside the mouth, the nerve was removed, the canal widened, and an implant pin placed through it to ensure proper fit. The endodontic stabilizer was removed from the tooth and the tooth was placed back into the socket. While holding the tooth firmly in place, a long endodontic spiral drill was placed inside the hollow root canal, and, with a slow-running contra-angle drill, a hole was made into the bone above the canal and as deep as possible without involving the floor of the nasal cavity. The drill was then removed and, with the use of Kri paste and oxyphosphate of zinc cement, the endodontic stabilizer was placed back in the tooth (Fig. 13-24). The pin was tapped deep into the bone to stabilize the tooth, and crowns were cemented over the reimplanted tooth and its abutments (Fig. 13-25). Fig. 13-26 is an x-ray of the finished case.

In another case of accidental injury, seven teeth were severely damaged in a car accident. Three teeth had been completely knocked out, and four others were so badly luxated that they were lying

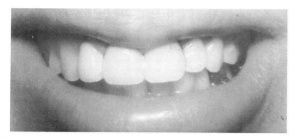

Fig. 13-25. The three-unit completed porcelain-fused-to-metal splint helped to support the reimplanted tooth.

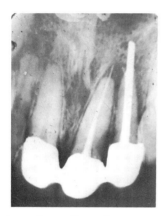

Fig. 13-26. Postoperative radiograph.

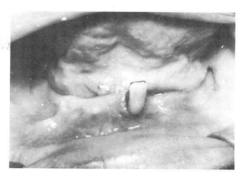

Fig. 13-27. The only teeth remaining were a loose lateral incisor and second molar.

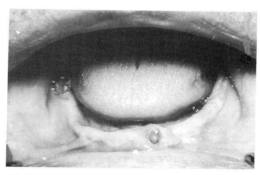

Fig. 13-28. The lateral incisor and molar were prepared for full coverage.

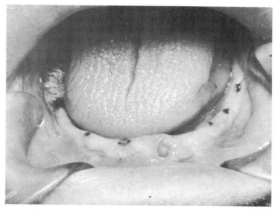

Fig. 13-29. All the contemplated implant sites were marked with indelible pencil.

horizontally below the tongue. Eighteen hours after the accident, the luxated teeth were realigned and the knocked-out ones reimplanted; all of them were stabilized with endodontic implants. No other splints were used. The patient was pain-free and could eat normally 1 hour after the operation. Some years later resorption started on the reimplanted teeth. Eventually the roots resorbed, leaving only the stabilizers. These were still firmly fixed in the bone without any roots around them. This apparently indicates that the diseased root acts as an irritant and is eliminated by the body, but the implant is tolerated even as nearby diseased tissues are resorbed.

So far it has not been possible to predict or to exclude the onset of root resorption, nor has it been possible to foretell the type of resorption. Two types of root resorption have been observed. One type commences at the apex and slowly destroys the root. This process is quite painless. The other type of resorption seems to be initiated by an aggressive metaplasia of the marginal gums, which eventually severs the tooth into two parts. Here the gums are painful and bleeding.

ENDODONTIC ROOT STABILIZERS COMBINED WITH PROSTHODONTIC IMPLANTS

In combination with endosseous and subperiosteal implants, endodontic pin implants are used primarily to stabilize loose teeth to serve as natural abutments for fixed dentures. As always, the

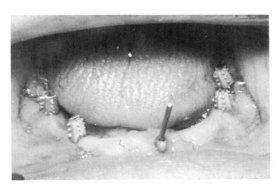

Fig. 13-30. An endodontic root stabilizer was set deeply into the bone existing below the loose incisor, immediately stabilizing it. All implants were set into the bone, and gold copings were placed over them.

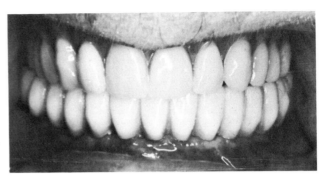

Fig. 13-31. A full arch fixed denture was cemented over the abutments.

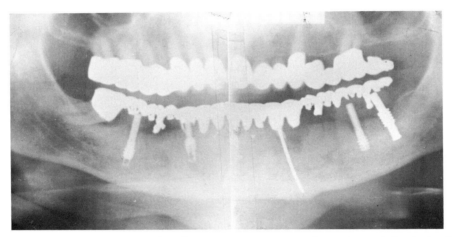

Fig. 13-32. A 3-year postoperative Panorex roentgenogram shows the endodontic implant stabilizer and the implants. Some bone resorption is evident around the left first implant extending downward from the alveolar crest. Also, an infrabony pocket exists along part of the mesial wall of the remaining right molar. The patient, however, has been enjoying eating and chewing for the past 3½ years. There is no mobility.

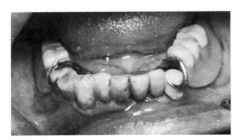

Fig. 13-33. The mouth of a 55-year-old physician.

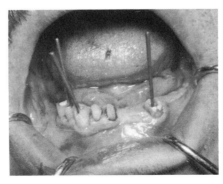

Fig. 13-34. Three loose teeth were supported with endodontic stabilizers.

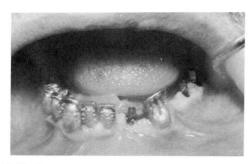

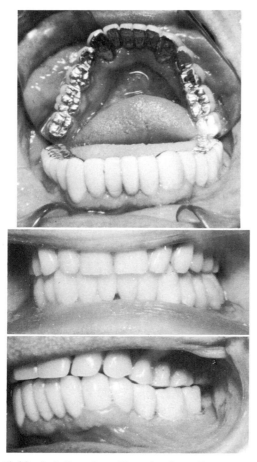

Fig. 13-35. Castings were fitted over the prepared abutment teeth and five vent-plants were set into the osseous structures, four of which were set in both posterior edentulous areas.

Fig. 13-36. A full arch gold occlusal-acrylic veneer fixed denture was cemented over the endodontically stabilized teeth, with implants adding more support to them.

choice of an endosseous or subperiosteal implant depends on the amount of remaining alveolar bone.

The patient pictured in Fig. 13-27 had only two natural teeth remaining in the mandible, a loosened lateral incisor and a mesially-tipped right second molar. These two teeth were first prepared (Fig. 13-28), and the sites for placing endosseous implants were marked on the fibromucosal tissue (Fig. 13-29). After four vent-plants were inserted, an endodontic stabilizer was placed through the lateral incisor and into the underlying bone, giving the tooth immediate stabilization (Fig. 13-30). A full arch, veneer crown, fixed denture was then cemented into position over the much tighter lateral incisor, remaining molar, and vent-plants (Fig. 13-31). A Panorex radiograph clearly demonstrates the final result (Fig. 13-32).

Another patient helped by the combined implant procedure is shown in Fig. 13-33. Here the patient, who had only a few remaining mandibular anterior teeth, was afflicted with a poorly functioning, removable, bilaterally free-end saddle partial denture. Endodontic root stabilizers were used to help stabi-

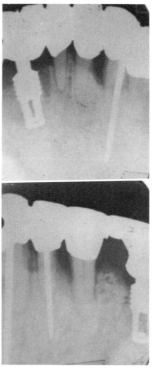

Fig. 13-37. Intraoral periapical radiographs show the stabilizers and a few of the vent-plants.

lize a few of his remaining weak anterior teeth (Fig. 13-34), and vent-plants were used posteriorly in both edentulous areas (Fig. 13-35). A full arch acrylic-and-gold fixed denture was then fabricated and cemented into position with hard cement (Fig. 13-36). Fig. 13-37 shows the intraoral radiographs.

Other cases of stabilizing anterior mandibular teeth with endodontic implants and using other types of endosseous implants laterally are shown in Fig. 13-38. Note that the type of prosthodontic implant selected is determined by the local anatomy of the site.

In cases where insufficient bone exists to use endosseous implants with endodontically stabilized natural teeth, subperiosteal implants may be suitable. Several unilateral, finger type subperiosteal implants have been used successfully in combination with endodontic root stabilizers to help support a fixed denture (Fig. 13-39).

Another unique combination of endodontic pin implants with other types of implants is seen in the case of a woman well into her seventies. This patient had been wearing a partial denture that utilized her remaining two lower bicuspid teeth as the abutments. She was in constant pain because the denture rested on an extremely thin knife-edge

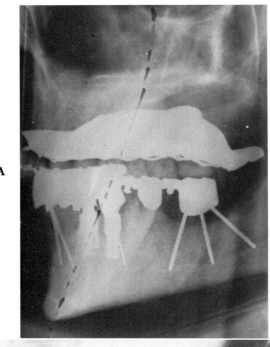

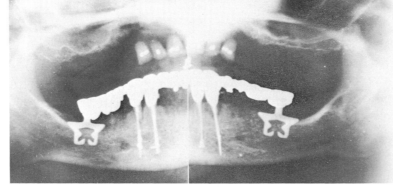

Fig. 13-38. A, A lateral plate roentgenogram shows another case of anterior endodontic root stabilizers in combination with vent-plants and a posterior triplant. B, A Panorex showing four stabilized anterior teeth working in symbiosis with two posterior blades, all of which support a full arch restoration.

ridge, which was really the remaining mylohyoid ridge.

The two bicuspid teeth were prepared to their cementoenamel junctions, and endodontic stabilizers were used as additional support (Fig. 13-40). A

uniquely designed scalloped template with a specially chosen spring-type stress-breaker attachment was included posteriorly on either side. Anteriorly, an inverted U-shaped bar of gold, with its vertical portion fused to the base of the template, was included (Fig. 13-41). The template was cemented over the gold post copings, which already had been cemented over the two remaining bicuspid teeth (Fig. 13-42).

Three pin type implants were drilled through predetermined holes in the anterior part of the

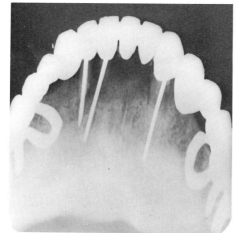

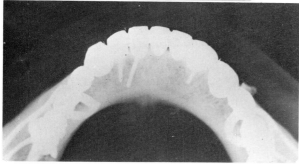

Fig. 13-39. Anteriorly are endodontic stabilizers. Posteriorly are bilaterally placed subperiosteal implants that were used for the endentulous areas because there was not enough alveolar bone for endosseous screws or blades.

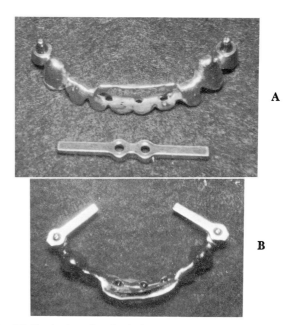

Fig. 13-41. A, A uniquely designed scalloped template with Gerber spring type attachments was cast. Below the template is seen the female attachment bar, which is processed to the prosthesis. B, An occlusal view of the template with both female attachments in place over the male attachment.

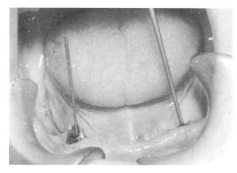

Fig. 13-40. Two remaining strategically situated roots were further supported with endodontic stabilizers.

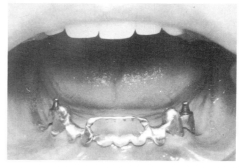

Fig. 13-42. The template was cemented into position, supported only by two gold post copings that were cemented over the two bicuspid roots after the stabilizers were set.

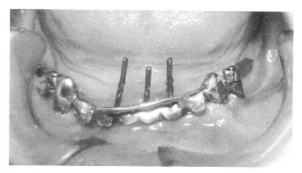

Fig. 13-43. Three pin type implants were then drilled through predetermined holes made in the anterior portion of the template. They were driven as deeply as possible, ending on top of the cortical plate of bone that lay at the inferior border of the mandible.

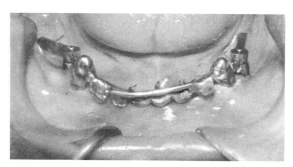

Fig. 13-44. The excess length of the extending pin implants was cut away so that the pins could be bent underneath the inverted U-shaped bar extending superiorly from the scalloped template.

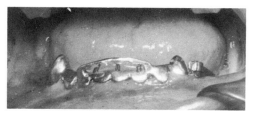

Fig. 13-45. The pins were then bent so that they fell within the confines of the inverted U-shaped bar.

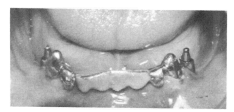

Fig. 13-46. The pins were fused to each other and locked between the inverted bar and template with cold cure acrylic. When the acrylic hardened it was prepared so that no undercuts remained. The vertical acrylic bar was then polished.

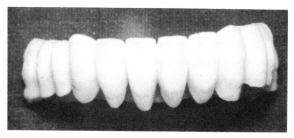

Fig. 13-47. The acrylic full arch splint. It can be worn either with temporary cement or with no cement at all, allowing it to be taken off and placed back on at will.

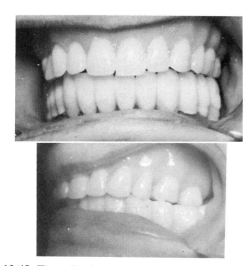

Fig. 13-48. The splint in position.

template (Fig. 13-43). These pins were extended deep into the bone, down to the cortical plate in the inferior portion of the mandible. The three pins were shortened to the height of the horizontal portion of the U-shaped bar (Fig. 13-44) and then bent anteriorly so that they fitted flush to, but underneath, the horizontal bar (Fig. 13-45). The three pins were fused together (using the brush-on technique) and to the entire inverted U-shaped bar with cold cure acrylic, thereby becoming an integral part of the template (Fig. 13-46). An all-acrylic-over-gold full arch denture was then processed (Fig. 13-47). The bridge was used as a fixed removable denture and was set buccal to the mylohyoid ridge, instead of on it, to avoid further pain (Fig. 13-48). A Panorex shows the implants and prosthesis (Fig. 13-49).

For a patient requiring a unilateral fixed partial denture, it was necessary to avoid using previously jacketed anterior teeth. Therefore an endodontic pin implant was planned to stabilize an upper left cuspid

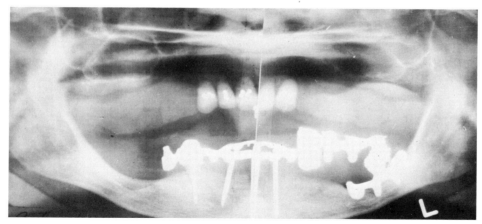

Fig. 13-49. A 5½-year postoperative Panorex showing completed case. The left bicuspid had been removed and replaced with a unilateral subperiosteal implant.

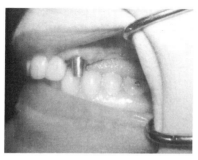

Fig. 13-50. A left cuspid with a completely horizontal fracture of its root midway between its apex and cementoenamel junction was fitted for a gold post prior to further supporting it with an endodontic root stabilizer.

whose root was completely fractured horizontally halfway down its length. The cuspid was first prepared (Fig. 13-50) and then a vent-plant was placed behind it (Fig. 13-51). After impressions were made, the apical half of the cuspid root was removed through the buccal plate of bone and the endodontic pin implantation performed (Fig. 13-52). A gold post was cemented over the cuspid root and a veneer casting placed over it. Then a gold coping was placed over the vent-plant post. An alginate impression of the opposing jaw, a wax interocclusal record of centric relation, and a plaster index picking up the cuspid casting and implant coping were made for completing the bridge. The bridge was tried and cemented (Fig. 13-53) and a triplant added posteriorly for additional support (Fig. 13-54). The superstructure was then cemented (Fig. 13-55).

Radiographs of the case show how each type of implant uniquely serves its particular purpose (Fig. 13-56).

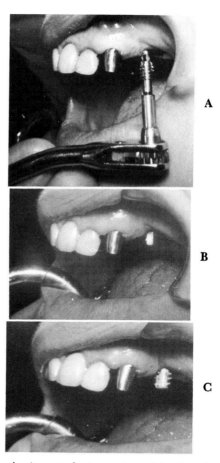

Fig. 13-51. A, A vent-plant was tapped in the edentulous second bicuspid region behind the cuspid post. **B,** The shaft of the vent-plant extended 4 mm. out of the fibromucosal tissue. **C,** An interchangeable prefabricated gold coping was placed over the implant post and its occlusal clearance carefully checked.

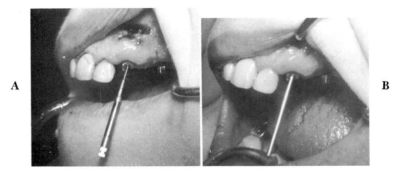

Fig. 13-52, A, The gold post was removed from the fractured cuspid, and the apical half of the root was removed through the labial cortical plate. Rotary reamers were then used to widen the intact portion of the root. B, The endodontic root stabilizer was then fitted accurately inside the root, extending deep beyond the void left by the removed root.

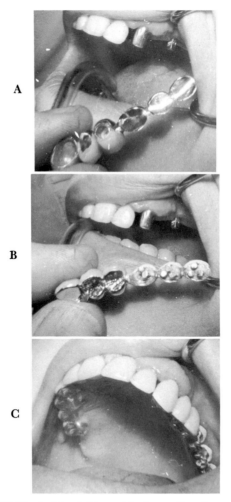

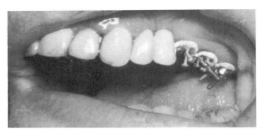

Fig. 13-54. Pin implants were driven through the openings in the template.

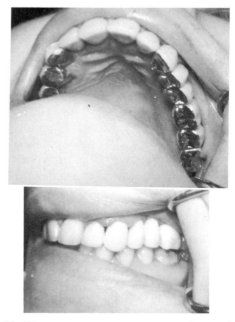

Fig. 13-53. A, The bridge with the scalloped template was fitted into position. B and C, The prosthesis was cemented with hard cement.

Fig. 13-55. The superstructure was cemented over the template after the triplant pins were affixed with acrylic.

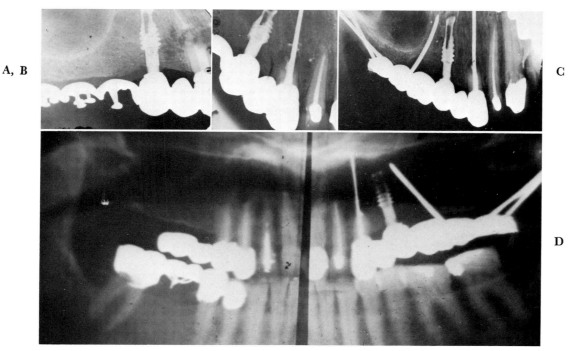

Fig. 13-56. A, Roentgenogram shows broken cuspid root prior to its removal. The vent-plant is seen in the bicuspid region. B, The endodontic implant stabilizer as seen 6 months after apicoectomy. C, A cross-sectional occlusal x-ray taken 2 years after initial insertions shows the endodontic implant stabilizer, the vent-plant, and the triplant. Notice the regeneration of bone resembling a lamina dura around the mesial wall of the vent plant and the circumvention of the sinus with the triplant. D, A Panorex x-ray illustrating the bridge and implants 5 years postoperatively.

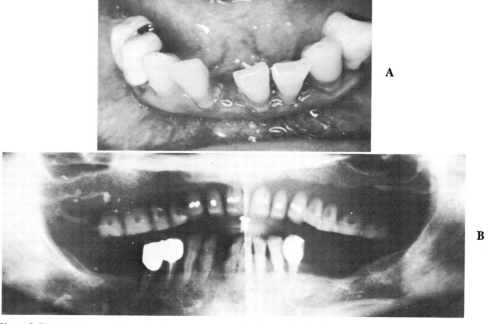

Fig. 13-57. A, The existing teeth were extremely loose. B, A Panorex shows very little supporting bone.

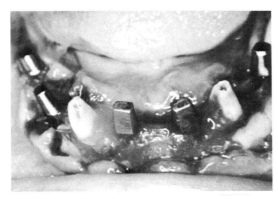

Fig. 13-58. Four blade implants were tapped into the bone.

Since the addition of the blade type implants, with their extremely retentive and self-supporting qualities, many loosened teeth that would previously have been supported by endodontic stabilizers are now extracted and replaced with the endosseous blades.

The following case illustrates this clearly. The patient, an attractive woman in her early forties, had extremely loose teeth in her mandibular arch (Fig. 13-57). The two cuspid teeth were prepared for full crown restorations, and their nerves were removed. The remaining teeth were extracted.

Two narrow blade implants were placed mesially to the two cuspids, and two double-posted blades

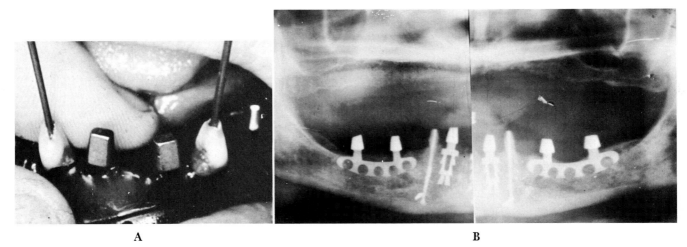

A   B

Fig. 13-59. A, Endodontic stabilizers were introduced into the cuspids. The teeth and implants are protected from the saliva with the use of rubber dams. B, An immediate postoperative radiograph.

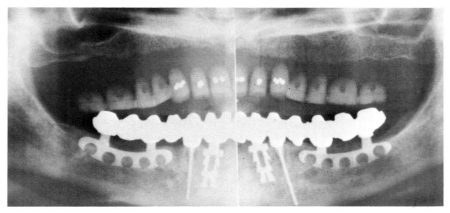

Fig. 13-60. Six months later than Fig. 13-59. Notice that the Kri paste seen around the apices of the stabilizers in Fig. 13-59 has been completely resorbed.

were set into the bone distal to the cuspids (Fig. 13-58). Rubber dam* with built-in flexible frame was applied over the cuspids and implant posts during the endodontic stabilizer insertion procedures (Fig. 13-59, *A*) and a Panorex radiograph was taken (Fig. 13-59, *B*). The Panorex film shows that the Kri paste is easily absorbed by the time the fixed full arch prosthesis was completed (Fig. 13-60).

REASONS FOR FAILURE

As with any other type of operation, all kinds of accidents can occur during an endodontic stabilizer implant procedure. No matter how careful or skillful an operator is, occasional incidents occur. Here the

*Webber Rapi Dam, Isaac Mosel Co., Inc., Philadelphia, Pa.

discussion will be limited to the more frequent accidents occurring during the implant part of the operation.

One of the most frequent accidents before the development of the Kri paste barrier technique was filling the borehole with cement. If more than just traces of cement went into the borehole, the cement had to be removed by a curetting operation (Fig. 13-61).

Overshooting the target depth and perforating the bone can easily happen; it can be avoided only by careful occlusal radiography during drilling and implanting the pin (Fig. 13-62). If the implant has been set too deeply, it should be withdrawn to its proper depth. The patient will be unaware of the accident and the bone wound will heal within a very

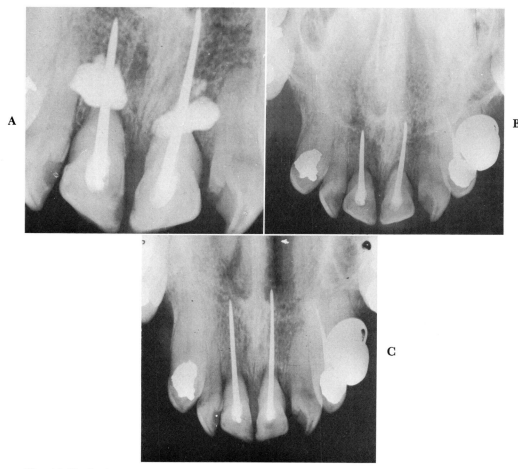

Fig. 13-61. A, A great amount of excess cement was pushed apically beyond the bore holes. In order to prevent irritation and severe inflammation, the cement had to be removed immediately by incising the mucoperiosteal tissue, reflecting it, and curetting it. **B,** Eighteen months later. **C,** Five and a half years later. (From Orlay, H. G.: Endodontic implants, J. Oral Implant Transplant Surg., pp. 44-53, 1965.)

short time. In the mandible, the perforation is invariably on the inner aspect of the bone, and it is palpable only by bimanual examination. Perforation into the maxillary sinus, although not dangerous, results in any unstably set pin (Fig. 13-63). In the nose, not only may the pin be unstable, it will also irritate (Fig. 13-64). If the pin is unstable, it should be removed. If there is enough of the pin in bone to give good support, the protruding part must be removed by cutting it below the nasal mucosa at the nasal bone level. This is accomplished like an apicoectomy.

When injury to the mandibular nerve during implantation is suspected and a proper diagnosis cannot be made because of too deep anesthesia, the canal should be temporarily sealed with a short post. Later the post can be removed and the implantation completed. Usually no anesthesia is needed at this point. At most, instilling a few drops of an anestheticum will be enough to make the operation painless.

If the operator is reasonably certain that no accident occurred during implantation and yet the patient complains of mandibular nerve irritation,

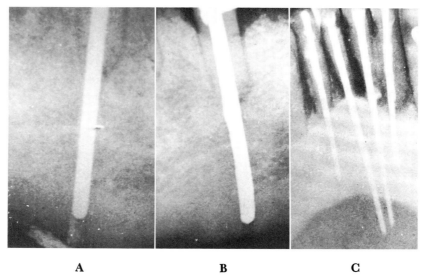

A   **B**   **C**

Fig. 13-62. Overshooting accidents. **A,** The post overshot a lower premolar and went through the jaw. It was immediately withdrawn into the bone and this radiograph taken. **B,** Five weeks later. **C,** In this case, overshooting was detected only after cementation. Radiograph taken 1 year after the operation. (From Orlay, H. G.: Endodontic implants, J. Oral Implant Transplant Surg., pp. 44-53, 1965.)

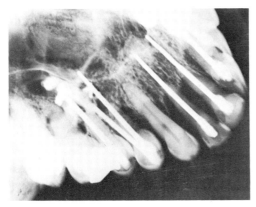

Fig. 13-63. Pins perforating the maxillary sinus. Although usually no problems arise for the patient, the pins become more unstable. (Courtesy H. G. Orlay.)

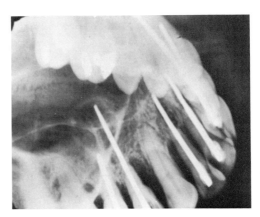

Fig. 13-64. Pins perforating the nasal vestibulum as well as the sinus. The pin in the nose will be very irritating. (Courtesy H. G. Orlay.)

the trouble probably has been induced by a hemorrhage around the nerve. Immediate extraction of the implant is not recommended. Paresthesia will usually disappear slowly and gradually. Only if it persists more than 1 week should steps be started to correct the situation.

If a stabilizer loosens in its tooth, it should be reinserted after cleaning and disinfecting the root canal. The reinsertion is almost painless.

In a few cases, the implants broke after insertion. This was probably a result of bubbles in the cast metal. An implant must be cast in a vacuum and/or be checked by industrial radiography. It is also important, therefore, to seal the apices with chlorpercha or some other soft type of filling material. It is imperative to widen the canals of the maxillary and mandibular anterior teeth toward the palatal and lingual surfaces respectively, so that the endodontic stabilizer pins will enter the bone in these directions. If the pins are made to follow exactly the direction of the canals, they would often end up perforating the concave labial surfaces of the maxillae and mandible.

CHAPTER 14 Causes of implant failure

An implantologist must be familiar with many kinds of implants. He must not only know the various types of screw, pin, blade, and subperiosteal implants but also when to use each and how to insert it most advantageously. The experiences of skilled operators using well-designed implants have provided ample, well-documented evidence that implants function in accordance with the biomechanical principles typical of the site and are compatible with the tissues. Not only are they functionally and scientifically acceptable, they have provided thousands of patients with esthetically superior replacements for lost teeth.

Despite the obvious advantages of dental implants, strong opposition persists. Because of the number of failures, resistance to the widespread use of implants has been considerable. Granted, there have been numerous failures. Many of these can be explained by the facts that early implant designs were unsuitable, operative techniques were not perfected, and the many considerations in candidate evaluation were unknown or overlooked. Today, however, the skillful operator is well aware of these factors. Most experienced implantologists freely admit that if an implant intervention fails, the fault lies not in the idea of using a dental implant but in inaccurate patient evaluation, inappropriate choice of implant, or poor operative technique.

Without discussing the often obvious errors resulting from inexperience, this chapter will concentrate on the major areas wherein a skilled operator might make a mistake. These areas concern preoperative evaluation, implant design and instrumentation, and operative techniques.

PREOPERATIVE EVALUATION

The value of accurately diagnosing both systemic and local conditions cannot be underestimated. The difference between a relatively uncomplicated, logically sequential implantation and a disrupting series of patch and repair efforts often begins here. A few minutes reviewing a patient's general health and examining his remaining teeth and gums can set the initial stages for success or failure. Careful radiographic studies, in addition to examination by eye and hand, will help the evaluation.

Poor health

Naturally any chronic, severe systemic condition, such as blood or bone dyscrasias, uncontrolled diabetes, or severe allergies, contraindicates an implantation. Some conditions, such as a history of heart disease, make the patient a risky candidate. The obvious dangers here, difficulties in anesthetizing the site or overexcitability during the operation, are not the only considerations. Possible postoperative infection and its consequences should also be estimated.

After explaining the procedure, which should be done with any presenting candidate, the patient's reactions should be evaluated. The neurotic patient, particularly one tending to hypochondria, should perhaps be avoided. His fears, although imaginary, may actually provoke adverse physiologic reactions. He can "worry" the implant by unnatural biting, probing, poking, and "testing." Even the best-seated implant will not heal under such treatment.

The patient whose mouth bears evidence of poor oral hygiene might also be an unsuccessful candidate. If such a patient, despite prior warnings that poor oral hygiene could result in severe periodontal problems or the eventual loss of his natural teeth, presents himself for implantation with problems arising from these forewarned conditions, he should be rejected as a candidate. If he did not care enough to prevent the problems, it is overly optimistic to assume that he will take proper care of his implants. Those patients who are unaware that their problems were initiated by poor oral hygiene and who show a

608

sincere desire to correct their detrimental habits may be acceptable candidates.

Whatever the reason for implantation, the role of good oral hygiene after implantation and the reasons for it should always be explained to any candidate. The dentist who knowingly performs an implantation on a candidate with consistently poor oral hygiene habits or the dentist who fails to stress the importance of proper hygiene should not be surprised if postoperative complications arise.

Periodontal disease should be cured, or at least controlled, before implantation and its causes corrected or alleviated. If poor occlusion has resulted in pockets or abscesses around remaining natural teeth, it certainly will not help a dental implant. Here common sense dictates: periodontal problems leading to the eventual loss of natural teeth will also lead to the loss of dental implants.

Poor site selection

Many of the problems arising during endosseous implant interventions can be avoided by proper selection and evaluation of the implant site. The following observations generally hold true.

There must be sufficient alveolar bone in which to bury the implant. If there is not, the implant may impinge upon the mandibular canal, maxillary sinus, or nasal vestibulum. Errors here will cause, at the very least, sensitivity or pain. At most, facial paresthesia caused by nerve damage can occur.

When too little alveolar bone height remains and if post type implants are used, the implants may

eventually fail because of soft tissue invagination. A 2- or 3-mm. invagination is harmless, providing that the narrow abutment post, *not* the open spirals, is embedded in the area. Otherwise a rapid invagination of the epithelial tissue occurs in and between the spirals, preventing the regeneration of bone or

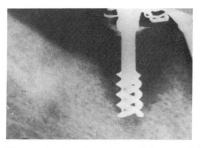

Fig. 14-2. The typical V-shaped breakdown of bone associated with soft tissue invagination is exemplified by this case.

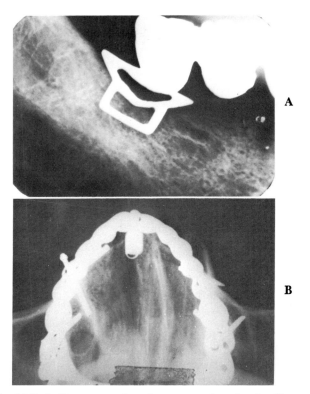

Fig. 14-3. A, Bone resorption also occurs when the shoulder of the blade implant is not buried below the alveolar crest of bone. B, A cross-sectional x-ray reveals perforation of the labial and buccal plates of bone with pin implants, which often can occur. (From Linkow, L. I.: The era of endosseous implants, J. D. C. Dent. Soc. 42[2]:14-19, 1967.)

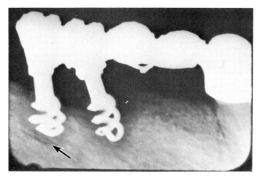

Fig. 14-1. Bone resorption rapidly occurs where the open spirals are not deeply buried in the bone. In this case, a rapid invagination of the epithelium through the spirals that were near the alveolar crest took place, preventing the bone regeneration from growing closer to the implants. (From Linkow, L. I.: Clinical evaluation of the various designed endosseous implants, J. Oral Implant Transplant Surg. 12:35-46, 1966.)

dense connective tissue close to the implant. Within 2 or 3 months, a large radiolucent area can be seen around the spiral portion of such an implant (Fig. 14-1).

As a rule, when less than 5 mm. of alveolar bone height exists, it is inadvisable to use a post type implant. A blade-vent, whose stability depends on its anteroposterior length rather than its depth, can be often used in a shallow area. However, enough bone must remain to bury the implant's shoulder, or epithelial invagination does occur (Fig. 14-2).

In addition to adequate bone height, there must be adequate bone width. Narrow ridges are unsuitable for post type implants, since there also must be sufficient bone *around* an implant to hold it secure. Fortunately, blade implants can now be used in such situations.

When faced with a case where little bone exists between the alveolar crest and a sinus or the mandibular canal, a triplant is often recommended. Be-

cause the stability of such an implant depends on diverging the legs as far apart as possible, the danger of perforation is particularly great (Fig. 14-3). Great care must be taken in evaluating the most advantageous positions for triplant pins. If one of the pins perforates the bone, the triplant becomes less stable.

Unhealed extraction sites

Unhealed extraction sites, or open sockets, should be avoided. The bone in such an area is in a state of flux. Unless the implant can extend beyond the apex of the socket into an artificially made one and can be splinted to a tooth on each side, which would provide the stability needed for normal healing, an open socket is an undesirable site. Post type implants in open sockets usually fail (Fig. 14-4). Implants placed too near sockets also tend to fail (Fig. 14-5).

When desiring to substitute a recently lost tooth,

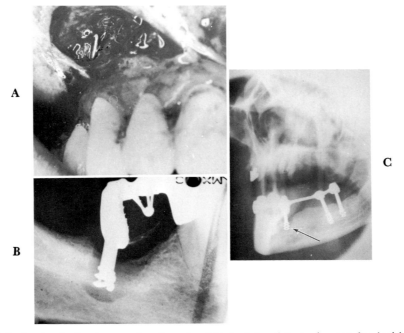

Fig. 14-4. A, A pin implant perforating the labial plate of bone is seen by incising and retracting the mucoperiosteal tissue. B, Post type implants must not be placed into recent sockets unless they can be set beyond the floor of the socket into a deeper artificial one and immediately stabilized with a prefabricated fixed denture. Otherwise a rapid epithelial invagination takes place directly into the sockets, preventing future bone regeneration. (From Linkow, L. I.: Alloplastic implants. In Goldman, H. M., Forrest, S. P., Byrd, D. L., and McDonald, R. E.: Current therapy in dentistry, vol. 3, St. Louis, 1968, The C. V. Mosby Co., pp. 335-356.) C, Another post type implant failing in an open socket. If no bone in the floor or the walls of the socket is available for some part of an implant, the intervention should be delayed until the bone heals.

two choices are possible. If the operator wants to use a post type implant, he should allow the site to heal before performing the implantation; or, and this is now a very practical alternative, he could use a blade-vent.

IMPLANT DESIGN AND INSTRUMENTATION

One of the most basic considerations in implantology is using an implant design compatible with the biomechanical and physiologic forces typical of the site. Examples of failures caused by inappropriate implant design or excessively difficult operative procedures have been extensively covered elsewhere, particularly in Chapter 5. The following list summarizes the characteristics of a successful endosseous implant.

1. The implant must be made of an inert, biologically acceptable material.
2. It must be lightweight but strong, ductile, and difficult to break or fracture.
3. It must be radiopaque on x-rays.
4. It must be easy to insert.
5. It must be prefabricated for standardization and coordination of operative procedures.
6. Both the design and material of the implant must be able to withstand functional stress.
7. In design, the implant must be restricted at its neck, where it exits the alveolar bone and fibromucosal tissues.
8. The deepest portions should contain openings or vents, both to allow for the possibility of the bone growing through the openings and to permit the normal flow of blood and lymph, which aids healing.
9. The insertion of the implant should require a minimum of armamentarium.
10. The implant should be architecturally designed to provide immediate retention upon insertion.

Poorly designed implants

How just one uncompensated divergence from the list of implant design and insertion requirements can result in failure is summarized in Fig. 14-6. In *A* several implant designs are shown just after insertion. All are screw-type implants. Most are made of metal, but one is made of synthetic sapphire, all of which are known to be biologically inert materials. All were splinted for security, but *B* and *C* show what usually happens when a solid screw type implant with an unrestricted neck is used. Even though

broad-necked implants may be successful in some cases, there is a tendency for bone breakdown to occur with this type of design, no matter of what material it is constructed.

Proof that an unrestricted neck and a solid body in an implant can cause bone breakdown is shown in Fig. 14-7. To ensure that these particular design features, not the material of which the implant was made, caused the failures, Linkow coated several of his implant designs with synthetic sapphire. Bone breakdown did not occur.

Fragile implants

Fragility of the material of which the implant is constructed or the design itself can lead to implant breakage during insertion. The majority of failures caused by implant breakage have occurred with those spiral-post implants made of Vitallium (Fig. 14-8). Vitallium is a brittle metal. The unique double-helical design, so advantageous to retention and fluid drainage, makes this type of implant weaker than some other, more sturdily constructed models. Because the spiral-post implant is not self-tapping, it must be inserted gently or it will fracture or break. In situations where resistance is met and the operator is sure that the implant has not been set deeply enough, the hole should be widened

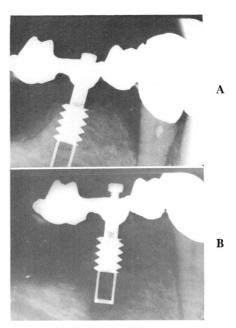

Fig. 14-5. A, A vent-plant placed too close to an open socket. **B,** The bone flanking the socket nearest the implant became undermined and resorption was the result.

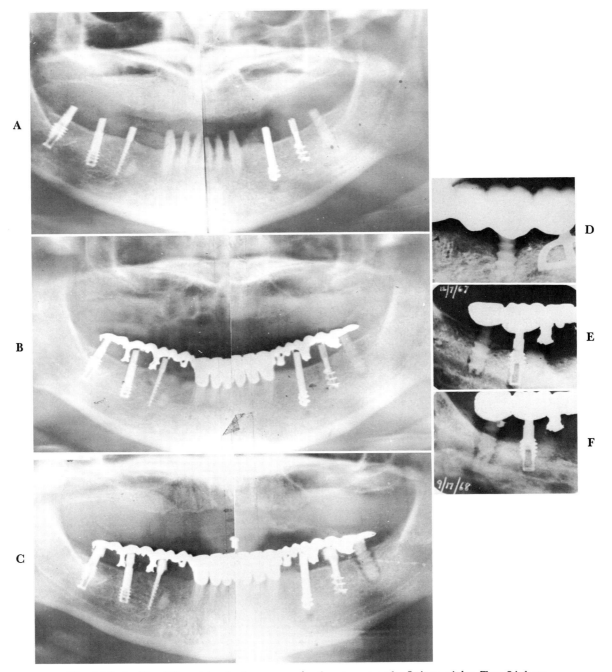

Fig. 14-6. A, Six different implants are seen in the same mouth. *Left to right:* Two Linkow titanium vent-plants, a narrow ridge (M. Cherchève) implant, a Cherchève spiral-shaft implant, a Muratori spiral implant, and a Sandhaus crystalline bone screw (aluminum oxide). The picture was taken immediately after the implants were placed. B, Three months later a breakdown of bone had started around the synthetic sapphire implant. C, Fourteen months postoperatively, the continued breakdown around the crystalline bone screw, but not around any of the others, is clearly shown. D, A blade-vent is acting as anchor tooth while the crystalline bone screw is anterior to it. Evidence of osteolysis is seen only around the anterior implant. E, Poorly trephined bone shows the holes around both implants made larger and deeper than their diameter. F, Two years later the bone has filled in around the deep portions of the vent-plant but not around the synthetic sapphire.

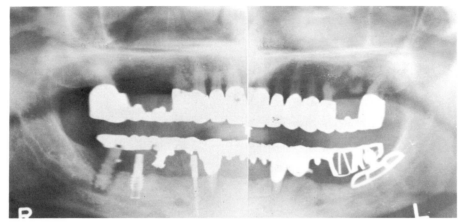

Fig. 14-7. The crystalline bone screw could be failing for two reasons other than poor design: it was screwed too deeply and could have sunk slightly through the superior wall of the mandibular canal, thus loosening the implant; or the hole made with the tap could have been too large, causing the failure.

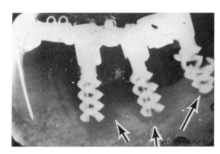

Fig. 14-8. A broken posterior implant occurred by trying to screw it deeper while the bone resisted. Osteolysis is caused by insufficient depths of implant and not by the broken screw. (From Linkow, L. I.: Alloplastic implants. In Goldman, H. M., Forrest, S. P., Byrd, D. L., and McDonald, R. E.: Current therapy in dentistry, vol. 3, St. Louis, 1968, The C. V. Mosby Co., pp. 335-356.)

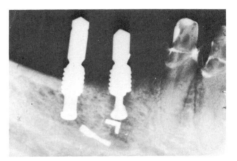

Fig. 14-9. The uprights joining the threads with the apical ring of the vent-plant broke during its insertion because of improper use of the helical burs. A helical bur was used that had a narrower diameter than the apical ring (thereby placing a great deal of pressure and torque on the ring) that was smaller in diameter than the outer diameter of the implant threads.

so that the spiral-post can be inserted to its maximum depth.

The vent-plant, being self-tapping and stronger than the spiral-shaft implant because it is made of titanium rather than Vitallium, has much less chance of breakage when forced into position. Occasionally, however, vent-plants have broken (Fig. 14-9).

Another candidate for easy breakage is the narrow ridge implant (Fig. 14-10). If its site has not been properly prepared, it can be snapped while forcing it into the bone.

Breakage, which may be expected if the operator persists in forcing the implant into the site, is usually detectable. When it occurs, the implant should be removed. Whether or not the immediate reinsertion of another implant into the site is possible depends on the damage. If too much bone has been destroyed removing the broken implant, reinsertion should not be attempted until the bone has healed.

Dull instruments

The burs and taps used in dentistry can be used only a certain number of times before they become dull or fracture or break. As the tools become dull, the bone's resistance increases. This causes a great deal of friction that heats the bone, and heat can destroy bone.

The operator should always be sure that he has

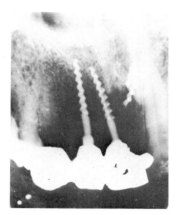

Fig. 14-10. A broken narrow ridge implant is seen leaning toward the neighboring tooth. Broken pieces of implants, although not usually the cause of any problems, should be removed at the same time breakage happens.

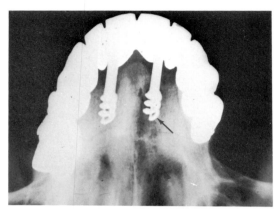

Fig. 14-11. The upper left implant perforated the labial plate of bone *(arrow)* during its insertion without the dentist being aware of it. A 6-month postoperative cross-sectional radiograph reveals the great amount of bone resorption caused by the perforation.

on hand enough of each sized bur and tap so that he can constantly interchange them. This is particularly wise when working on patients with excessively dense mandibles, a not uncommon characteristic. Tools should be sharpened as often as necessary to avoid friction-induced heat damage.

As a further safeguard against burning, water spray attachments should always be used, even with the sharpest rotary instruments. Also recommended is that a dental assistant use an independent water spray to doubly ensure adequate coolness.

OPERATIVE PROCEDURES

Most of the mistakes leading to failure in performing an implant intervention occur during the operative procedures. The operative procedures can be divided into two major groups, surgical and prosthodontic. Although these procedures vary according to the type of implant used, some general rules prevail.

Surgical procedures

Surgical procedures deal with making a site for the implant and inserting it. Each type of implant has its own particular method of insertion, and undoubtedly some implants are easier to use than others. Ease and simplicity of insertion, of course, produce fewer complications. However, the choice of an implant is dictated by the suitability of its design, as well as by its method of insertion.

Although generally applicable to all implants, the following problems commonly encountered during surgery may be more significant in dealing with

one kind of implant than another. For this reason recommendations for the proper use of the implant or alternative approaches are included in the discussion.

Overdrilling. Careless or overenthusiastic drilling with burs or taps can lead to perforation of the buccal, labial, lingual, or palatal plates of bone (Fig. 14-11). In the maxilla, a sinus may be entered (Fig. 14-12) or the nasal vestibulum penetrated (Fig. 14-13). In the mandible, the inferior alveolar nerve may be affected (Fig. 14-14). In addition to actually penetrating these structures and others, such as the pterygoid plexus of veins and the incisive foramen, the sites may be approached too closely, resulting in pain and other complications.

During surgery the depth and direction that the burs and taps are being driven must be continually checked with as many types of x-rays as necessary, such as periapical, intraoral, cross-sectional, occlusal, lateral plate, lateral head, profile topographic, cephalometric, and Panorex roentgenograms—whichever most accurately reveals the true picture of the operation's progress.

Although initial x-rays may reveal enough alveolar bone between an anatomic landmark and the alveolar crest, continual checking to see that the operator is well within his limits is essential. Many operators, to ensure that they truly know the shape of the bone as well as its height, routinely incise the fibromucosal tissue and reflect it to expose the underlying bone before any type of implant is inserted.

Improperly seated implants. When any type of post implant is being inserted, the operator may feel

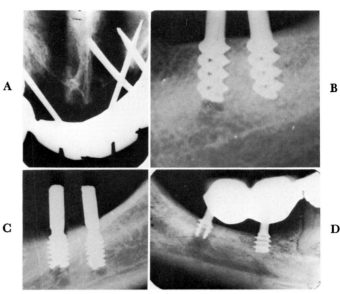

Fig. 14-13. A, Pin implants are deeply embedded in the nasal vestibulum. B, A number of operative mistakes caused failure with the implants. The trephining of bone below the first implant perforated the mandibular canal. Also, the spirals were too close to the alveolar crest. A two- to three-spiraled implant should have been used insted of the four-spiraled one. (Arrow points to area of canal perforation.) C, Both helical burs penetrated the canal, causing temporary paresthesia. However, the most posterior implant was also set into the mandibular canal and had to be removed. D, The posterior implant was not firmly anchored because the underlying bone was overtrephined with the helical bur. In most situations where the canal is involved either by the instrumentation prior to the implant insertion or by the implant itself, a paresthesia is usually the result.

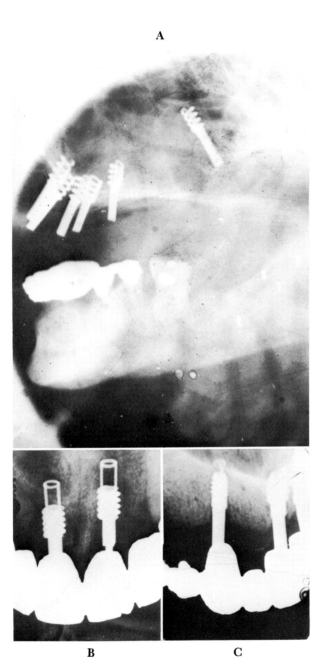

Fig. 14-12. A, A Cherchève type of spiral implant that was pushed into the maxillary sinus. It must be removed as quickly as possible. (From Linkow, L. I.: Alloplastic implants. In Goldman, H. M., Forrest, S. P., Byrd, D. L., and McDonald, R. E.: Current therapy in dentistry, vol. 3, St. Louis, 1968, The C. V. Mosby Co., pp. 335-356.) B and C, Radiographs showing various vent-plants perforating the nasal vestibulum.

resistance from a spicule of bone and assume that the bottom of the prepared hole has been reached. He thus leaves the implant too high, causing the invagination of epithelial tissue into the spirals.

Setting the implant as deep as the prepared hole is usually a problem only with the spiral-shaft implant, and a number of failures—particularly by a timid, inexperienced operator—may result (Fig. 14-15). The operator should always carefully check his x-rays and review his previous estimates as he seats the implant. When he is sure that the implant has not been set deeply enough and yet he feels resistance, the hole should be widened so that the spiral-post implant can be inserted to its maximum depth. As has been previously mentioned, forcing an implant—particularly a spiral-post implant—into its site may result in the implant's breaking.

There is less chance of incorrectly seating an implant when using the vent-plant or the blade-vent.

Because the vent-plant is self-tapping, it is screwed directly into the bone to the desired depth. The blade-vent is tapped to its proper depth with a mallet; thus, the implant makes its own path in bone. However, mistakes do occur (Fig. 14-16).

Lack of parallelism. Implants should be seated so that they are parallel to each other and to the remaining prepared teeth. When they are not set into the bone so that they are perpendicular to the occlusal plane or in a direct line parallel to the occlusal forces, they will not be able to withstand the masticatory pressures brought to bear upon them (Fig. 14-17). Also, it is very difficult to fabricate a fixed partial or complete bridge that will fit passively over nonparallel posts. Telescopic copings may be used, but it is better to avoid this complication.

Insufficient number of implants or natural teeth. Any structure, natural or man-made, needs a strong enough foundation to stabilize it. This is particularly true when dealing with the number of implants needed to support a full arch fixed denture. For example, if sufficient alveolar bone exists only in a few scattered areas of an edentulous maxilla or mandible and only a few implants can be placed, in time the case will fail (Fig. 14-18). If five or six implants are indicated and if there is alveolar bone

available for only three, it is obvious that the three cannot do the job as well.

The positions of the implants are also important. They must be functionally spaced across the span, not clumped together (Fig. 14-19). When situations arise where clumping of implants or using too few is the only solution, the entire case may be contraindicated. Frequently, however, a combination of endosseous and subperiosteal implants can successfully solve the problem.

Improper placement of triplant pins. There are very few areas of bone in either the maxilla or man-

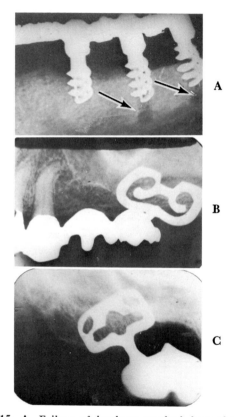

Fig. 14-15. A, Failure of implants resulted from the fact that the implants met too much resistance from the bone and therefore could not be screwed as deeply as the preceding bone burs. As a result, the spirals were not buried deep enough under the fibromucosal tissue, which led to bone resorption. (From Linkow, L. I.: Alloplastic implants. In Goldman, H. M., Forrest, S. P., Byrd, D. L., and McDonald, R. E.: Current therapy in dentistry, vol. 3, St. Louis, 1968, The C. V. Mosby Co., pp. 335-356.) **B and C,** Although sufficient bone existed, a portion of the shoulders of each one of the blade implants was not buried under the alveolar crest. Although these implants are still functioning satisfactorily in the mouth, this error could lead to failure.

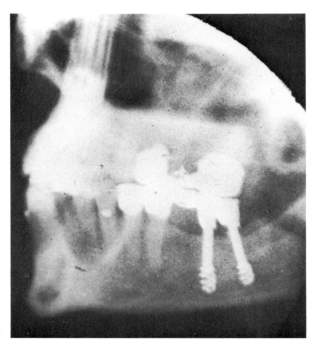

Fig. 14-14. The spiral-shaft implants were set through and below the inferior border of the mandibular canal, causing a paresthesia.

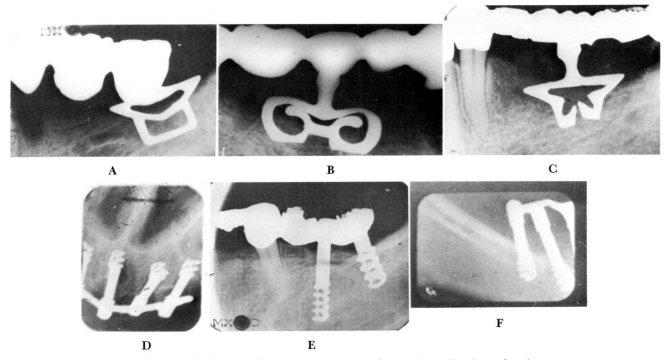

Fig. 14-16. **A to C,** These radiographs reveal resorption of bone directly under the superficially placed shoulders of the blade implants. **D to F,** Implants that are not parallel to each other and to the remaining teeth can cause difficulty in seating the bridge. Also, and even more important, is that if they are not placed vertical to the occlusal forces, bone breakdown can occur as a result of unequal destruction of the forces that are brought to bear upon them.

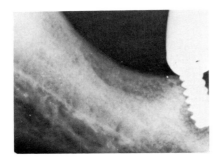

Fig. 14-17. A Lew screw failing for several reasons: the implant was not set parallel to the remaining teeth, and since it was distally tipped, the forces brought to bear upon it caused the distal proximal surface of the bone to resorb. The trephining may have been made larger than the screw threads. The neck is not reduced.

dible where a truly three-dimensional triplant can be formed without perforating a cortical plate of bone. Therefore a great many pin implants must be placed in one plane, rather than in three or even two planes. As a result, many times the entire bridge with the pins attached can be easily removed (Fig. 14-20). A triplant placed in one plane is far less

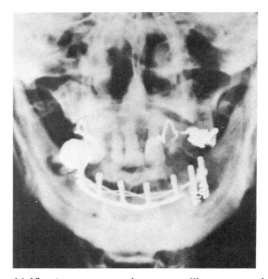

Fig. 14-18. A posteroanterior x-ray illustrates a large periapical rarefaction underneath the right molar and the left posterior two spiral-shaft implants. Since an entire prosthesis was supported by only these three remaining abutments, resorption had to occur. There must always be enough abutments present, whether they are natural teeth or implants.

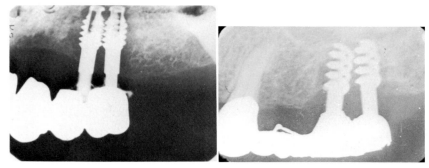

Fig. 14-19. These two radiographs reveal a rapid resorption of bone because of the proximity of the implants. They should be set at least 4 mm. away from one another.

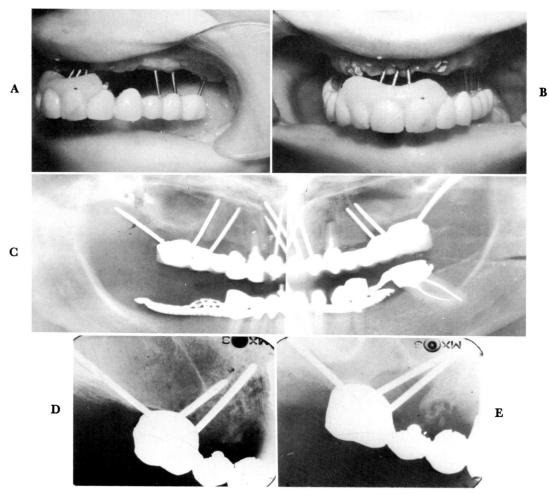

Fig. 14-20. A and B, Often a bridge can be removed with all of the triplant pins still attached to it and still diverging from each other. Very seldom will any fibrous tissue be attached to the pins, such as is usually the case with the post type and blade implants, indicating the lack of a physiologic pseudomembrane attachment. **C,** A Panorex showing the entire prosthesis and the diverging pins just prior to its removal. **D,** Periapical radiograph taken immediately after pins were inserted. **E,** Six months' postoperative radiograph reveals large breakdown of bone around the two mesially directed pins, which were placed too close together and too close to the buccal plate of bone.

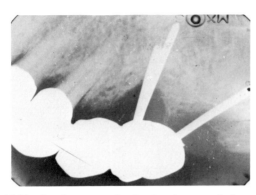

Fig. 14-21. Another case clearly showing osteolysis around the two mesial pins that were not directed at different angles.

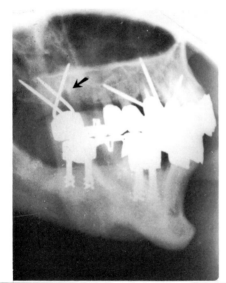

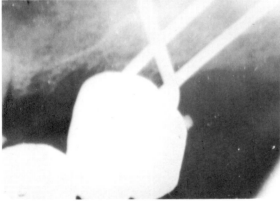

Fig. 14-22. A lateral plate roentgenogram and an intraoral periapical x-ray illustrate bone resorption in the areas where the pins are crossing over one another in the bone.

functional and resists lateral forces far less than does a three-dimensional triplant.

The deeper the triplant pins are set into bone and the more divergent they are, the greater the chance of success. The pins should diverge from one another, wherever possible, at least at a 45-degree angle. When they are too close to one another, bone resorption occurs (Fig. 14-21). Also, the pins should not cross one another in bone (Fig. 14-22).

To prevent bone loss at the crest of the alveolar ridge, the pins should converge at an angle that leaves a few millimeters of bone between each pin (Fig. 14-23). This is tricky, because the pins must also be close enough to one another so that a moderately sized acrylic core can be built to carry a normal tooth restoration. The solution in most cases is to angle the pins to leave enough space between them and to bend them together where they emerge into the oral cavity.

Improperly stabilized triplants. Triplant pins

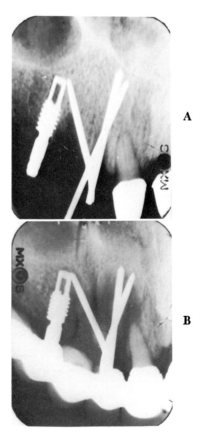

A

B

Fig. 14-23. A, Immediate postoperative x-ray showing that two of the three pins are much too close to one another. B, In only 6 months' time a great deal of bone resorption is clearly evident.

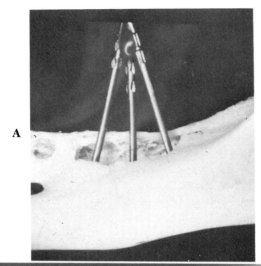

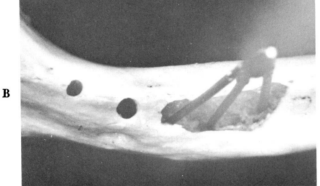

Fig. 14-24. **A,** A good portion of the alveolar bone was removed from a mandible and a triplant was placed into the open cavity. **B,** A lateral view showing the pins in the void and the labial and lingual cortical plates of bone still intact.

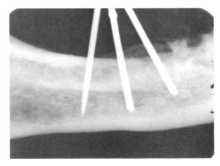

Fig. 14-25. The dried specimen was radiographed and the x-ray shows the pins to be buried in bone. The true situation was camouflaged by the buccal and lingual plates of cortical bone.

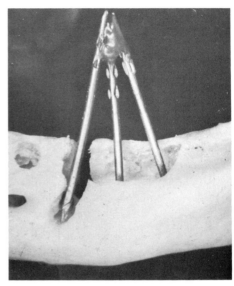

Fig. 14-26. The buccal and lingual cortical plates were then perforated a few millimeters in width and ½ inch in length, and once again the pins were placed inside.

are characterized by their smooth surfaces. This means that, unlike the post type implants and the blade-vent, no pseudoperiodontal membrane is found to encourage osteogenesis. Collagenous tissue does grow up to and encircle the pins, but it forms a kind of sleeve through which the pins can slip without pulling on the bone. As the bone around the pins is not stimulated, a certain amount of resorption occurs. This tendency becomes severe if the triplant is not securely stabilized.

Formerly, when patients complained of pain or mobility, the implantologist could find little reason for it on x-ray studies. The following studies show that diagnosis solely by x-ray can be misleading. Linkow demonstrated experimentally with mandibular and maxillary jaws that the density of the buccal, lingual, or palatal cortical plates of bone can disguise the true resorption picture taking place in alveolar bone flanking a narrow pin. Scooping out alveolar bone, he placed the pins inside the hole (Fig. 14-24). Then he x-rayed the dried specimen (Fig. 14-25). Because the cortical plates of bone camouflaged the lack of alveolar bone, bone appears to completely encapsulate the triplant. He then cut away portions of cortical plates (Fig. 14-26) and once again radiographed the area (Fig. 14-27). In this way he established the fallibility of x-rays in diagnosing bone resorption in triplants.

It is now known that each triplant used in long

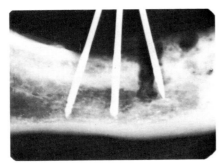

Fig. 14-27. The bone around the mesial pin now revealed the true picture.

edentulous spans or in totally edentulous jaws should be stabilized by a thin metal plate set directly over the bone, wherever possible.

Using the old operative method, each and every triplant exhibits what in a natural tooth would be considered to be a trifurcation involvement concerning the fibromucosal tissue lying between the bony alveolar crest and the tissue-bearing surface of the acrylic core. As the fibromucosa moves during normal activities of the jaw, it tugs on the emerging triplant pins. As a result, they move and cause bone resorption (Fig. 14-28).

Triplants may be stabilized in such a way as to eliminate potential soft tissue trifurcation involvement. This can be done by incising and retracting the tissue over the site and by driving the pin implants directly through a thin metal plate adapted over the bone. The pins are then fused together right over the plate (Fig. 14-29). The incised tissues are sutured around the protruding acrylic core.

In addition to the thin metal plate fitted over the bone with each triplant, a template should be placed over the fibromucosal tissue to act as a stress-distributing bar. Together, these should complement one another and resolve the movement problems that encourage bone resorption (Fig. 14-30).

When a triplant is anticipated in an edentulous area between natural teeth, neither the plate nor a template is necessary if the implant is secured to the teeth on either side with a fixed splint.

In long edentulous spans or in the totally edentulous jaw, the addition of a fourth pin—making the triplant actually a quadraplant—has been found helpful. The problem here is that all the legs should diverge. If this is difficult with a triplant, it is even harder with a quadraplant.

Improper acrylic fusion of triplant pins. Unless the acrylic used to fuse the triplant pins together is brushed on layer by layer, air bubbles may be

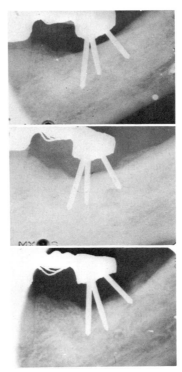

Fig. 14-28. Three serial radiographs show the steady bone resorption around a mandibular triplant.

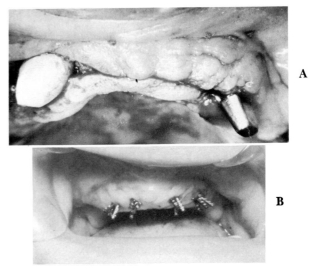

A

B

Fig. 14-29. A, The acrylic core was built over a thin metal plate adapted to the bone. The core included the triplant pins, which were driven through the plate. **B,** In a completely edentulous maxilla, placing pin implants directly through the fibromucosal tissue and into the bone without the use of a metal rigid template could easily lead to failure.

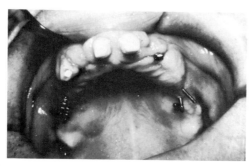

Fig. 14-30. When other teeth as well as other post type implants are used as abutments for the support of a full arch fixed denture, the longevity of triplants used without a template is increased. However, success is more assured with a template.

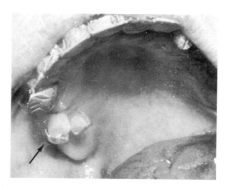

Fig. 14-31. An aluminum shell previously filled with cold cure acrylic and placed over the ends of the pins was disked open after the acrylic hardened. However, the core *(arrow)* fabricated in this method might contain air bubbles. Therefore it is necessary to always build the core with the brush-on technique.

trapped inside the acrylic core. This weakens it, and it may crack or the pins may loosen inside the core. The core should be built by starting at the most gingival portion of the pins and gradually building up in an occlusal direction until the ends of the pins, which were previously notched with a fissure bur for added retention, are completely encapsulated with the acrylic core. In this way no bubbles should be included in the core. This is the most successful method known so far (Fig. 14-31).

Excessively thick fibromucosa. In those cases where the fibromucosal tissue in the maxillary molar and tuberosity areas is very flabby or mobile or is as much as 6 to 7 mm. thick, it may have to be removed. Before deciding, the operator should determine the type of implant to be used. If triplants and a stress-distributing template are to be used, the tissue should be removed at least 2 to 3 months prior to the implant intervention. Otherwise, the template will not be anchored to firm, immovable tissue and it can move up and down, loosening the implants through improper support (Fig. 14-32).

If using a spiral-post implant, vent-plant, or blade-vent, provision may be made for excessively thick tissue by using post implants or blade-vents with extra long necks. This will prevent their occlusal ends from being completely buried in the tissue and is often preferable to cutting away the excess tissue (Fig. 14-33). If excess tissue is to be removed, only the submucosal tissue is scooped out, leaving the mucosa intact.

Prosthodontic considerations

Included in this section are the prosthodontic procedures applicable to implantology. Most opera-

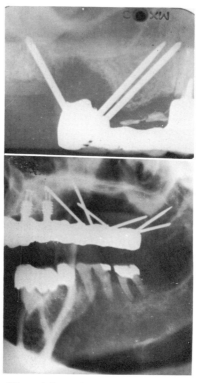

Fig. 14-32. The triplants in these two cases are failing as a result of excessively thick fibromucosal tissue that restricted the depth of the pins into the bone.

tors are familiar with these procedures or variations of them as they are used in other aspects of dentistry. Their role in the success or failure of an implant intervention is obvious in most cases. If a miscalculation occurs in any prosthodontic phase of the opera-

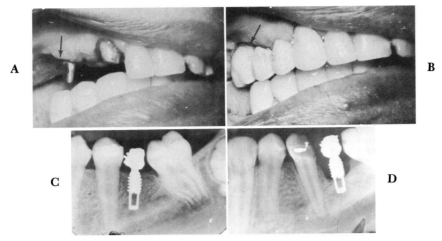

Fig. 14-33. A and B, Using a blade with an extra long neck is frequently preferable to cutting away a good portion of the tissue. Here the processed fixed partial denture had to be fitted to the atypical and irregular gum line because of the tissue removal. Arrows point to areas where the fibromucosal tissue was excessively removed, resulting in overlengthening of the molar crowns. **C,** Immediate postoperative x-ray shows bone around an unsupported single tooth implant. **D,** The bone damage is evident 12 months later around the unsupported vent-plant. Also, this was an earlier designed implant, which also contributed to its failure.

tive procedure, the result may be immediately evident or develop over a period of weeks. The following considerations are common prosthodontic causes of implant failure.

Unsupported implants. Normal movements of the tongue, cheeks, and lips are enough to dislodge an implant with a protruding post. Immediate splinting protects the protruding post and also protects the soft parts of the mouth from the post's sharp edges. Although the internally-threaded vent-plant and Muratori's internally-threaded spiral screw implant do not protrude as far into the mouth as a nonthreaded implant, it is advisable to use a splint to ensure immobility.

Single tooth implants unsupported by neighboring teeth will fail (Fig. 14-34). They must be immediately stabilized by a splint or the implant can move and prevent healing. No matter what type of implant is used, a temporary splint is needed unless a permanent one has been prepared beforehand.

Cementing implants to the temporary splint. In securing a temporary splint to either natural or implant abutments, no cement of any sort should ever be used inside the crowns that will cover the implants. Because the protruding shafts of the implants are square with no taper, it is difficult to remove a temporary splint without dislodging the implants unless some provision to ease removal has been made. For this reason, the protruding shafts are

covered with gold copings. These are cold cured with acrylic resin into lumens in the splint. The lumens should be slightly larger than the copings so that no interference can occur in seating the temporary splint over the copings. When securing the splint, the gold copings should be lubricated with Vaseline. The crowns that will fit over the natural tooth abutments can be filled with a temporary cement. However, care should be taken; if any cement slips around the implants and sets there, the strain exerted on the implants during splint removal may loosen them or pull them out (Fig. 14-35).

If difficulty is encountered in removing a temporary splint, those portions over the implants should be severed with rotary disks so that the splint can be easily removed without disturbing the implants.

Prolonged seating of a temporary splint. A temporary acrylic splint should not be seated too long because it tends to change in dimension. The resulting unbalanced splint may pull on the implants and dislodge them. Also, the temporary cement used to secure the splint may give way, causing the splint to loosen and move the implants (Fig. 14-36).

As soon as possible a permanent prosthesis should be set over the abutments to permanently stabilize them. As the operator becomes more experienced, the temporary splint stage can be avoided. Instead a prefabricated fixed denture, properly occluded and balanced, can be cemented over the implant

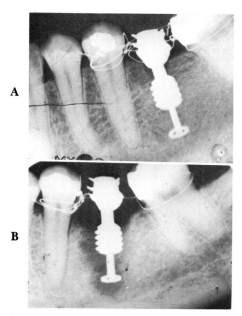

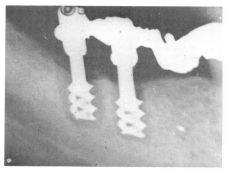

Fig. 14-36. Bone resorption is seen around these two spiral posts because the temporary acrylic splint was worn much too long and loose, thereby loosening the implants.

Fig. 14-34. **A,** Another single tooth implant, stabilized only by wiring to neighboring teeth. **B,** A few months later, the mobility allowed by this method has caused a great deal of bone resorption.

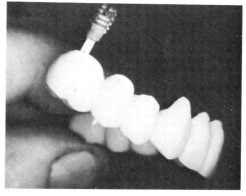

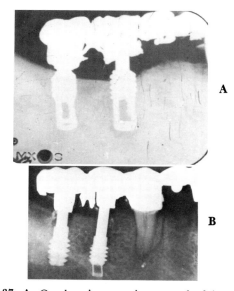

Fig. 14-35. Cements, whether of a temporary or more permanent type, should never be used inside the crown that covers the implant. In this case, the cement stuck to the implant post, pulling it out with the splint.

Fig. 14-37. **A,** Overhanging margins cause food impaction, which leads to bone resorption. Also, impingement of the overhanging crowns can cause severe pain, inflammation, and swelling to the soft tissue in the areas of the implants, which can lead to bone resorption. **B,** Also shows perforation of the mandibular canal with the anterior vent-plant.

shafts and natural tooth abutments immediately after the implants are inserted. In many cases this eliminates possible complications.

Pontic impingement on the soft tissues. Severe pain can be caused by the impingement of the pontics or implant crowns on the fibromucosal tissue (Fig. 14-37). The most bothersome areas are where the buccogingival line angles meet the underlying mucosal tissue.

A prefabricated appliance, particularly its bucco-

gingival line angles, should be checked carefully prior to an implant intervention by having the patient wear the prosthesis temporarily for a day. Impingement marks can easily be seen on the soft tissue (Fig. 14-38) and the offending areas removed from the tissue-bearing surface of the involved pontics. If any adjustments have proved necessary, permanent cementing of the prosthesis in place should be postponed until the patient wears the prosthesis temporarily for a few more days. After the prosthesis proves

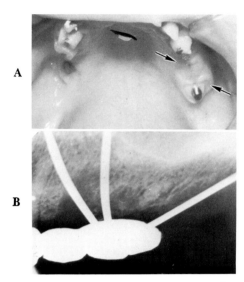

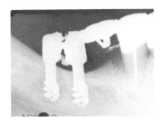

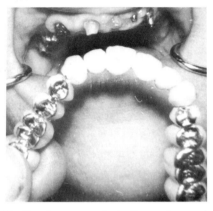

Fig. 14-39. A broken solder joint can lead to an increased load and stress on the isolated implant leading to bone resorption. The solder joint could have also broken because of a poorly fitted bridge that caused excess stress on the solder joints as well as on the implants themselves.

Fig. 14-38. **A,** The soft tissue directly surrounding the blade implant is compressed *(arrows)* because of poor pontic relationship. The tissues can become mutilated and inflamed if this is not alleviated. **B,** Triplants were forced through improperly sized and directed holes in the template (the holes were too small). This caused a torque action on the template and on the pins themselves (notice how pins are curved in bone), which led to bone destruction.

Fig. 14-40. Poorly prepared teeth—such as short teeth used without adequate steps to lengthen their clinical crowns with well-fitted telescopic copings or pin-ledge type of restorations—can lead to loosening of the bridge, with eventual loosening of the implants.

to be comfortable, it may be seated with oxyphosphate of zinc cement.

Poorly fitting permanent splints. A permanent splint must fit passively over the implants or else it will act as an orthodontic appliance. To ensure a passive fit, the protruding implant posts and abutments should be parallel and the impressions made of them extremely accurate. Tension or pressure between the abutments of a fixed denture can cause excessive strain on both the implant and the prosthesis (Fig. 14-39).

Misuse of modeling compound copper tube impressions. Copper tube impression compound should never be used in taking an impression of an acrylic core over a triplant or over a blade implant. Removing such an impression can sometimes dislodge the implant. Any one of the elastic impression materials is preferable for such purposes. However, compound impressions can be used without coolants. To eliminate "drag," the impression is removed and replaced over the implant post a few times. When it is removed the last time it is placed in cold water.

Poor crown preparation. If the length and degree of taper of a crown are not carefully shaped, the crown may be of little value as an abutment (Fig. 14-40). The supposedly permanent cement

seal may break, leaving the still-sealed implants to bear alone the stresses upon the bridge. Such undue pressure will cause implant failure.

Improper use of cement. Temporary cement should not be used for the final cementation of the completed prosthesis. Because the abutment teeth have usually been tapered and their line angles eliminated, temporary cement can easily wash away between the crown and the tooth. Temporary cement inside the crown covering the square-shafted, untapered implant is far less likely to wash away. As a result, not only is undue strain placed on the still cemented implants, but tooth decay eventually occurs inside the empty crowns (Fig. 14-41). Again, if the implants have been cemented to the prosthesis, there is a good chance of loosening them while removing the bridge to repair the broken cement seals. Therefore all fixed dentures should be sealed to the implants and teeth with oxyphosphate of zinc cement, which should be trimmed to avoid irritation

(Fig. 14-42). It should be noted that Linkow now prefers the carboxylate cements.

Failure to immobilize implants when using a removable prosthesis. If a removable prosthesis is desired either by the dentist or the patient, some provision must be made to keep its movements from eventually loosening the implants and remaining teeth. The typical removable appliance derives some of its retention from its soft tissue adaptation. Because of this it rides up and down over the fibromucosa. If a mesostructure splint consisting of copings soldered together by a dolder bar is not prepared to connect all the implants and remaining teeth, the movements of the removable appliance as it rides up and down will eventually dislodge the implants. Therefore a removable prosthesis should be fabricated over a mesostructure.

In planning such an appliance for an edentulous mandible, usually post type implants or blade-vents secured with a full arch, fixed mesostructure are all that is necessary.

Poor choice of prosthesis material. In planning

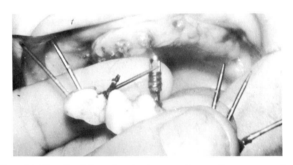

Fig. 14-41. Cavities developing underneath crowns that support fixed dentures also lead to eventual loss of the bridge as a result of cement seal leakage that loosens the prosthesis, thereby increasing the load on the implants and resulting in their eventual mobility. Here are seen two triplants and a vent-plant pulled out of the mouth still attached to the bridge.

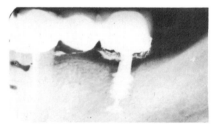

Fig. 14-42. Any hard cement left underneath crowns covering implants can cause irritation of the soft tissue, which can lead to bone resorption.

a full arch prosthesis for an edentulous maxilla, a porcelain-fused-to-metal prosthesis should never be used. This type of appliance is very heavy, and the effect of gravity on a maxillary prosthesis should be considered. For a full arch maxillary restoration, an all-acrylic splint, an acrylic-built-over-gold splint, or an all-acrylic palateless type denture are suitable. Very recently, a new metal formula for the fusion of porcelain to it has been developed. Platinum is replaced with palladium mixed with gold, resulting in an extremely lightweight prosthesis.

Poor occlusion. One of the most important considerations in the long-term security of implants is proper occlusion (Fig. 14-43). Occlusal disharmony can cause the implants to loosen by increasing the shock of premature or interfering contacts on the implants. It is vitally important to take accurate impressions for both temporary and final splints. These splints must be carefully fabricated, inserted, occluded, and balanced.

REASONS FOR SUBPERIOSTEAL IMPLANT FAILURES

A subperiosteal implant may fail for anatomic, systemic, or operative reasons. These include:

Poor choice of site. Subperiosteal implants are indicated only for a mandible where sufficient alveolar bone resorption has occurred. Otherwise, as the bone resorbs, the implant will fit inaccurately and move, causing complications (Fig. 14-44).

Inaccurate impression of site. To get a true impression of the bone's landscape, the site must be surgically exposed. When planning a full mandibular restoration, the impression must include the external oblique ridges, mylohyoid ridge, symphysis, genial

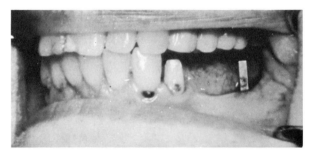

Fig. 14-43. Poor judgment in restorative procedures could lead to failure. The upper bridge should have first been constructed longer so that the torque action would be decreased on the lower implant, which would then have been made shorter. The bridge should also have been fabricated with shorter clinical crowns.

tubercles, and neurovascular bundles of nerves exiting the mental foramina. If these are not properly exposed for a good impression, there is an excellent chance that the implant framework will be inadequate.

Poor fit of the implant. The implant must fit its site exactly (Fig. 14-45). This can be ensured not only by taking an accurate impression over exposed bone but also by availing oneself of the best possible laboratory.

Improper incision of the soft tissues. The mucosal and submucosal tissues must be incised cleanly and accurately right down to the bone, and the tissue must be retracted without tearing it in order to reduce postoperative edema. Tearing or mutilating

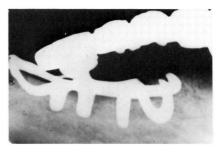

Fig. 14-44. Periapical radiograph reveals resorption underneath unilateral subperiosteal implant, since it was seated in an area where much alveolar bone still existed.

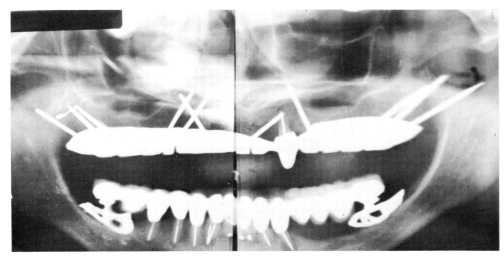

Fig. 14-45. A Panorex shows poor adaptation of the bilateral subperiosteal implants to the bone caused by a poor fit.

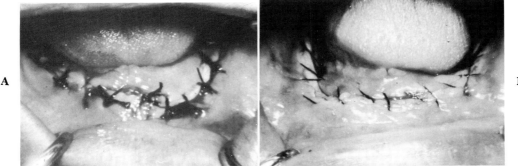

Fig. 14-46. A, Poor suturing. The sutures were made too far lingually, excessively stretching the buccal tissue. The knots also lie over the wound, irritating it and retarding healing. B, The sutures are too few, too irregular, and too far apart. Compare with Fig. 14-47, *A* and *B*.

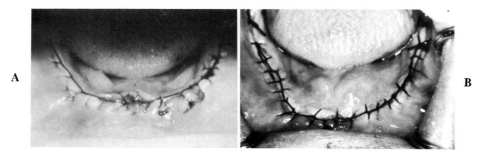

Fig. 14-47. A, Suturing must be done carefully to cover the underlying bone completely. Interrupted sutures or a combination of interrupted and mattress sutures are usually indicated. B, Sometimes continuous suturing is preferred. However, enough sutures should always be used so that no open spaces exist between the incised tissues.

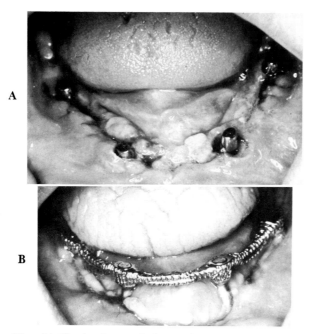

Fig. 14-48. A, Severe inflammation of the fibromucosal tissue, which was "squeezed" between the implant's substructure and the denture. B, The anterior struts of the substructure have become exposed. Such a situation can rarely be compensated.

the periosteum will result in excessive bone resorption and the bone's healing by secondary intention.

Incomplete healing. At least 3 to 6 weeks should be allowed for the healing of the soft tissues before inserting the implant. (If, however, the implantation is done as a 1-day procedure, this is not neces-

sary.) By waiting this period of time, the tissues should have healed completely and be fairly elastic. Thus when they are stretched and sutured over the implant, they will not tear. Any tearing would expose the substructure of the implant, leading to eventual failure.

Poor suturing techniques. Suturing must be done carefully to avoid stretching and tearing the tissues (Fig. 14-46). As many sutures as are necessary to completely cover the bone should be used. Not even a minute amount of bone should be left exposed. The sutures—whether they be interrupted, mattress, or continuous—should be neat, close together, and accomplished with a fine silk suture (Fig. 14-47).

Poor occlusion. Undue stress on the prosthesis will be transmitted to the implant. The consequences will cause the implant to fail.

Improper stress distribution. The denture should rest on the posts, not on soft tissues. Otherwise the denture will compress the tissues between it and the underlying substructure of the implant, causing inflammation and irritation (Fig. 14-48). The tissue may also be rubbed away from one of the underlying struts, leaving it exposed and creating a pathway for infection.

As can be seen with all types of implants—endosseous or subperiosteal—the failures were largely caused by errors in patient evaluation, choice of implant, or operative technique. Clinical experience will teach the reasons why one type of implant will fail and another type will succeed. Experience, together with continual careful evaluation and good craftsmanship, will radically reduce the number of failures.

CHAPTER 15 Atypical implant situations

Today most partially or completely edentulous patients can be helped by one or a combination of several endosseous techniques. Linkow has been able to perform at least one type of implant intervention on from 80% to 95% of his presenting patients, enabling them to avoid removable prostheses.

The following cases are unusual; most patients do not have such debilities nor is insertion of the implant normally so difficult. Yet the results of endosseous procedures on these patients seem to promise their wider use in atypical situations. Masticatory function has been restored by various endosseous techniques to patients suffering from congenital deformities such as cleft palate, severe malocclusion, and deformities caused by traumatic injury or diseases. The temporary use of endosseous implants in prosthodontics has also been successful.

Case 1
A full mouth restoration for a patient with a cleft palate

The patient, a 17-year-old boy, was depressed and despondent because of his cleft palate and hare lip. His remaining mandibular teeth were three right atypically shaped molars, a left second molar, and three anterior peg-shaped incisors that were severely malpositioned (Fig. 15-1). His upper teeth on the left side consisted of an atypically peg-shaped second bicuspid and two tapered molars, and on the right side a tapered second bicuspid and a molar (Fig. 15-2). The patient had been wearing a full upper acrylic denture with holes in it corresponding to the remaining molar teeth (Fig. 15-3).

The mandibular teeth were prepared for full crown coverage. Compound tube impressions, a wax interocclusal record of centric relation, and other necessary records were taken. On the second visit platinum copings were fitted over the lower teeth (Fig. 15-4), and once again a wax interocclusal record of centric relation was taken. A plaster index of the entire lower arch was made, picking up the copings (Fig. 15-5). From this, the final full arch, porcelain-fused-to-metal prosthesis was fabricated (Fig. 15-6). This was cemented into place (Fig. 15-7).

The remaining maxillary teeth were then prepared for full crown coverage. Plastic copings were fabricated with a bite block (Fig. 15-8). The copings were placed in the patient's mouth, and a bite registration and a plaster index were made. The models were articulated and metal copings cast (Fig. 15-9).

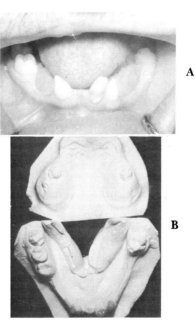

Fig. 15-1. A, The lower teeth were peg-shaped and flared out from one another. **B,** Maxillary and mandibular study casts. No teeth existed in the maxilla anterior to the atypically shaped molars on each side.

629

Another bite and index were then taken of the copings in the mouth.

Five porcelain-fused-to-metal crowns were fabricated to fit over the atypical copings. These were flared out buccally to meet with the lower posterior teeth.

A final wax interocclusal record of centric relation was taken (Fig. 15-10), followed by a plaster index of the entire maxilla. The five porcelain-fused-to-metal crowns were picked up with the plaster. The master stone model was then poured and articulated, with the stone model duplicating the lower full arch splint.

A specially designed template was waxed up. Extending from the template were predetermined hollow copings in the region of the central incisors and two internally threaded systems. This latter feature allowed the dentist to easily replace the anterior prosthetic appliance by screwing it on and off the template as the patient matured.

The wax template with its internal threaded at-

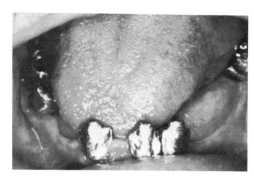

Fig. 15-4. All lower teeth were prepared parallel to each other, without any nerve exposures, and castings were made and fitted over the prepared teeth.

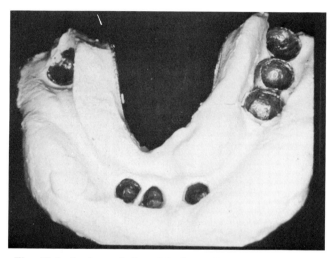

Fig. 15-5. A plaster index picked up all of the mandibular copings.

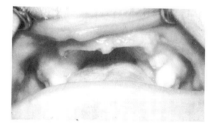

Fig. 15-2. Clinical view of the maxilla.

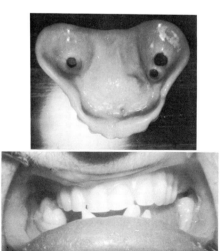

Fig. 15-3. A, The denture that the patient utilized for most of his life. B, The upper denture and peg-shaped teeth with which the patient had no function.

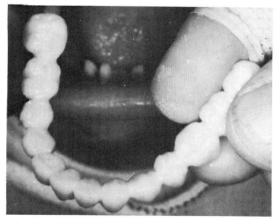

Fig. 15-6. A full arch porcelain-fused-to-metal prosthesis was fabricated.

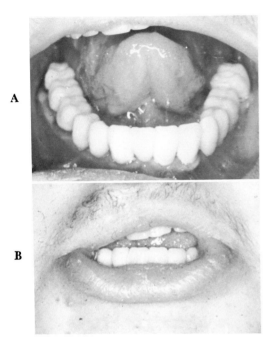

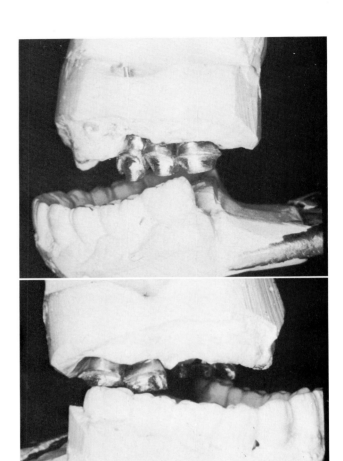

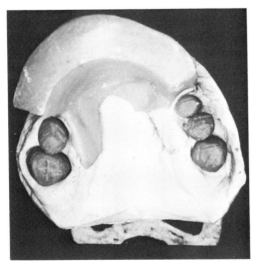

A

B

Fig. 15-7, A, The fixed denture is cemented with oxyphosphate of zinc cement. B, The incisal edges of the mandibular restoration were parallel to a horizontal plane, fabricated completely independently of the upper denture.

Fig. 15-9. Metal copings are seen on articulated master casts. Note the extreme prognathic appearance from the limited anterior growth of the maxilla.

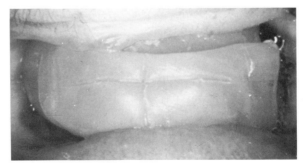

Fig. 15-8. Duralay copings were made to accurately fit over the prepared maxillary teeth. Anteriorly a tray and wax bite rim are also seen.

Fig. 15-10. A wax interocclusal record of centric relation is taken with the castings in the mouth.

tachments were then cast in gold. After polishing, the template was soldered to the glazed porcelain-fused-to-metal crowns, which had all been soldered to each other (Fig. 15-11).

A removable anterior quadrant consisting of individually waxed teeth and a pink saddle area conforming to the anterior gold template contour was waxed (Fig. 15-12). It was fitted into the mouth, and all necessary adjustments were made.

A processed acrylic anterior quadrant of teeth with a pink acrylic portion resembling the patient's gums was then fabricated (Fig. 15-13). This was fused to the gold connecting bar that contained the

screws for attaching the anterior quadrant to the metal template.

The occlusion was once again checked and balanced in the mouth and the upper prosthesis removed. The two areas on the gingiva corresponding to the prefabricated hollow copings on the template were marked with indelible pencil. Because the alveolar bone in this area had resorbed to a knife-edge ridge and blind drilling seemed unwise, an incision was made to expose the bone. Then the implant sites were prepared (Fig. 15-14).

Two narrow ridge implants were carefully screwed into the ridge (Fig. 15-15) and positioned

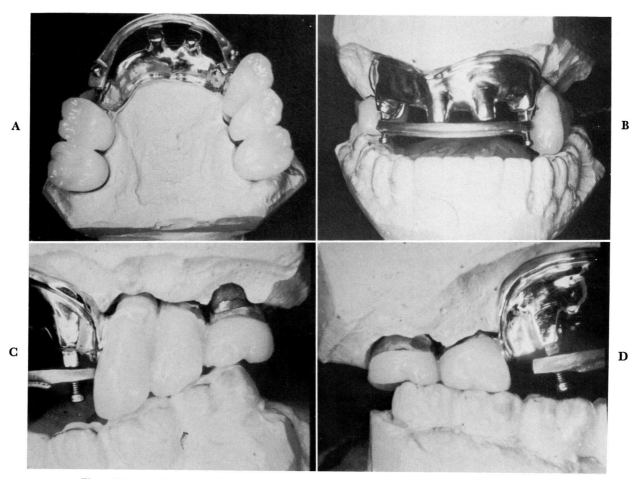

Fig. 15-11. A, The posterior castings are soldered together and porcelain is glazed to them. Also seen is an anterior gold template soldered to the copings. **B,** The anterior view shows two anterior pontics, which are hollow inside to cover two implants that will be placed into the bone anteriorly, protruding from the template. The rounded bar is attached to the template by means of two screws seen. The bar will be processed into the anterior quadrant of acrylic teeth. **C,** Close-up view from the left side showing the three porcelain-fused-to-metal crowns soldered to the anterior metal template. A portion of the bar with the screw that fixates it to the template also is seen. **D,** Same view from the right side.

to fit exactly into the hollow cores of the prefabricated metal template. Interrupted sutures were used to close the tissues over the exposed bone, and the maxillary prosthesis was temporarily placed over the five remaining posterior teeth. The anterior quadrant was screwed into the female threadings of the template.

Five days later the sutures were removed. The bridge containing the five porcelain-fused-to-metal crowns and template was cemented with oxyphosphate of zinc cement over the posterior teeth and anterior implants (Fig. 15-16). The anterior quadrant was then screwed into the template (Fig. 15-17), and the occlusion was adjusted (Fig. 15-18).

Healing took place uneventfully. Upon completion of the case, the patient enjoyed a fixed instead of a removable partial denture. Esthetically his mouth, teeth, and lips exhibit a more natural appearance than previously (Fig. 15-19), and functionally the patient is more than satisfied.

A posteroanterior roentgenogram (Fig. 15-20) and two lateral plate radiographs (Fig. 15-21) show

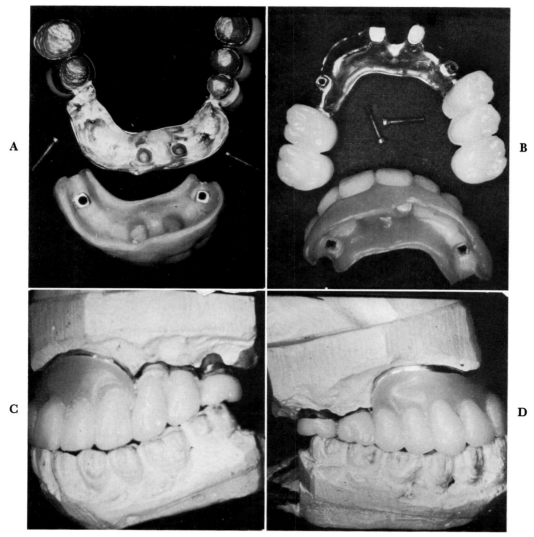

Fig. 15-12. A, The tissue-bearing side of the template and castings are seen with the waxed anterior quadrant of teeth. The bar with its two sets of internal threadings is waxed inside. **B,** The occlusal view of the porcelain and template is seen with the anterior wax-up. **C,** The waxed anterior quadrant is fitted over the template on the master cast (left side view). **D,** The right side showing the wax-up and posterior porcelain restorations.

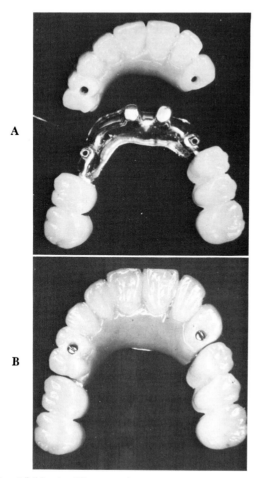

Fig. 15-13. A, The anterior quadrant is completed with heat-curing acrylic technique. B, The finished acrylic anterior quadrant is screwed into the template.

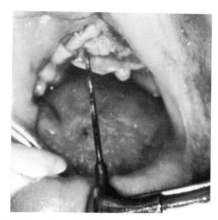

Fig. 15-14. The tissue in the anterior portion of the maxilla is incised and reflected and a narrow sized twist drill is carefully rotated into the narrow bone ridge to its proper depth.

the finished prosthesis and narrow ridge implants in position.

Case 2
Restoring centric occlusion by occlusal reconstruction with the aid of vent-plants

The most striking form of mandibular malposition is prognathism, sometimes called functional mesiocclusion. In this condition the mandible has been shifted to a forced, protruded position that is the only comfortable relationship of the jaws. The lower anterior teeth are labial to the uppers, sometimes completely covering them, and usually the lower posteriors are buccal to the upper posterior teeth. Temporomandibular joint disturbances can occur in conjunction with prognathism.

In some cases of mesiocclusion the anterior teeth can be restored to an edge-to-edge relationship. This

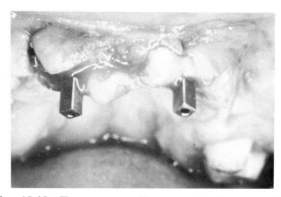

Fig. 15-15. Two narrow ridge type implants are then screwed into position.

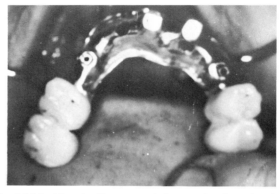

Fig. 15-16. After healing around the two implants has been completed, the framework is cemented into position with hard cement.

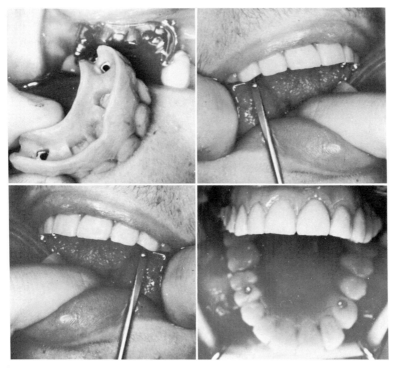

Fig. 15-17. The anterior quadrant of teeth is then fitted over the anterior portion of the framework and screwed into position.

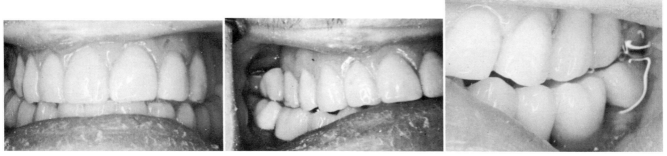

Fig. 15-18. The completed case.

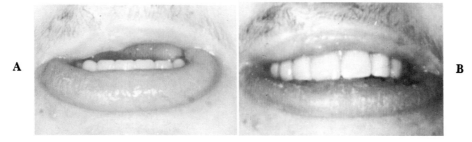

A   B

Fig. 15-19. A, The patient without the new upper teeth. **B,** The upper teeth in position.

means that the condyles are able to retrude comfortably, and a more correct centric position can be established. In such cases, which are often referred to as false Class III mesiocclusions, the anterior maxillary and mandibular incisors and cuspids can be shortened until posterior contact is produced. However, the approach to such a procedure must be conservative. If the anterior teeth cannot be brought edge-to-edge, grinding alone will not correct the condition. If the underbite is extreme, the

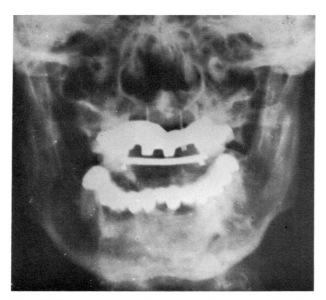

Fig. 15-20. A posteroanterior view of the case showing the full arch lower fixed denture as well as the maxillary anterior narrow ridge implants, template, and bar. The acrylic teeth cannot be noticed on the radiograph.

degree of grinding necessary to establish freeway space will be prohibitive. Therefore grinding by itself is not indicated. Where occlusal contact of the posterior teeth cannot be achieved, grinding alone should not be attempted. In these instances, if orthodontia is not feasible, prosthetic or surgical procedures should be employed in combination with grinding and occlusal rehabilitation to obtain the desired occlusion.

If posterior contact cannot be obtained by conservative grinding of the anterior teeth, the posterior crowns can be raised to meet the new occlusal heights. All missing teeth should be included in the fixed bridgework, and all malformed, malpositioned, or unattractive teeth in the anterior region should be individually restored with full crown coverage. If, however, posterior contact was attained by anterior grinding, all crown restorations can be constructed at the same occlusal height.

In all bite-raising cases, the freeway space must be carefully determined before any attempt is made to increase the crown lengths of the teeth. At rest position a physiologic freeway space must remain after the bite-raising has been completed; 1 to 2 mm. will suffice.

In this case a 43-year-old male patient appeared to have a severe Class III malocclusion (Fig. 15-22). However, when the mandible was retruded, contact was made between his upper and lower incisors (Fig. 15-23).

Using the incisal contacts as a guide, the patient's upper teeth were prepared, and the laboratory fabricated posterior veneer crown castings and

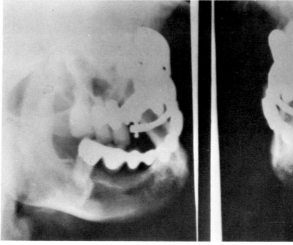
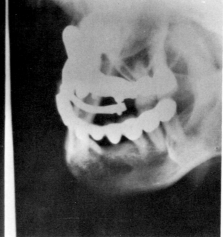

Fig. 15-21. Two lateral plate views.

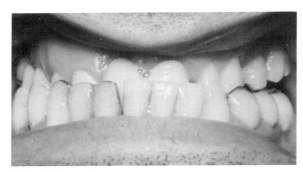

Fig. 15-22. The patient before treatment closed in this position—a Class III relationship.

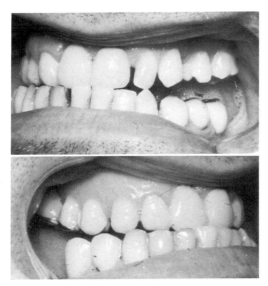

Fig. 15-23. Upon further observation, the incisal edges of the anterior upper and lower teeth almost met when the lower jaw was retruded.

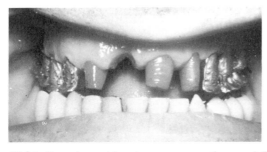

Fig. 15-24. Posterior gold veneer crown castings and Duralay anterior acrylic transfer copings are seated.

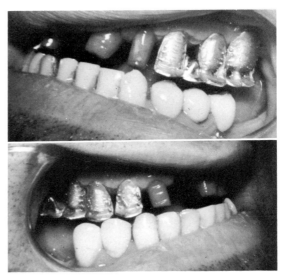

Fig. 15-25. The intermaxillary space was posteriorly divided equally by first lengthening the maxillary castings to one-half the distance.

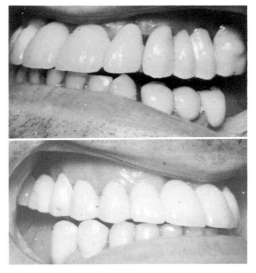

Fig. 15-26. The completed maxillary prosthesis included two posterior quadrants constructed of gold occlusal acrylic veneers and the anterior quadrant, which consisted of porcelain fused to metal. The posterior quadrants engaged with the anterior quadrant with gold dovetail interlocks. The interocclusal space between the new bridgework and the old lower restorations will then be closed by lengthening the lower restorations.

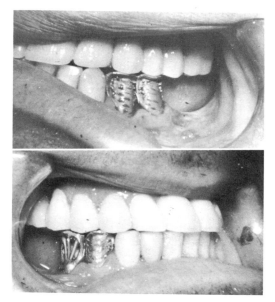

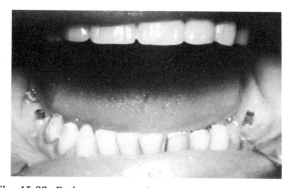

Fig. 15-27. Lower veneer crown castings are to meet the remaining interocclusal space.

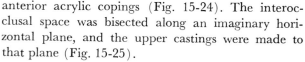

Fig. 15-28. Endosseous vent-plants are set bilaterally in the edentulous posterior areas.

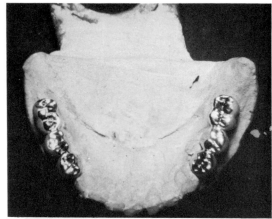

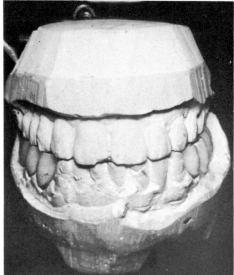

Fig. 15-29. Bilateral fixed partial dentures are completed.

anterior acrylic copings (Fig. 15-24). The interocclusal space was bisected along an imaginary horizontal plane, and the upper castings were made to that plane (Fig. 15-25).

A wax interocclusal record of centric relation was made, and a full arch maxillary plaster index was taken for the fabrication of a full arch splint constructed in three quadrants (Fig. 15-26). The two posterior acrylic-and-gold veneer bridges were interlocked with gold dovetails into deep rest seats that existed in the cuspid restorations of the anterior porcelain-baked-to-metal restoration. Lower castings were processed to close the "gap" that existed by bisecting the imaginary plane (Fig. 15-27).

Endosseous vent-plants were then set into the

bone distal to the last abutment tooth on each side of the mandibular arch (Fig. 15-28). Two unilateral acrylic-and-gold bridges were fabricated from the impressions (Fig. 15-29). These were tried in the mouth, balanced for proper occlusion, and then cemented with oxyphosphate of zinc cement (Fig. 15-30).

Case 3
Restoring a Class III malocclusion to a Class I relationship with maxillary and mandibular blades

In Linkow's opinion, the transition from a Class III to a Class I relationship should be accomplished by using the prostheses to restrict the closure of the mandible and by leaving a freeway space between

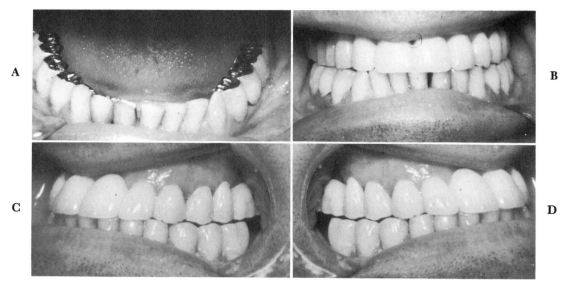

Fig. 15-30. **A,** The two mandibular unilateral partial dentures are cemented into position with hard cement. **B** to **D,** The completed case shows the elimination of the Class III malocclusion.

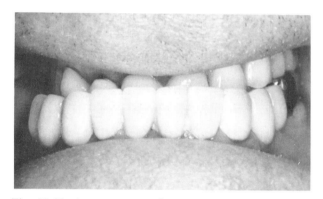

Fig. 15-31. A severe cross bite relationship.

both jaws at rest. This does not necessarily mean increasing the vertical dimension. An illustrative case is shown beginning with Fig. 15-31. The patient had previously undergone bite-raising procedures that opened his bite with removable appliances but that caused great discomfort and pain in his temporomandibular joints. His preoperative Panorex revealed very few maxillary teeth (Fig. 15-32).

Using the patient's removable denture as a platform, the operator molded a thick mix of acrylic over the denture and over the existing prepared teeth while the patient's jaw was in the most retruded position. It was imperative to maintain as close a bite as possible during this procedure in order not to increase the patient's true vertical dimension. Thus the bite was opened just enough to allow the molded max-

illary acrylic teeth to come edge to edge with the mandibular incisors. Once this had been accomplished, the temporary teeth were trimmed and polished. The physiologic rest position was immediately checked. If no rest position existed, it would have been necessary to shorten the acrylic teeth.

The patient wore the provisional splint for about 4 weeks, with no pain or discomfort. Using the "built-up" acrylic teeth on the removable denture as a bite guide, the operator fabricated impressions and castings for the teeth on the right side of the arch (Fig. 15-33). Blade implants were then placed on both sides of the maxillary arch (Fig. 15-34). All remaining mandibular teeth were prepared, and blade implants were placed in both posterior endentulous areas (Fig. 15-35).

A full arch fixed porcelain-baked-to-metal prosthesis was completed for each arch, placing the jaws in a Class I relationship (Fig. 15-36). A Panorex of the completed case shows the blade implant supports (Fig. 15-37).

Case 4
Restoring centric occlusion by occlusal reconstruction and a blade-vent

Another case of extremely poor occlusion restored with the help of an endosseous implant is that of a 46-year-old male patient. The patient, because of a traumatic injury during his childhood, was missing half of his left condyle. His maxillary

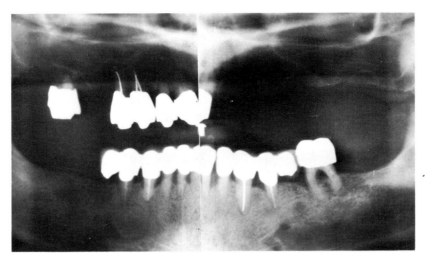

Fig. 15-32. A preoperative Panorex.

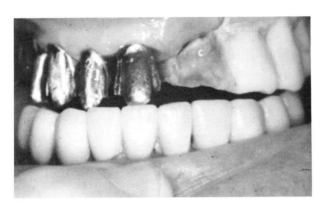

Fig. 15-33. Using the "built-up" acrylic teeth on the left side as a bite guide, metal copings were cast and fitted over the teeth on the right side.

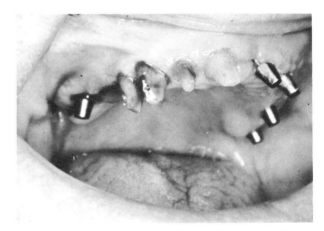

Fig. 15-34. Blade implants were implanted on both sides of the maxillary arch.

anterior quadrant of teeth had an extreme labial flare and exhibited an overjet of at least 5 mm. (Fig. 15-38). It was almost impossible for him to find his true centric relation; every time his teeth closed, they closed differently (Fig. 15-39). If it had not been for the introduction of a blade-vent into the maxillary tuberosity area to act as the posterior abutment for a full arch prosthesis, the prognosis for a fixed full arch denture would have been hopeless.

The supporting bone in both jaws, except for the bone around the left maxillary bicuspid tooth, was good. However, there was an extremely long edentulous area on the left side and an extremely wide sinus that dropped to the limit of the alveolar

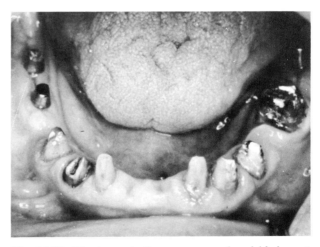

Fig. 15-35. The lower teeth were prepared and blade-vents were placed in both edentulous areas.

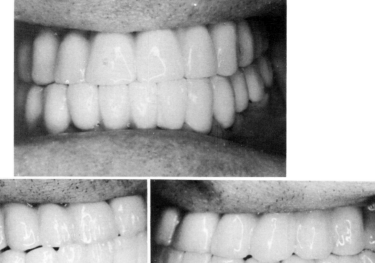

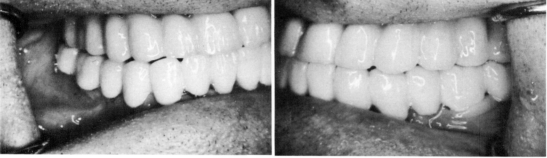

Fig. 15-36. The completed case, showing the teeth to be in a Class I relationship.

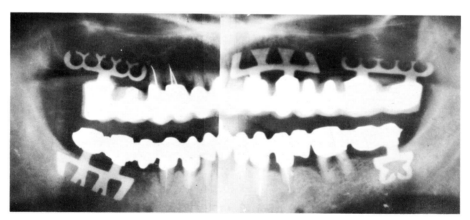

Fig. 15-37. The final Panorex.

crest. The only available bone was distal to the maxillary sinus in the maxillary tuberosity.

After careful evaluation of the radiographs, study casts, and the patient's mouth, the anterior quadrant of teeth were prepared to drastically reduce the overjet. This involved removing a great deal of the labial surfaces of these teeth, exposing the nerves and removing them, and filling the canals (Fig. 15-40).

The remaining teeth in the maxillary arch and the four lower posterior teeth on each side of the mandible were prepared. The lower anterior six teeth—being in good condition, free from caries, and with excellent bone support—were left alone.

Copper tube modeling compound impressions were taken of all the prepared teeth, as well as plaster indices and a wax interocclusal record of centric relation. The vertical dimension was not to be increased. The castings were placed on the master stone models (Fig. 15-41).

At the next visit, all metal copings were fitted over the prepared teeth (Fig. 15-42). Once again a wax interocclusal record of centric relation was made, and plaster indices were taken to pick up the copings. The laboratory procedures involved soldering the copings together and adding the pontics to fill the edentulous area on the left side of the maxilla. The last pontic was hollowed out and fitted passively over the soft tissues covering the maxillary tuberosity. The two unilateral lower pros-

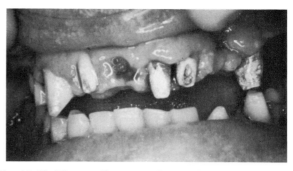

Fig. 15-40. The maxillary anterior quadrants of teeth were prepared at the expense of their labial surfaces to bring in the final tooth restorations. Root canal therapy was completed by filling the canals from the labial surfaces. The two posterior quadrants in the mandible were also prepared for full crown restorations.

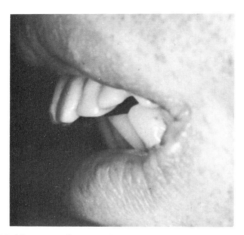

Fig. 15-38. A patient exhibiting an extreme overjet and flaring out of the anterior quadrant of teeth.

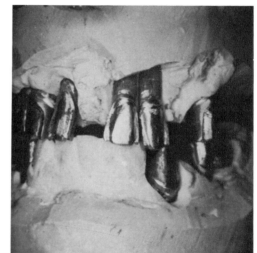

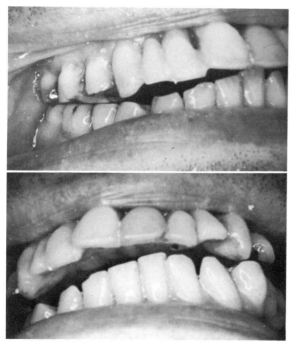

Fig. 15-39. The asymmetry of both arches is clearly visible.

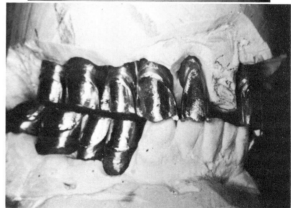

Fig. 15-41. The master articulated stone casts showing the metal copings in position over the dies. The copings were able to be lined up properly to afford a good final result.

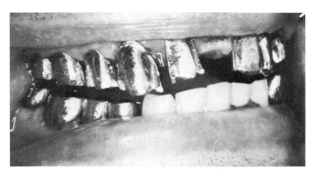

Fig. 15-42. The copings were placed over the prepared abutment teeth in both arches.

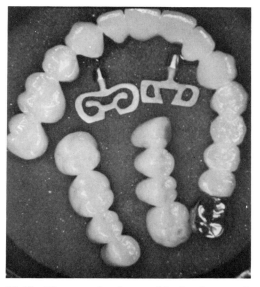

Fig. 15-43. The completed porcelain-fused-to-metal prostheses and two implants are seen.

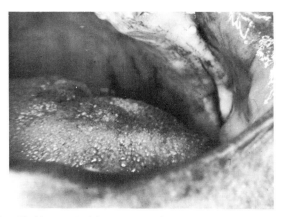

Fig. 15-44. An incision was made along the fibromucosal tissue at the crest of the ridge.

theses were then biscuit-baked with porcelain, tried in the mouth, and glazed to completion (Fig. 15-43).

The fibromucosal tissue covering the maxillary tuberosity was incised with a scapel (Fig. 15-44), the tissue reflected, and a thin groove made in the exposed bone with a No. 700L fissure bur. The blade implant was placed into the groove (Fig. 15-45) and tapped to its proper depth with a plastic-headed mallet and inserting instrument. The tissue was closed with a few interrupted sutures.

The sutures were removed (Fig. 15-46), and the full arch maxillary porcelain-fused-to-metal prosthesis was cemented with oxyphosphate of zinc cement (Fig. 15-47). The two lower posterior uni-

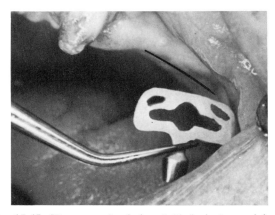

Fig. 15-45. The properly designed blade is inserted in its groove.

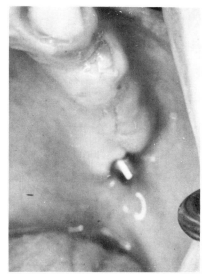

Fig. 15-46. Ten days after insertion of implant showing uneventful healing.

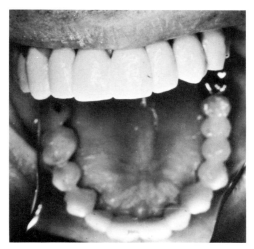

Fig. 15-47. The upper prosthesis is cemented with hard cement.

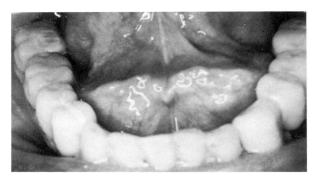

Fig. 15-48. Both lower partial dentures are also cemented into position.

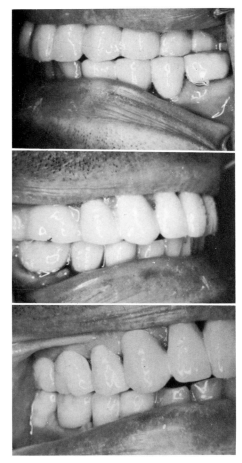

Fig. 15-49. The occlusion and overjet were greatly improved.

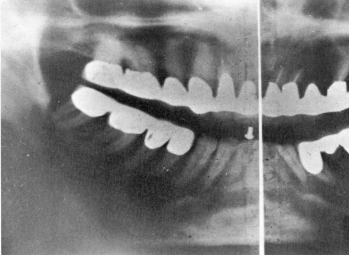
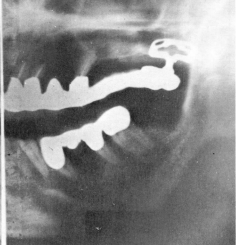

Fig. 15-50. A Panorex of the completed case.

lateral fixed partial dentures were cemented over the lower abutment teeth (Fig. 15-48).

As a result of the procedure, the patient's overjet was greatly reduced and his bite was much improved (Fig. 15-49). The patient no longer had to search for a normal centric relation position because he now automatically retruded to it. The Panorex clearly demonstrates the results (Fig. 15-50).

Case 5
Performing an apicoectomy to create space for an implant

When a post type implant cannot be introduced into the bone in a posterior edentulous maxilla because of a low-flaring sinus, a triplant intervention may be necessary. Three extremely important considerations for the triplant technique are the density of the osseous structure in the area, the depth of bone available, and the anteroposterior extension of the sinus. It is also imperative that there be enough bone in the maxillary tuberosity area for the distal triplant pin or pins. Anteriorly, there must be enough osseous tissue separating the root of the most posterior natural abutment and the floor of the maxillary sinus so that the pin can be inserted with the proper angulation and depth. Unless there is at least 2 mm. separating these two landmarks, a properly executed triplant cannot be performed; thus, such an implant is usually contraindicated. Sometimes, however, it is possible to create a space between the floor of the low-hanging maxillary sinus and the apex of the root of the last tooth by reducing the length of the root with an apicoectomy. The following case describes such a procedure.

The patient, a healthy woman in her early fifties, desired a fixed rather than a removable partial denture to replace her missing maxillary molars.

Periapical intraoral radiographs of the maxillary right bicuspid teeth and of the edentulous posterior area were taken, as was a Panorex radiograph. The results disclosed that the anterior extension of the floor of the maxillary sinus was in direct contact with the apex of the root of the upper second bicuspid tooth. The x-rays also revealed that successful root canal therapy had been performed on the second bicuspid tooth.

Upon examining the mouth clinically, the two bicuspid teeth were found to have very short clinical

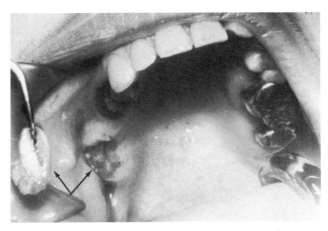

Fig. 15-52. Since there was no interocclusal space between the last lower molar and fibromucosal tissue in the maxilla that existed distal to the cantilevered molar, a large portion of the thickened fibromucosal tissue that was contacting the lower molar was removed surgically *(arrows)*.

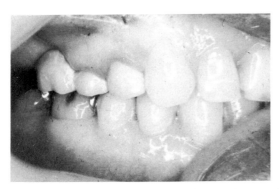

Fig. 15-51. The patient could not function any longer with her upper three-unit fixed partial denture using the two bicuspids and a cantilevered molar, which was driven into the fibromucosal tissue, as the abutments.

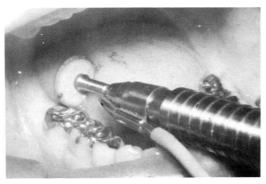

Fig. 15-53. The occlusal surface of the last molar inlay was also reduced.

crowns. Additionally, and most importantly, the mucoperiosteal tissue along the alveolar crest posterior to the second bicuspid tooth was so thick that it was in direct contact with the somewhat extruded lower right molar tooth (Fig. 15-51). This made it impossible to place any teeth in the area without treatment.

On the first operative visit, the short crowns of both maxillary bicuspid teeth were lengthened by electrosurgically removing the soft tissue. The two teeth were then prepared for veneer crown restorations. The thick and protruding fibromucosal tissue extending below the alveolar ridge in the posterior edentulous area was reduced almost to the underlying bone with a scapel and electrosurgery (Fig. 15-52). The partially exfoliated mandibular molar was also reduced occlusally by judicious grinding of the gold inlay covering it (Fig. 15-53).

Copper band impressions, a wax interocclusal record of centric relation, a plaster index, and an alginate (irreversible hydrocolloid) impression of the lower jaw were taken of the bicuspid teeth. Temporary crown forms were placed over the prepared abutment teeth, and the patient was dismissed.

To allow adequate healing of the treated soft tissues, almost 2 weeks lapsed between visits (Fig. 15-54). Then the temporary crown forms were removed, and the veneer castings were tried over the maxillary bicuspid teeth. All necessary occlusal and gingival adjustments were made.

A wax interocclusal record of centric relation and a plaster index, which included the two crowns as well as the entire edentulous area, were taken. The index was then articulated with the previously poured lower stone model, and from this master

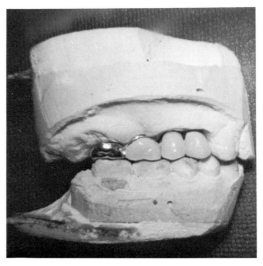

Fig. 15-55. A prefabricated unilateral four-unit veneer type bridge seen on the model.

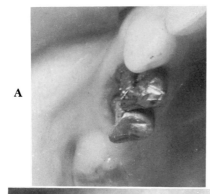

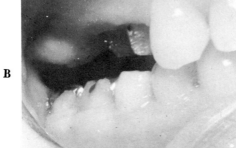

Fig. 15-54. The tissue as it appeared 2 weeks after surgery. Enough space was created to include an upper implant and second molar.

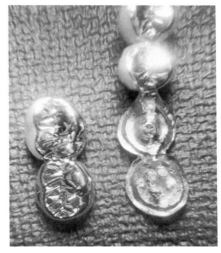

Fig. 15-56. Posteriorly, a scalloped template and two-unit superstructure are seen.

model the completed fixed denture was constructed (Fig. 15-55). The prosthesis contained the two veneer crowns and their acrylic facings. Distal to the second bicuspid crown and fixed to it was a scalloped template with a few protruding vertical pin heads (Fig. 15-56). The superstructure was also prefabricated. For this case, it consisted of two molar crowns cast in one piece, which fit exactly over the template (Fig. 15-57).

On the third visit, the bicuspid veneer crowns with the extended template were fitted over the prepared teeth, and the occlusion was checked. All adjustments were completed prior to inserting the superstructure. With the superstructure in place, the occlusion was carefully checked and corrected. It was then removed, leaving the template in position.

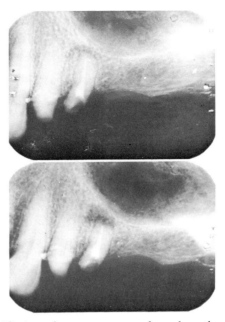

Fig. 15-59. An apicoectomy was performed on the root tip to make room between it and the antral floor. (From Linkow, L.I.: Atypical implantations for anatomically contraindicated situations, Dent. Concepts, Fall, 1967.)

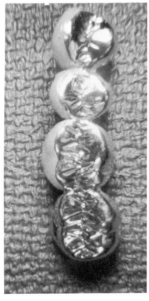

Fig. 15-57. The two-unit molar superstructure fits exactly over the underlying template.

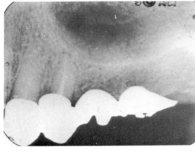

Fig. 15-58. The second premolar root is touching the floor of the maxillary sinus.

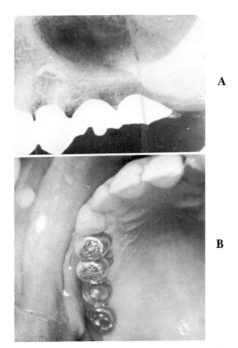

A

B

Fig. 15-60. A, The framework was fitted into position and radiographed in order to determine where to drill the holes in the template to accommodate the pin implants. B, The framework was cemented into position over the two anterior bicuspid preparations after the holes were made through the template outside the mouth.

An intraoral x-ray, which included the floor of the maxillary sinus and the apex of the second bicuspid tooth, was taken (Fig. 15-58). The scalloped template with its two anterior bicuspid crowns was then removed.

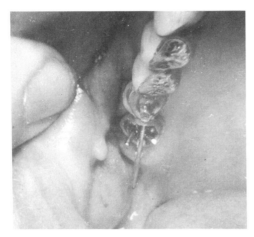

Fig. 15-61. The pin implants were then driven through the template one by one, circumventing the maxillary sinus in an anteroposterior direction.

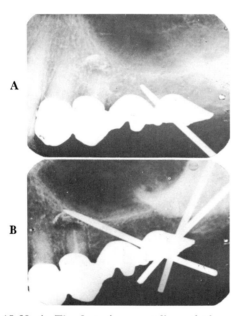

Fig. 15-62. A, The first pin was radiographed a number of times in order to be certain that it would be driven between the tooth apex and the floor of the sinus. B, The periapical radiograph showing the three pins in their proper positions. The ends protruding through the template were cut short so that they would not interfere with the fitting of the superstructure. (From Linkow, L. I.: Atypical implantations for anatomically contraindicated situations, Dent. Concepts, Fall, 1967.)

The positions of the three triplant pin holes to be made in the template were determined from the x-rays and were made with a No. 557 fissure bur. The holes were angled in the template in the same direction as the implant pins were to be directed. The holes were made large enough to avoid interference with the angulation of the pins. Otherwise the template, pins, or both could have become distorted, causing constant pressure in the area.

To make room for the triplant pin, the apicoectomy was then performed. Great care was taken not to injure the floor of the sinus (Fig. 15-59). The bicuspid crowns with the extending template were cemented with hard cement over the bicuspid preparations (Fig. 15-60). The implant pins were slowly driven through the template and deep in-

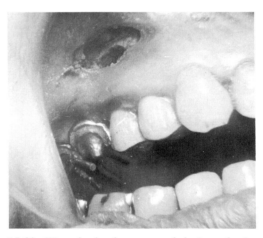

Fig. 15-63. The pin implants extended through the scalloped template. High up in the maxillary tissue is seen the exposed bone and area where the apicoectomy was performed.

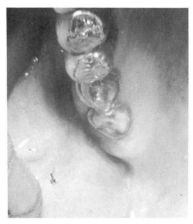

Fig. 15-64. The three pins were locked to each other and to the template with acrylic.

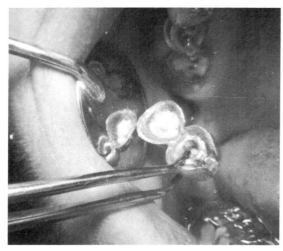

Fig. 15-65. The superstructure was then cemented over the built-up acrylic core and gold post extending from the template.

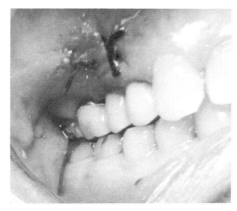

Fig. 15-66. The occlusion was once again checked. Sutures were used to close the wound.

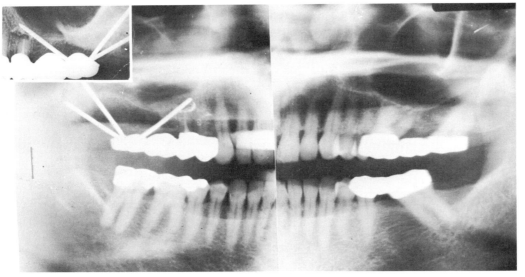

Fig. 15-67. A Panorex and intraoral radiograph showing the completed case. (From Linkow, L. I.: Atypical implantations for anatomically contraindicated situations, Dent. Concepts, Fall, 1967.)

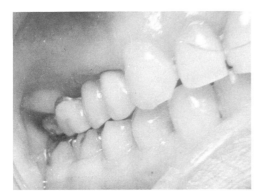

Fig. 15-68. Three weeks later, the tissue looks excellent.

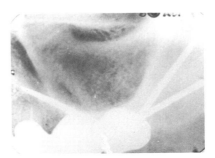

Fig. 15-69. An 18-month postoperative x-ray shows filling-in of bone and the implant in excellent condition.

to the bone (Fig. 15-61). During this procedure, radiographs were taken to guide the operator in directing the pins around the sinus (Fig. 15-62). By not suturing the soft tissue covering the area of the root resection, the anterior pin was clinically visible as it traversed the bone void separating the sinus floor from the shortened root (Fig. 15-63).

The excess was cut off the protruding pins, and the remaining ends were carefully notched with a fissure bur for added retention during their fusion with acrylic. The protruding pins were then fused together with cold cure acrylic, using the brush-on technique (Fig. 15-64). Only a minimum amount of acrylic was used, to avoid interference with the fitting of the superstructure. The superstructure was tried on before the acrylic hardened (Fig. 15-65). This ensured that only a minimum amount of adjustment was necessary when cementing on the superstructure.

The superstructure was then cemented over the template. Oxyphosphate of zinc cement was used

inside the crown covering the gold post extending from the template, and acrylic was used inside the crown fitting over the acrylic core. When the cement hardened, it was trimmed. Sutures were placed in the area of the apicoectomy (Fig. 15-66). Roentgenograms were taken (Fig. 15-67).

The sutures covering the area of the apicoectomy were removed a week later. Three weeks later the tissue had completely healed (Fig. 15-68). Eighteen months after surgery, x-rays showed the healed site (Fig. 15-69).

This case was an unusual approach to providing room for a proper triplant. The fact that the second bicuspid tooth had previous root canal therapy helped the operator decide on an apicoectomy. However, such an approach can become an almost routine procedure if the operator decides it is beneficial to the patient to devitalize a tooth in order to provide a fixed partial denture for a posterior edentulous area. An alternative, and better, approach for such a problem is to insert a blade-vent in the maxillary tuberosity. This involves no devitalization of teeth and gives added security for a fixed partial denture.

Case 6
Using the zygomatic arch as an implant site

There have been unique and uncommon situations in which a patient has no normal type of occlusion and cannot tolerate a removable appliance. In the following case, the woman had multiple anomalies that made conventional removable dentures impossible.

The patient had five remaining maxillary teeth—the left central incisor, the left second molar, and the right central, lateral, and cuspid teeth (Fig. 15-70). Furthermore, her right maxillary ridge was practically nonexistent; if teeth were constructed to

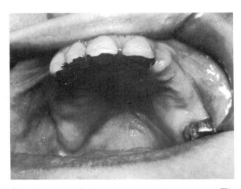

Fig. 15-70. The remaining upper teeth are seen. The alveolar bone in the right posterior quadrant was completely resorbed buccolingually to such an extent that the original ridge crest was so far lingual to the lower ridge that the upper teeth were completely lingual to the lower ones, with no contact.

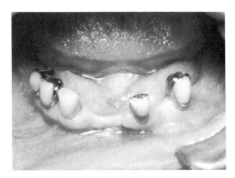

Fig. 15-71. The five remaining lower teeth.

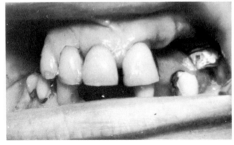

Fig. 15-72. From an anterior view both lower right bicuspids are seen to extend buccally far more than the resorbed opposing maxillary ridge.

contact the center of this ridge, they would completely fall lingually and not meet the opposing teeth.

The patient's remaining mandibular teeth included the right cuspid, first and second bicuspids, the left cuspid, and the second bicuspid (Fig. 15-71). When her lower jaw was retruded to centric occlusion, her right mandibular teeth were extend-

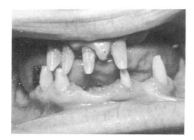

Fig. 15-73. Both arches of teeth were prepared together.

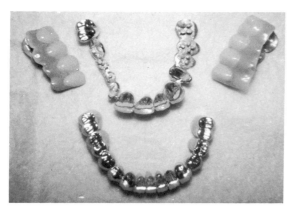

Fig. 15-74. A prefabricated lower full arch acrylic-facing-gold occlusal prosthesis was fabricated. The upper arch included bilateral templates and superstructures with pink acrylic saddles to build the arch out buccally.

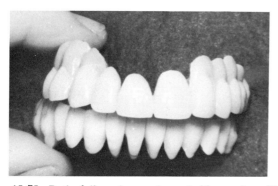

Fig. 15-75. Both full arch prostheses held together. The maxillary superstructures are seen fitted over the corresponding scalloped templates.

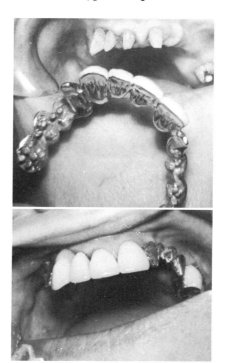

Fig. 15-76. The upper prosthesis was cemented into position.

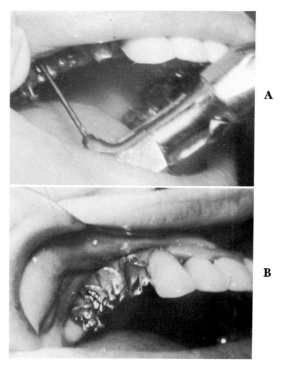

Fig. 15-77. A, Pin implants were carefully driven through the template and angulated in such a manner as to end deep in the zygomatic arch. B, The pins were then shortened and notched.

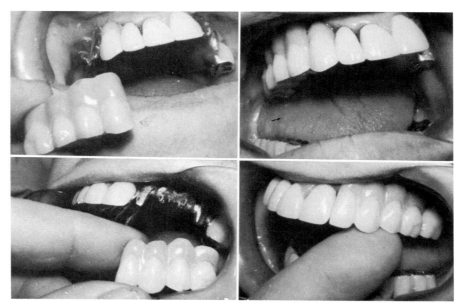

Fig. 15-78. The superstructures were tried.

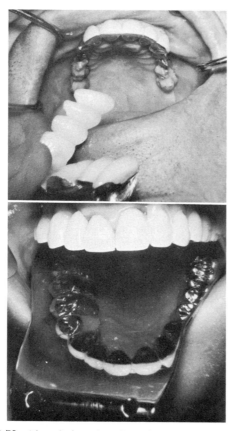

Fig. 15-79. After fusing the pins with acrylic, both super-structures were cemented with hard cement over the templates.

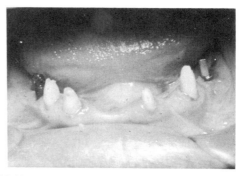

Fig. 15-80. Implant posts were placed in both posterior edentulous areas in the mandible.

ing buccally much further than her opposing resorbed and narrower maxillary ridge (Fig. 15-72). Obviously, an unusual approach was necessary.

The teeth were prepared for full crown coverage restorations (Fig. 15-73), and all necessary plaster indices and a wax interocclusal record of centric relation were taken for the completion of a prefabricated bridgework. This bridgework consisted of a lower full arch acrylic-and-gold splint, and an upper full arch splint including a bilateral scalloped template with two superstructures (Fig. 15-74). The template on the right side was built out buccally to contact the mucosal tissue covering the inferior portion of the zygoma. Its superstructure included an acrylic-and-gold veneer crown bridge with a buccal flange of pink resin to extend the right side of the

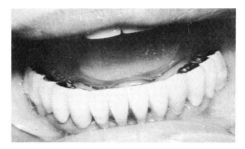

Fig. 15-81. The lower prosthesis was also cemented.

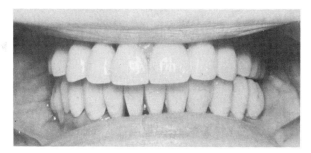

Fig. 15-82. The anterior view of the completed case.

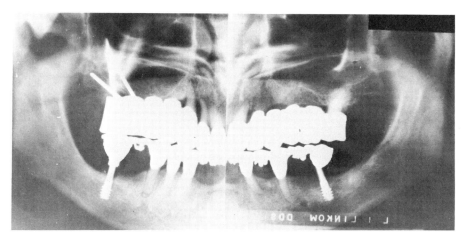

Fig. 15-83. A Panorex showing the pins extending into the zygomatic arch.

patient's face (Fig. 15-75). The left superstructure also included a pink acrylic buccal flange. The prosthesis was tried in the mouth.

The exact location of the zygomatic arch was determined. (In this case, study skulls and x-rays were used as determinants. Today, however, reflecting the soft tissues to expose the bone is the preferable approach.) Upon determination of the zygomatic arch, holes were made through the template in the direction the pins were to be driven. Then the prosthesis was cemented over the teeth with oxyphosphate of zinc cement (Fig. 15-76). Pin implants were slowly driven through the template in an acute buccal direction in order to enter the zygomatic arch (Fig. 15-77). During pin insertion, x-rays were taken at various intervals to ensure accurate placement.

The superstructures were tried in the mouth (Fig. 15-78) and articulated. Both superstructures were then removed. The pins were fused together with acrylic, and the superstructures were reinserted and cemented (Fig. 15-79).

Endosseous post implants were set into the man-

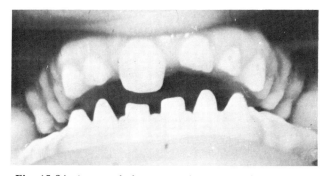

Fig. 15-84. A case of almost complete anodontia of the permanent teeth.

dible (Fig. 15-80) and the lower prosthesis cemented into position (Fig. 15-81). Final adjustments for proper articulation were accomplished in the mouth (Fig. 15-82). A Panorex shows the case in the mouth (Fig. 15-83).

To date, 5 years later, the fixed full arch denture has been more than satisfactory. The patient has had no pain or discomfort and is much happier than she was with her former restoration.

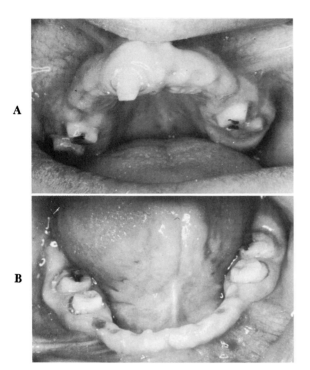

Fig. 15-85. A, The only remaining maxillary teeth were the right central incisor and both 12-year molars, which were prepared for full crown restorations. Also seen are two deciduous second molars that were to be kept. B, Only two deciduous second molars and two permanent 12-year molars remained in the lower arch.

Case 7
Full mouth fixed dentures for partial anodontia

A 17-year-old boy was extremely upset over the condition of his mouth. He had only five permanent teeth: the maxillary right central incisor and the mandibular and maxillary right and left 12-year molars. His other teeth were deciduous and beginning to loosen (Fig. 15-84). Radiographic examination revealed no other permanent tooth buds.

All the deciduous teeth, except the four deciduous E's, were removed. The reason for retaining the deciduous E's was to maintain the buccolingual width of the alveolar bone. The ridges where the other deciduous teeth were extracted were completely knife-edged but camouflaged with a thick covering of fibromucosa.

All remaining teeth were prepared for full coverage restorations (Fig. 15-85). Four blade implants were carefully set into the knife-edge ridges—two in each arch—and the sites sutured closed (Fig. 15-86).

After 5 days the sutures were removed (Fig. 15-87). The tissue-bearing surfaces of the pontics were checked for impingement and all necessary adjustments made. The prosthesis were cemented into position, and the occlusion was carefully checked and balanced (Fig. 15-88).

The preoperative Panorex compared with the postoperative film is a good summary of the case

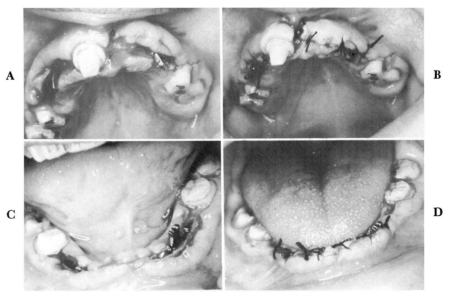

Fig. 15-86. A, Blade implants were placed into the bone on both sides of the maxilla. B, The tissues were sutured. C, Two blade implants were tapped into the mandibular bone. D, The tissues were sutured.

(Fig. 15-89). The formerly depressed and embarrassed boy is now thrilled, happy, and healthy.

Case 8
Orthodontia aided by implants

In this case, a young adult with a Class II malocclusion was restored to a normal Class I relationship without the bother of an extraoral head or neck appliance, which is not practical in public. This patient had lost her left posterior mandibular teeth (Fig. 15-90). The implant, a blade-vent, was inserted into the edentulous area (Fig. 15-91). The nearest remaining teeth, having been prepared for full crown coverage, were used as natural abutments

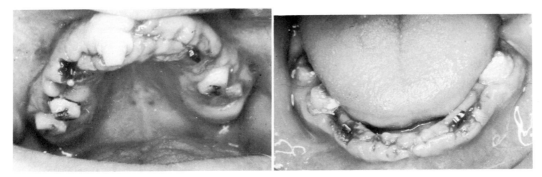

Fig. 15-87. Five days postoperatively, immediately after removal of the sutures.

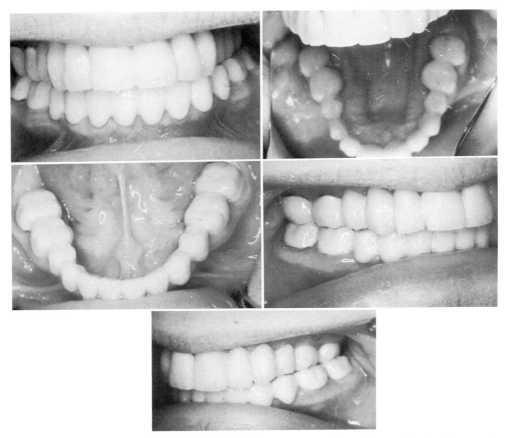

Fig. 15-88. The completed case included upper and lower full arch porcelain-fused-to-metal dentures.

for a fixed partial denture. A buccal tube was processed to the buccal surface of the crown covering the implant (Fig. 15-92).

The intermaxillary rubber band extended from the maxillary hook attached to the labial arch wire back to the buccal tube on the mandibular crown covering the implant (Fig. 15-93). It was worn 24 hours a day, thus speeding the reduction of the over-bite and overjet.

This case might also have been treated in the following manner. The implant could have been stabilized to the nearest natural tooth by banding both the tooth and the implant post and extending a .040 rigid wire between them, soldering it to the

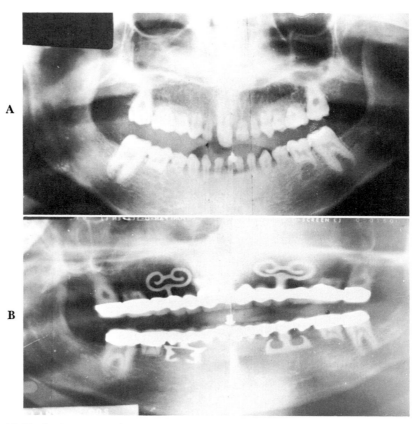

Fig. 15-89. **A,** A preoperative Panorex shows the only five permanent teeth. All others were deciduous. **B,** The Panorex of the completed case, showing the blades.

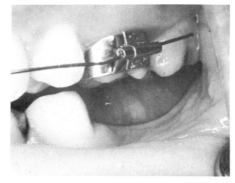

Fig. 15-90. A lower edentulous posterior area with an upper arch wire and molar band with buccal tube is seen.

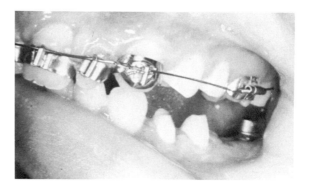

Fig. 15-91. The blade implant post is seen protruding through the fibromucosal tissue. The two bicuspid teeth were prepared for full crown restorations.

inside of buccal tubes (Fig. 15-94). The rest of the procedure follows that described previously.

Case 9
Using a single tooth blade implant supported by a labial arch appliance

A young girl undergoing orthodontic treatment for malocclusion lost her maxillary central incisor in an accident. Her orthodontist utilized the lost incisor as a space maintainer by removing the root at the cementoenamel junction and banding the remaining coronal portion with a twin arch band ligated to the labial arch wire (Fig. 15-95). This held the tooth in position for 3 years, at which time it became necessary to replace this temporary device since orthodontic treatment was nearing completion. Because the girl's anterior teeth were caries-free, her parents were reluctant to have them prepared for full crown coverage, especially at such an early age. Thus a single tooth implant intervention was discussed and agreed upon.

A specially designed single tooth blade implant was inserted, and the wound was closed with two small sutures. The coronal portion of the original tooth, which was exactly the same color as the other anterior teeth, was hollowed out to fit loosely over the implant post, thus permitting easy alignment in

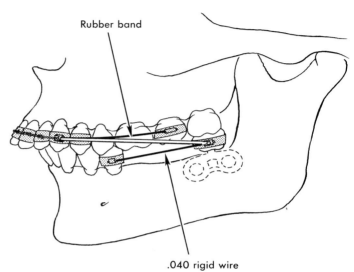

Fig. 15-94. A diagram of another way to accomplish the same results. The rubber band extends from the maxillary hook, which is attached to the labial arch wire in the region of the cuspid, to the buccal tube, which is attached to the buccal surface of the crown covering the implant in the edentulous molar area. In order to stabilize and splint the implant to the anterior abutment tooth so that it can be strong enough to serve as an anchor for the distal movement of the anterior and posterior quadrant of maxillary teeth, a rigid .040 wire is soldered to the inside of the buccal tubes of both abutments. In this case, the bicuspid tooth was also banded and the buccal tube soldered to it.

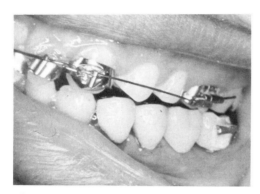

Fig. 15-92. A four-unit bridge was cemented over the two bicuspid teeth and implant post. The last crown had a buccal tube attached.

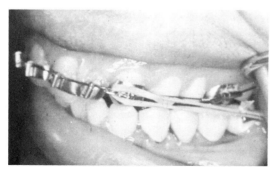

Fig. 15-93. Distal movement of the posterior quadrant of teeth can now be managed using the implant as the intraoral anchorage. In this manner the patient, being an adult, did not have to use an extraoral head or neck band.

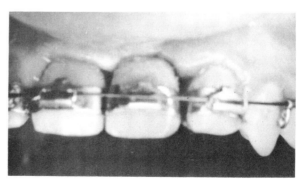

Fig. 15-95. The coronal portion of the left central incisor was attached to the labial arch wire. No root portion of the tooth existed. (From Linkow, L. I.: The endosseous blade implant and its use in orthodontics, Int. J. Orthodont. 8[4]:149-154, 1969.)

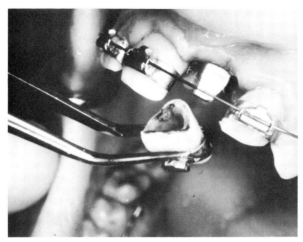

Fig. 15-96. The tooth was hollowed out to accept the protruding post. (From Linkow, L. I.: The endosseous blade implant and its use in orthodontics, Int. J. Orthodont. 8[4]:149-154, 1969.)

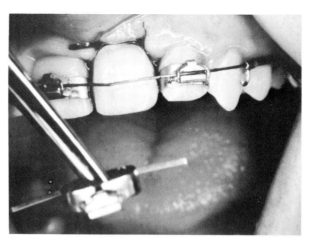

Fig. 15-97. A band containing a labial bracket and two rigid lingual arms was fitted to the left central incisor. (From Linkow, L. I.: The endosseous blade implant and its use in orthodontics, Int. J. Orthodont. 8[4]:149-154, 1969.)

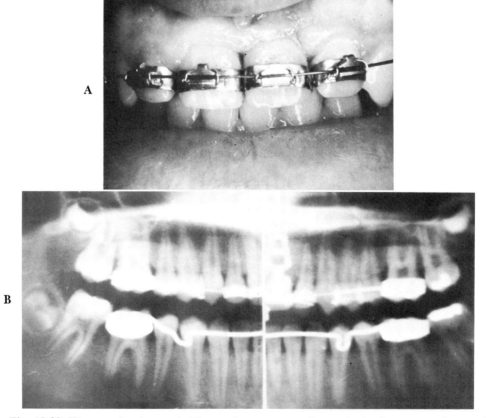

Fig. 15-98. The completed case. **A,** The tooth was cemented over the implant post and secured to the arch wire. **B,** The Panorex roentgenogram of the completed case. (From Linkow, L. I.: The endosseous blade implant and its use in orthodontics, Int. J. Orthodont. 8[4]:149-154, 1969.)

the arch (Fig. 15-96). After cleansing with peroxide, the hollowed-out interior was packed with a filling material that takes on the same shade as the tooth.* The crown was replaced, positioned properly, and removed before the material hardened. After hardening in hot water for 5 minutes, the tooth was refitted and readjusted. A twin arch band with a rigid wire extending lingually to the center of each neighboring tooth was provided by the orthodontist (Fig. 15-97).

*Adaptic, made by Johnson & Johnson, New Brunswick, N. J.

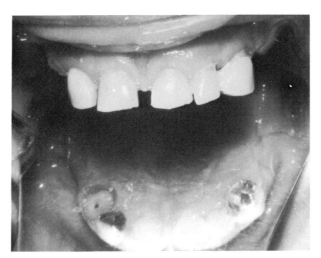

Fig. 15-99. A maxillary arch with six loose teeth and a large anterior diastema.

The band was cemented over the original tooth crown with hard cement, and the crown was cemented over the implant post. After removing the hardened excess cement, the natural tooth crown was ligated with .010 stainless steel to the labial arch wire for support during bone regeneration (Fig. 15-98).

Case 10
Restoring a maxillary arch with a large anterior diastema

Dealing with a large space between two maxillary incisors is particularly difficult when the few remaining anterior teeth are periodontally involved. A cumbersome removable appliance would seriously threaten such teeth. As for the diastema, the patient may be used to it and also fear that obliterating the gap will make the central incisors undesirably large and bulky. In such a situation, Linkow uses posterior blade type implants to permit full arch splinting and yet still maintain the anterior diastema.

In this case there are six anterior periodontally involved teeth, including only a root of the right cuspid, and a large diastema between both central incisors (Fig. 15-99). The teeth were prepared, and castings made with palatal extensions emanating from the lingual shoulders of the central incisor copings. The copings were not over-built to close the diastema.

The castings were fitted in the mouth and a wax

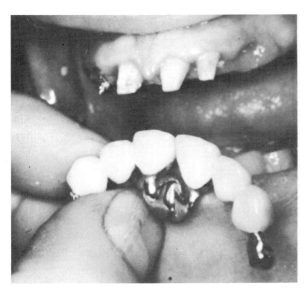

Fig. 15-100. The anterior restoration—both quadrants joined by a palatal plate—was fitted in the mouth. The diastema was still present.

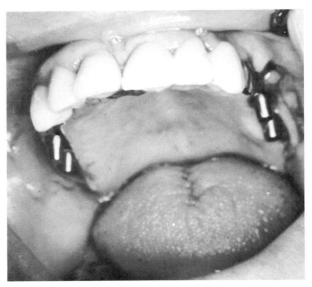

Fig. 15-101. Blade implants were set into the two posterior edentulous areas.

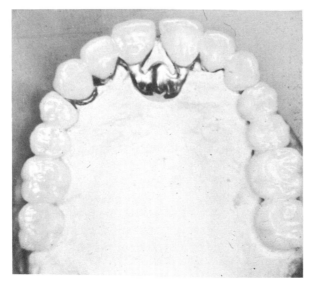

Fig. 15-102. The two posterior segments fit over the anterior cantilevered thimble posts and over the protruding implant posts. Note the palatal connecting plate.

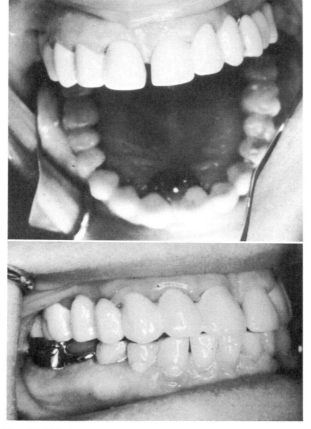

Fig. 15-103. The three sections were cemented in with hard cement, and the occlusion was carefully balanced.

bite taken. From the master stone model the anterior prosthesis was fabricated in porcelain baked to metal. The left and right quadrants were joined with a palatal plate soldered to both palatal extensions and designed to fit passively over the soft tissues. Two gold cantilevered, thimble type pontics extended distally from each side of the anterior restoration (Fig. 15-100).

The anterior prosthesis was fitted over the anterior tooth preparations, and then blade implants were placed into both posterior edentulous areas (Fig. 15-101). After healing, a full mouth, hydrocolloid impression was taken, accurately duplicating the implant posts and the cantilevered thimble pontics. The two posterior unilateral fixed partial dentures were processed (Fig. 15-102). The finished bridges were then cemented in the mouth and the occlusion carefully balanced (Fig. 15-103).

Several advantages are gained by the method described. The restored central incisors can be kept relatively narrow mesiodistally and the diastema maintained. All anterior teeth can be splinted to one another by the soldered castings and palatal connecting plate. The posterior implant abutments permit stabilizing the anterior quadrant of teeth with a full arch fixed prosthesis. The full arch fixed restoration also greatly reduces buccolingual movements of the posterior implants, as well as labiolingual movements of the anterior teeth.

Case 11
Designing restorations for a patient with a severe brux habit

The anterior mandibular teeth of a 57-year-old man were worn down well into the dentin from

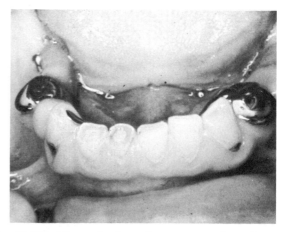

Fig. 15-104. The patient's teeth were worn down from severe bruxism.

severe bruxism (Fig. 15-104). The patient had been wearing a stainless steel lingual bar type removable denture to replace posterior teeth on both sides of his mandible. His completely edentulous maxilla was restored with his fifth conventional denture, the previous four having been broken by grinding.

The remaining mandibular teeth were prepared for full crown restorations, and blade implants were placed in both posterior edentulous areas (Fig. 15-105). A full arch fixed prosthesis was fabricated and cemented over the implants and teeth (Fig. 15-106).

Because there was not enough bone for implants, the new maxillary prosthesis was a full arch removable denture. This denture contained acrylic teeth and a cast gold palate to resist breakage.

It was decided to open the bite. Because some wearing away of the acrylic maxillary teeth was anticipated, the posterior maxillary teeth were made slightly longer than the anticipated distance that the bite was to be opened. Once wear patterns had been established, gold onlays were planned.

After approximately 4 months, facets appeared on the occlusal surfaces of the acrylic teeth of the maxillary denture. After taking an alginate impression of the entire denture, the occlusal surfaces of all maxillary teeth were reduced 1½ mm. To ensure that the onlays would be perfectly set, parallel vertical holes were made in each tooth to accept readymade plastic pins. The teeth were thoroughly lubricated and the pins inserted.

Melted blue inlay wax was poured into the alginate impression of the original occlusal surfaces, and the alginate impression was quickly placed over the denture with its newly reduced teeth. When the wax had cooled, the resulting pattern was an exact replica of the worn occlusal pattern of the teeth. The entire wax pattern with the attached plastic pins was removed, sprued, and cast in gold. It was then cemented into position over the prepared acrylic denture teeth (Fig. 15-107). The denture was fitted in the mouth, and the articulation was once again carefully checked for any prematurities (Fig. 15-108).

Case 12
Stabilizing a fixed bridge over a long edentulous span

When the terminal abutment tooth or teeth supporting a fixed bridge have lost a great deal of bone

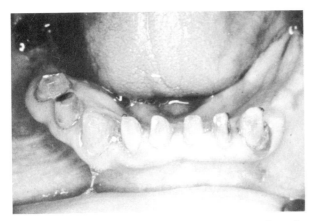

Fig. 15-105. The mandibular teeth were prepared, and a blade implant was placed posteriorly on each side of the mandible.

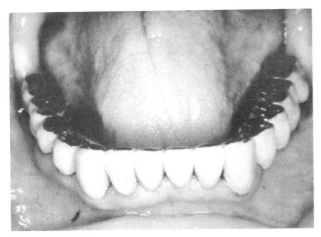

Fig. 15-106. The full arch fixed prosthesis cemented in position.

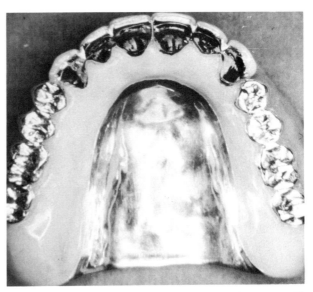

Fig. 15-107. The maxillary denture contained a cast gold palate and acrylic teeth with gold occlusal surfaces.

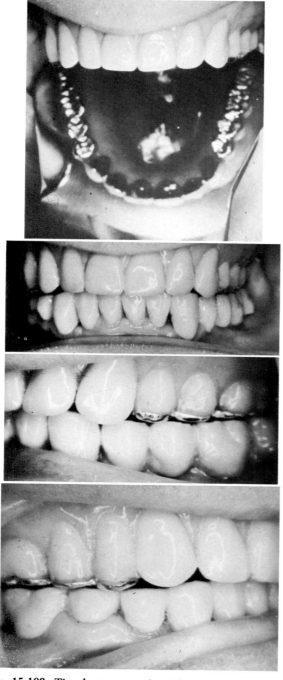

Fig. 15-108. The denture was fitted in the mouth and articulated with the lower prosthesis.

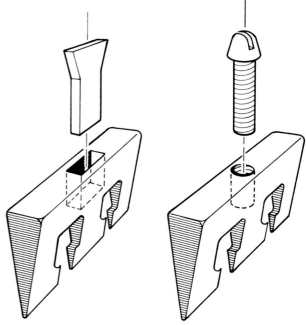

Fig. 15-109. Two different types of bridge-stabilizing blade implants. After the body of the blade has been seated in bone, the post—either a rectangular slip-in shaft (left) or a modified screw (right)—is inserted.

and loosened, it may be possible to stabilize the bridge without removing it. Two things are needed: a fairly long edentulous span and a specially constructed blade. This blade differs from other blade designs primarily in that its abutment post is removable (Fig. 15-109). Because a blade without a post is short, it is relatively easy to maneuver in tight spots.

The basic bridge stabilizing technique is accomplished in the following manner, as exemplified by a mandibular case (Fig. 15-110). First, the fibromucosal tissues are incised just inferior to the tissue-bearing surface of the pontics and retracted to expose the bony ridge. Second, a groove is made to accept the entire depth of the blade, and the blade is tapped in until its shoulder is buried 1 to 2 mm. below the alveolar crest. At this stage it may be necessary to remove the buccogingival third of the pontic for better access to the implant site.

Third, the tissue-bearing surface of the pontic is hollow-ground with a round or fissure bur, taking care not to cut through the occlusal surface. Fourth, the abutment post is inserted into the body of the blade. Fifth, cold cure acrylic resin is brushed into the pontic to fill the hole and secure the post. The

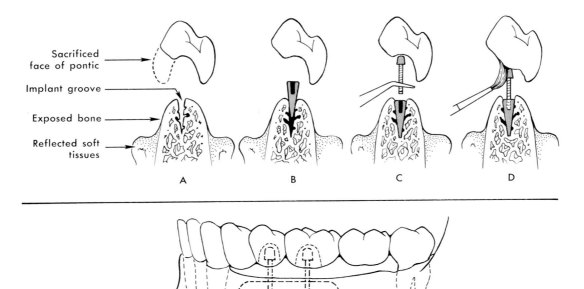

Sacrificed
face of pontic

Implant groove

Exposed bone

Reflected soft
tissues

A   B   C   D

Fig. 15-110. Fixed bridge stabilization procedure when a terminal abutment tooth has loosened. **A,** The groove has been prepared for the implant. It was necessary to remove the bucco-gingival third of the pontic to approach the bone properly. The pontic was also hollowed out at the same time. **B,** The special blade is set into the prepared groove. **C,** After the blade has been tapped into the bone, its abutment post (in this case, a screw) is inserted. **D,** Cold cure acrylic resin is brushed on to secure the post and to rebuild the pontic. *Lateral view* shows a double-posted implant used as a fixed bridge stabilizer.

face of the pontic, if removed, is also restored. When the acrylic hardens, it is carefully trimmed and polished. Finally, the incised tissues are cleansed and rejoined with sutures, which are removed in about 1 week. The loose terminal abutment teeth—as well as the bridge—are now stabilized.

FUTURE APPLICATIONS FOR ENDOSSEOUS IMPLANTS

Because endosseous implant techniques have been so successful in fixed denture situations and in providing the only solution in some atypical cases,

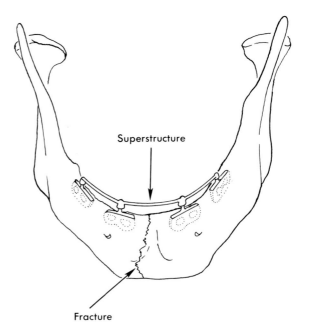

Fig. 15-111. Diagram of a proposed method of stabilizing a fracture in an edentulous mandible. After blades are placed on both sides of the fracture, it is reduced. An elastic impression of the implant posts is taken while the fractured elements are held firmly in their proper relationship. From the impression a fixed superstructure is fabricated and cemented with hard cement over the posts. The superstructure splint holds the joined ends of the fracture and immobilizes them until healing takes place, 6 to 8 weeks later.

Superstructure

Fracture

it is hoped that more and more operators will expand the horizons of these useful devices. Among some of the areas currently being investigated are the following.

Pedodontics. The child who has just lost his central or lateral incisor as a result of traumatic injury can be helped by an endodontic root stabilizer. The tooth may be replaced in its socket and stabilized by the endodontic pin. The pin gives immediate support and also may help retain the tooth, if and when its root resorbs. A long and narrow single tooth blade can be used where an incisor tooth had been lost for several months, after the socket has healed.

Tripod implants may be used as space maintainers, thereby involving no other teeth, as is the case with routine space-maintaining procedures. If used for such a purpose, the operator should be very careful that the deepest portions of the triplant pins completely circumvent the crowns of unerupted permanent bicuspid teeth.

Periodontia. Unfortunately, when only two or three loose teeth are all that remain in a dental arch, the periodontist is at a disadvantage. After he treats these teeth, eliminates the inflammatory tissue, and reduces existing infrabony pockets, he knows that a removable prosthesis will only promote the future loss of these teeth. Even if the few remaining teeth are splinted to one another, the removable appliance will eventually cause the splinted teeth to loosen. If,

however, these teeth can be splinted with a full arch fixed denture supported by strategically placed implants firmly embedded in bone, the long-term prognosis would certainly be more optimistic.

Oral surgery. Endosseous implants of the blade type can be strategically placed on both sides of a fracture in a completely edentulous jaw. After the fracture has been reduced, the implants can be stabilized with a fixed superstructure to immobilize it (Fig. 15-111). By this technique it may not be necessary to inconvenience the patient with an external fixation method.

Miscellaneous uses. The psychologically disturbed patient who cannot tolerate the thought of a removable complete denture or partial prosthesis may be satisfied with implants combined with a fixed denture or palateless removable maxillary dentures with internal "clip-on" attachments. Feelings of self-assurance, confidence, and youthfulness are just a few of the benefits derived from the introduction of implants.

Implants may also play a very important role in the lives of those unfortunate patients who, either from birth or later, were striken with some debilitating disease. Since they are unable to insert or care for a removable appliance, their comfort and health may be improved by the introduction of endosseous implants utilized as abutments for fixed bridgework.

Bibliography

Abata, A.: The study of tissue reaction to a magnetic metal implant, University of Chicago, 1961, Dissertation.

Abel, H.: Die Befestigung implantierten Porzellan, Zbl. Rundschau. 22:869, 1934.

Abrezol, R. P.: Système d'attachement pour fixation des prosthèses complètes du bas sur deux piliers implantés, Rev. Implant., No. 3, April, 1958.

Achard and Benaim: Implant tubulaire endo-osseux, Rev. Franc. Odontostomat., 1961.

Achdjian, A.: Modified implant technique, Lebanese Dent. Mag. 5:139-143, 1955.

Ackermann, F.: Le mécanisme des machoires, Paris, 1952, Masson & Cie, Editeurs.

Ackermann, F.: Biostatica delle protesis totali su impianti metallici sottopriostali, Actualities Odontostomat., No. 46, 1959.

Ackermann, F.: Equilibrium with subperiosteal complete denture implants, J. Prosth. Dent. 9:1049-1055, 1959.

Ackermann, F.: La prosthèse complète non implantée; les solutions et ses impassés actuelles, Rev. Franc. Odontostomat. 7(5):707, 1960.

Ackermann, F.: Principe et technique à la base des prosthèses á prolongement, Actualites Odontostomat., 1960.

Ackermann, H.: Un nouveau moyen de retention pour prosthèses à cavaliers, Rev. Suisse Odont., November, 1957.

Ackermann, R.: Résultats après un an de pratique hôpitalière des implants aiguilles, Rev. Odontostomat. 7(5):707, 1960.

Ackermann, R.: Un cours d'implantologie-aiguille, Rev. Odontoimplant., No. 2, June, 1966.

Adams, D. F.: Implant therapy of infrabony pockets, J. West. Soc. Periodont., Vol. 14, 1966.

Adisman, J. K.: The internal clip attachment in fixedremovable partial denture prosthesis, New York J. Dent. 32(4):125-129, 1962.

Agnew, R. G., and Fong, C.: Histological studies on experimental transplantation of teeth, Oral Surg. 1:18, 1956.

Agon, C.: A proposito della tolleranza dei corpi estranei intratissulari a livello del cavo orale, Arch. Stomat. (Roma) 4:219, 1952.

Agren, E.: Apparatur for registrering av rodnad, svullnad och blodning, henagenhet i tandkottet vid gingiviter, Svensk. Tandlak. T. 46:39-44, 1953.

Ahnert, W.: Subperiostale Gerustimplantationen zur Verankerung von Zahnersatz—Klinische Erfahrungen mit Gerust-implantaten, Zahnaerztl. Welt. 62(22):739-744, 1961.

Albrecht, J.: Implantation Kunstlicher Zahne, Deutsch. Mschr. Zahnheilk. 12:254, 1894.

Albright, F.: Hyperparathyroidism; its diagnosis and exclusion, New Eng. J. Med. 209:476-480, 1933.

Albright, F., Aub, J. C., and Bauer, W.: A case of osteitis fibrosa cystica (osteomalacia) with evidence of hyperactivity of the parathyroid bodies, metabolic study II, J. Clin. Invest. 8:229-248, 1930.

Albright, F., Aub, J. C., and Bauer, W.: Hyperparathyroidism, common and polymorphic condition as illustrated by seventeen proved cases from one clinic, J.A.M.A. 102:1276-1287, 1934.

Albucasis, and Da Gros, V. G.: L'art dentaire chez les arabes, Odontologie, 1899.

Alcira, C. P.: Zehn Jahre Erfahrungen mit endossosen Implantaten, Tribuna Odont. 51:4-6, 1967.

Alessandri, M.: Skin and bone banks, Ann. Med. Nav. (Roma) 67:757, 1962.

Alvez de Souze, and Daher Saad, A.: Bioestatica dos implantes aloplasticos sobperiosticos totals dos maxilaries, J. Estomat. 11:33-44; ibid. Acta Stomat. Belg. 63(1):95, 1966.

American College of Surgeons: Manual of pre-operative and post-operative care, Philadelphia, 1967, W. B. Saunders Co.

Amler, M. H., and others: Bone degeneration following grafts with polyvinyl plastic sponge, Oral Surg. 11: 654-661, 1958.

Amodeo: Modo di consolidamento dei denti impiantati, 1895.

Amodeo: Deux cas d'implantation dentaire consolidée, Odontologie, August, 1899.

Amodeo: Deux implantations consolidée faites dans un cas de pyorrhée, Rev. Stomat., 1900.

Anderson, H. B.: Chronic focal infection of the mouth and tonsils in relation to life insurance, Proc. Ass. Life Insurance Med. Directors America, 1922.

Anderson, K. J., LeCocq, J., Akeson, W., and Harrington, P.: End-point results of processed heterogenous, autogenous and homogenous bone transplants in the human; a histologic study, Clin. Orthop., No. 33, 1964.

Anderson, K. J., LeCocq, J. F., and Mooney, J. G.: Clinical evaluation of processed heterogenous bone transplants, presented at the Annual Meeting of Western Orthopedic Association, San Francisco, October, 1962.

Anderson, K. J., LeCocq, J. F., and Mooney, J. G.: Clinical evaluation of processed heterogenous bone transplants; a preliminary study, Clin. Orthop. 29:248, 1963.

Anderson, K. J., Kingwall, J. A., Schmidt, J., LeCocq, J. F., and Clawson, D. K.: Induced connective tissue metaplasia: I. Heterogenous bone extract implants in the rat anterior eye chamber, Transplant Bull. 7:399, 1960.

Anderson, K. J., Schmidt, J., and LeCocq, J. F.: The vascularization and cellular response induced by homogenous deproteinized bone transplants in the anterior chamber of the rat eye, Transplant. Bull. 24: 97, 1959.

Anderson, K. J., Schmidt, J., and LeCocq, J. F.: The effect of particle size of the heterogenous bone transplantation on the host tissue vascular penetration, J. Bone Joint Surg. 41-A: 1455, 1959.

Anderson, L. D.: Compression plate fixation and the effect of different types of internal fixation on fracture healing, J. Bone Joint Surg. 47-A(1):191-208, 1965.

Anderson, L. D., Gilmer, W. S., Jr., and Tooms, R. E.: Experimental fractures treated with loose and tight fitting medullary nails, Surg. Forum 13:455-457, 1962.

André, R. S., Sloviter, H. A., and Groff, R. A.: The use of fetal calf bone for repair of skull defects in dogs, Plast. Reconstr. Surg. 28:378, 1961.

Andreas, M.: Statistiche Betrechtungen zu Implantationsgerusten, Deutsch. Zahnaerztl. Z. 15(4):424-427, 1960.

Andrei, G., and Ravenne, P.: Ricerche sulle infezioni focali; la produzione sperimentale di lesioni simili a quelle dei reumatismo articolare acuto, Sieroterapico Milanese (Milano) 13:804, 1934.

Andres, C.: Implants heteroplasticos endomaxilares con el torrillo Formiggini, Protesis Dent., No. 2, 1957.

Andrews, R. R.: Evidence of prehistoric dentistry in South America, Trans. Pan. Amer. Med. Congress. 35:102, 1893.

Andrews, R. R.: Prehistoric crania from Central America, Int. J. 3(14):914, 1893.

Andrysek, K.: Uber den Einfluss der Versteifung gegossener und gepragter Implantate, Zahnaerztl. Welt. 61(24):783-787, 1960.

Andrysek, K.: Untersuchengen uber des Verhalten gegossener und gepragter Implantate bei Belastungen, Zahnaerztl. Welt. 61(5):129-131, 1960.

Andrysek, K.: Impianti sottoperiostali in tantalio secondo Marziani, Rev. Ital. Stomat. 1:83, 1960; ibid. Schweiz. Mschr. Zahnheilk. 70(10):1007, 1960.

Angulo, A.: Protesis implantadas, Venezuela Odont. 12(3): April, 1958.

Anosova, K. G.: Current status of bone homoplasty of defects of the cranial vault, Vestn. Khir. Grekov. 89: 86, 1962.

Apfel, H.: Transplantation of unerupted third molar tooth, Oral Surg. 1:96, 1956.

Applegate, O. C.: The rationale of partial denture choice, J. Prosth. Dent. 10:891-907, 1960.

Applegate, O. C.: An evaluation of the support of the removable partial denture, J. Prosth. Dent. 10:112-123, 1960.

Archer, W. H.: Cirurgia bucodental, versao castelhana, tomo 1, Buenos Aires, Editorial Mundi, pp. 214-217.

Archer, W. H.: Implantatzahnersatz: Chirurgisch-ungüsntigqualifiziert, J. Prosth. Dent. 10(6):1127-1131, 1960.

Arnaudow, M.: Gibt es subperiostale implantate? Forsetzung: die versenkten Implantate, Deutsch. Zahnaerztl. Z. 17(4):336-339, 1962; ibid., 18(6):312-314, 1963.

Arnemann: Système de chirurgie, Gotinga, 1802.

Arrow, W.: Glossary of implant dentistry, Dent. Survey 29:760-762, 1953.

Arrow, W.: Laboratory aspects in the construction of implant dentures, Dent. Dig. 59:254-256, 1953.

Arturo, B.: Il moncone artificiale individuale fuso per implanti ad ago, Convegno Italiano di Implantologia III, June, 1966; Seminaire des Implants Aiguilles di Parigi, November, 1966.

Aschoff, L.: Tratado de anatomia patologica, Buenos Aires, 1934, Editorial Labor X/A.

Atterbury, R. A.: Organization and duties of the hospital team, Dent. Dig. 70:262-263, 1964.

Atterbury, R. A., McNabb, W., and Lekan, G.: Admission records and operating room techniques for the dentist, Dent. Dig. 71:156-160, 1965.

Atterbury, R. A., and Vazirani, S. J.: Operating room decorum in oral surgery, Oral Surg. 14:1161-1164, 1961.

Atterbury, R. A., and Vazirani, S. J.: Suture material: an important accessory in the art of oral surgery, Dent. Dig. 74:258-261, 1968.

Aubry, M.: Discours d'ouverture au Troisième Congrès

Intérnational des Implants Dentaires, tenu à la Faculté de Médecine, July, 1961, Rev. Odontostomat., 1962.

Aubry, M.: Chirurgie et implantologie, Promotion Dent., 2ᵉ trimestre, No. 1, 1967.

Audoire, P.: Une technique d'empreinte pour implant aux elastomeres par injection, Rev. Franc. Odontostomat., No. 9, 1956.

Audoire, P.: Observations on subperiosteum plants (abstract), Int. Dent. J. 7:538-540, 1957.

Audoire, P.: Presentation clinique de proteurs d'implants, compte rendu à la Société Française d'Implantologie, January, 1958.

Audoire, P.: Conference sur le thème des implants au cercle d'études odontostomatologiques de la Côte d'Azur, 1959.

Audoire, P., and Pelletier, M.: Amelioration des conditions chirurgicales par l'emploi des anti-inflammatoires, Ass. Odontostomat. Implant., 1961.

Audoire, P., and Pelletier, M.: Rapport sur les implants juxta-osseus au Congrès Intérnational, July, 1961, Rev. Franc. Odontostomat. 9:659-670, 1962.

Avellanal, C. D.: Diccionario odontologico, 1955, Ediciones Ediar, p. 465.

Avery, J. K.: Possible ectodermal origin of the odontoblast, J. Dent. Res. 29:663, 1950.

Azoulai, R.: Autogenous transplantation and implantation, Inform. Dent. 48:1687-1691, 1966.

Azoulai, R.: Les états métastables de l'eau dans les tissus dentaires et leur incidence sur les hétérogreffes, Thèse pour le doctorat en chirurgie dentaire, Faculté de Médecine, Paris, 1969.

Bablick, L.: Studies on the fine tissue behavior of autoplastic and homoplastic bone chips in plastic surgery of the bone, Arch. Ohr. Nas.-Kehlkopfheilk. 180: 383, 1962.

Backlund, N., and Akesson, N. A.: A follow-up examination of crown and bridge prostheses, Odont. Rev. 86: 121-133, 1957.

Bader, J.: Induced fibrogenesis and intraosseous implants, Dent. Cadmos 33:1097-106, 1965.

Bader, J.: La serocytotherapie en implantologie, Rev. Trim. Implant., No. 3, April, 1968.

Baetzner, K.: Plastic surgery of the acetabular roof with heterologous ampulla transplantation, Arch. Orthop. Unfallchir. 52:194, 1960.

Bahn, S. L.: An investigation into the use ot plaster of Paris in filling defects in membranous bones, Master's thesis, Boston, 1962, Boston University School of Medicine.

Bahn, S. L.: Plaster: a bone substitute, Oral Surg. 21:672-681, 1966.

Balogh, K.: Support of lower dental prosthesis by implanted mental roots, Dent. Dig. 70:312-313, 1964.

Bandettini, R.: Considerazioni sugli impianti sottoperiostei, Clin. Odont. 3:82, 1951.

Baptista, P.: Osso anorganico, material para implante no rotina odontologica, Rev. Paule. Cir. Dent. 15:113, 1961.

Baratieri, C.: Gli implanti juxta ossei, Rass. Trim. Odont., No. 1, 1959.

Barladjan, J.: Replantation und Implantation, Zahnaerztl. Prax. 19:1954.

Barr, C. E.: Osteogenic activity following bone and sponge implantation, J. Dent. Res. 43:26-34, 1964.

Barrelle, J. J.: Contribution de la parodontologie aux implants, Rev. Odontoimplant., No. 2, June, 1966.

Barrelle, J. J.: Implantology in occlusal dontology and functional occlusal restoration, Rev. Trim. Implant., No. 7, May, 1969.

Barri, F.: Amelioration des conditions de tolerance des implants par traitement hormonal, Communication à la Société Française d'Implantologie, March, 1958.

Barri, F.: Les implants metalliques sous periostes comme supports de bridges; amelioration de condition de tolerance et de fixation, Atti II Simposio Internazionale Degli Impianti Sottoperiostei, Naples, 1958.

Barri, F.: Bridges fixés sur implants metalliques sousperiostes, Rev. Franc. Odontostomat. 10:1241, 1963.

Barri, F.: Complications des implants juxta-osseux, leur causes et leur traitements, Ass. Odontostomat. Implant., 1961.

Barri, F.: Initial intolerance of an implant: clinical observation of a case; subsequent denture construction using phonetic impression method, Rev. Franc. Odontostomat. 10:1504-1505, 1963.

Barsoum, W. M.: Implant dentures, Egyptian Dent. J. 3: 36-40, 1957.

Bartels, H. A., and Blechman, H.: Survey of the yeast population in saliva and an evaluation of some procedures of identification of *Candida albicans*, J. Dent. Res. 41:1386-1390, 1962.

Barth, A.: Histologische Untersuchungen uber Knochenimplantationen, Deitr. Path Anat. 17:65, 1895.

Barthlelemy de Maupassant, P.: Indications and contraindications for implants, Chir. Dent. France 24:31-36, 1964.

Baschkirzew, N. J., and Petrow, N. N.: Beitrage zur freien Knochenuberflanzung, Deutsch. Z. Chir. 113:490, 1912.

Bassett, C. A. L.: Environmental and cellular factors regulating osteogenesis, bone biodynamics, Boston, 1964, Little, Brown & Co.

Bassett, C. A. L., and Becker, R. O.: Generation of electric potentials by bone in response to mechanical stress, Science 137:1063, 1962.

Bassett, C. A. L., Becker, R., and Pawluk, R. J.: Effects of electric currents on bone, Nature 204(4959):652-654, 1964.

Bassett, C. A. L., and Creighton, D. K., Jr.: A comparison of host response to cortical autographs and processed calf heterografts, J. Bone Joint Surg. 44-A:842, 1962.

Bassett, C. A. L., and Creighton, D. K., Jr.: A possible substitute for the preserved homograft, Surg. Forum. **12:**445, 1961.

Bassett, C. A. L., Creighton, D. K., Jr., and Stinchfield, F. E.: Contributions of endosteum, cortex, and soft tissue to osteogenesis, Surg. Gynec. Obstet. **112:**145, 1961.

Bassett, C. A. L., and Herrmann, I.: Influence of oxygen concentration and mechanical factors of differentiation of connective tissues in vitro, Nature **190:**460, 1961.

Bassett, C. A. L., Hudgins, T. F., Jr., Trump, J. G., and Wright, K. A.: The clinical use of cathode ray sterilized grafts of cadaver bone, Surg. Forum **6:**549, 1956.

Bassett, C. A. L., and Lindecker, R. A.: Bibliography of bone transplantation, vol. 12, Baltimore, 1964, The Williams & Wilkins Co.

Bassett, C. A. L., and Packard, A. C., Jr.: A clinical assay of cathode ray sterilized cadaver bone grafts, Acta Orthop. Scand. **28:**198, 1959.

Bataille, R.: Le problème medical des implants, Actualites Odontostomat., No. 46, 1959.

Batt, H.: Considerazioni sugli impianti sotto-periostei, Schweiz. Mschr. Zahnbeilk. **1:**50, 1959.

Bauer, S.: Indicazione degli impianti alloplastici, Atti Simposio (Pavia), 1955.

Bauermeister, A.: Treatment of cysts, tumors and inflammatory processes of the bone with the "Kiel graft," Burns. Beitr. Klin. Chir. **203:**287, 1961.

Bechtol, C. O., Ferguson, A. B., Jr., and Laing, P. G.: Metals and engineering in bone and joint surgery, Baltimore, 1959, The Williams & Wilkins Co.

Beck, C., and Franz, H.: Behavior of implanted autoplastic and homoplastic bone grafts in the middle ear in animal experiments, Arch. Ohr. Nas. Kehlkopfheilk. **179:**111, 1961.

Becker, R. O.: The bioelectric factors in amphibian limb regeneration, J. Bone Joint Surg. **43-A:**643, 1961.

Becker, S. C.: Clinical procedures in occlusal rehabilitation, Philadelphia, 1958, W. B. Saunders Co., p. 214.

Becks, H.: Systemic background of paradentosis, J.A.D.A. **28:**1447-1459, 1941.

Beder, O. E.: Study of tissue reaction to titanium implants (a preliminary report,) J. Dent. Res. **34:**787, 1955.

Beder, O. E., and Ploger, W. J.: Intraoral titanium implants, Oral Surg. **12:**787-799, 1959.

Behrman, S. J.: Dental implants: a clinical pathologic evaluation, Ann. Dent. **20:**33-41, 1961.

Behrman, S. J.: Dental implants, Dent. Dig. **67:**333, 1961.

Behrman, S. J.: Magnets implanted in mandible: aid to denture retention, J.A.D.A. **68:**206-215, 1964.

Bell, W. H.: Use of heterogenous bone in oral surgery, J. Oral Surg. **19:**459, 1961.

Bello, B. V.: Maxillary implant denture, J. Implant. Dent. **5:**17-20, 1959.

Bello, B. V., and Areal, P. G. E.: Dentaduras implantadas, Rio de Janiero, 1956, privately published.

Benagiano, A.: L'Impianto endosseo in protesi dentale, Ann. Stomat., February, 1959.

Benagiano, A.: Impianti alloplastici, stottoperiostei o juxta-ossei, trattato di odontostomatologia e protesi, vol. IV, Russo, 1962, Rome, pp. 1-7.

Benaim, L.: Presentazione di un impianto tubulare endosseo, J. Stomat. Inf. Dent. **16:**7, 1959.

Benaim, L.: Impianto tubulare e intervento durante il 3, Rev. Franc. Odontostomat., 1961.

Benaim, L.: Implants viewed realistically, Inform. Dent. **44:**519-528, 1962.

Ben-Bassat, N.: Replacement of missing teeth by an implant and porcelain jacket crowns, Refuat Hashinaim. **9:**10-13, 1955.

Benoit, P. Q.: Transosseous implants, J. Oral Implant Transplant Surg. **10:**28, 1964.

Benoit, P. Q.: The transosseous supported implant and retention of complete lower prosthesis, J. Med. Bordeaux **142:**1031-3, 1965.

Benque, E. P.: Original considerations on implants into bone; stabilization of the gingival mucosa with therapeutic fibrosis, Inform. Dent. **46:**1070-1076, 1964.

Benque, E. P.: Valeur clinique de la fibrogenesis en implantologie, Inform. Dent., No. 6, 1965.

Benque, E. P.: Reimplantations et auto-transplantation des dents perdues par transfixation: methode personnelle, Rev. Trim. Implant., No. 3, April, 1968.

Berham, S. J.: Implantation: principles, practices and predictions, J. Dent. Med. **10:**116-23, 1955.

Berliner, A.: Ligatures, splints, bite planes and pyramids, Philadelphia, 1964, J. B. Lippincott Co.

Berman, N.: Implant technique for full lower denture, Washington Dent. J. **19:**15-17, 1950.

Berman, N.: Physiologic and mechanical aspects of the implant technique and its application to practical cases, Dent. Dig. **58:**342-347, 1952.

Berman, N.: Implant dentures vs. conventional dentures, Washington Dent. J. **21:**31-37, 1953.

Berman, N.: Implant dentures may be vindicated, New York Dent. J. **19:**250, 1953.

Berman, N.: Is the magnetic denture an asset? Washington Dent. J. **22:**19-20, 1953.

Berman, N.: Methods for improving implant dentures, Oral Surg. **8:**227-236, 1955.

Bernier, J., and Land Camby, C.: Histologic study on the reaction of alveolar bone to Vitallium implants, J. Amer. Dent. Ass. **30:**188, 1943.

Berry, A.: Radici di piomo per impianti dentali, J. Dent. Soc. **7:**549, 1888.

Bertelsen, A.: Experimental investigations into postfoetal osteogenesis, Acta Orthop. Scand., Vol. 15, 1944.

Bertolini, A. M.: Il futuro degli impianti, Inform. Odontostomat., No. 1, 1969.

Bertolini, A. M., and Malizia, E.: Gli elettroliti in biologia e in medicina, Milan, 1951, Edizioni Ambrosiana.

Bertolozzi, F. Z.: Radiology with points of reference in dental implant practice, Dent. Cadmos **31**:81-86, 1963.

Beube, F. E.: A study on reattachment of the supporting structures of the teeth, J. Periodont. **18**:55, 1947.

Bianconi, X. L.: Impianti endossei e sottoperiostei, Comunicazione al XXXIII Congress Italien Stomatoligia, Bologna, 1959.

Bienstock, J. B.: Implants: a review of research as regards tissue reaction to metal, plastic, and dental implants, Oral Surg. **8**:430-437, 1955.

Billings: Focal infection, New York, 1921, Appleton and Co.

Binder, R.: Impianti sottoperiostali in tantalio: metodo di pressatura, Comun. Sulla Relz. del Prof. Marziani. XXIX Congress Italien Stomatologia, Venice, 1954.

Bjork, A.: Facial growth in man, studied with the aid of metallic implants, Acta Odont. Scand. **13**:9-34, 1955.

Bleicher, S. H.: Lower implant denture: a review of the literature, J.A.D.A. **53**:310-315, 1956.

Blocksma, R.: Silicone implants for velopharyngeal incompetence: a progress report, Cleft Palate J. **1**:72-80, 1964.

Blumenthal, E. E.: Abstract of denture implants lecture, Bull. Hudson County Dent. Soc. **23**:16-17, 1954.

Bochenek, M., and Pachalski, A.: Use of bone grafts in the treatment of delayed union and false joints in the long bone, Chir. Narzad. Ruchu. Ortop. Pol. **26**:697, 1961.

Bodansky, M.: Nutritional vs. endocrine factors in bone metabolism during pregnancy, Texas J. Med. **34**:339-343, 1938.

Bodine, R. L., Jr.: Implant denture, Bull. Nat. Dent. Ass. **11**:11-21, 1952.

Bodine, R. L., Jr.: Experimental subperiosteal dental implants, U. S. Armed Forces Med. J., March, 1953.

Bodine, R. L., Jr.: Construction of the mandibular implant denture superstructure, J. Implant Dent. **1**:32-36, 1954.

Bodine, R. L., Jr.: Evaluation of the bicuspid single-tooth subperiosteal implant for fixed crown, J. Implant Dent., Vol. 3, No. 1, 1965.

Bodine, R. L., Jr.: Canine experimentation with subperiosteal prosthodontic implants, J. Implant Dent. **2**:14-19, 1955.

Bodine, R. L., Jr.: Prosthodontic essentials and an evaluation of the mandibular subperiosteal implant denture, J.A.D.A. **51**:654-664, 1955.

Bodine, R. L., Jr.: Implant denture bone impression: preparations and technique, J. Implant Dent. **4**:22-31, 1957.

Bodine, R. L., Jr.: Research with implant dentistry, Int. Dent. J. **7**:425-426, 1957.

Bodine, R. L., Jr.: Implant dentures today, J. Implant Dent. **4**:22-27, 1958.

Bodine, R. L., Jr.: Implant dentures: prosthodontic-favorable, J. Prosth. Dent. **10**:1132-1142, 1960.

Bodine, R. L., Jr.: Implant dentures; follow-up after 7-10 years, J.A.D.A. **67**:352-63, 1963.

Bodine, R. L., Jr., and Kotch, R. L.: Mandibular subperiosteal implant denture techniques, J. Prosth. Dent. **4**:396-412, 1954.

Bojanow, B.: On the unsolved problem of subperiosteal implants, Deutsch. Stomat. **15**:48-54, 1965.

Bonwill, W. G. A.: Implantation of metal tubes or pins of gold or iridium into the solid alveolar process, Dent. Cadmos **37**:611, 1895.

Borg, J. F.: Hyperthyroidism, a new consideration for the dentist, J.A.D.A. **22**:1683-1693, 1935.

Borghesio, A.: Considerazioni su alcuni casi di impianti sottoperiostale in Vitallium, Riv. Ital. Stomat. **1**:34-38, 1955.

Borghesio, A.: A proposito di interventi ravvicinati nella tecnica operatoria per impianti sottoperisteal, Rastrin. Odont., April-June, 1955.

Borgo, E.: Amortiguadores en implantodontologia, Rev. Venezuela Odont. Vol. 29, No. 6, 1965.

Borimechkov, L.: The osseous repair of mandibular defects by means of bone transplantation (experimental research), Nauch. Tr. Vissh. Med. Inst. Sofiia. **41**(3):35, 1962.

Borroni, M.: On the favorable action of calciferol on the take of homoplastic bone grafts, Arch. Ortop. **74**:370, 1961.

Boucher, C. O.: Implant dentures: prosthodontic-favorable, J. Prosth. Dent. **10**:1143-1148, 1960.

Boucher, L. J.: Injected Silastic for tissue projection, J. Prosth. Dent. **15**:73-82, 1965.

Boyne, P. J.: Treatment of oral bony defects in man with anorganic heterogenous bone, Oral Surg. **11**:322-329, 1958.

Boyne, P. J., and Losee, F. D.: Response of oral tissues to grafts of heterologus "anorganic" bone, I.A.D.R. **35**:89, 1957.

Brash, J. C.: Chapters in growth of jaws, normal and abnormal, in health and disease, Dental Board of United Kingdom, 1924.

Brauer, J. C., and Bahador, M. A.: Variations in calcification and eruption of deciduous and permanent teeth, J.A.D.A. **29**:1373-1387, 1942.

Bremm, K.: On the possibilities of the use of Rabl's method of induced osteomalacia, Z. Orthop. **97**:196, 1963.

Bridges, J. B., and Pritchard, J. J.: Bone and cartilage induction in the rabbit, J. Anat. **92**:28-38, 1958.

Brill, E.: Impianti di radici artificiali in porcellana, J. Dent. Belg. **6**:725, 1936.

Brill, N.: Adaptation and the hybrid prosthesis, J. Prosth. Dent. **5**:811, 1955.

Broadbent, B. H.: Face of normal child, Angle Orthodont. **7**(4):183-209, 1937.

Brock, V. W.: Mucosal inserts, J. Alabama Dent. Ass. **44:** 4-7, 1960.

Brodie, A. G.: On growth pattern of human head: from third month to eighth month of life, Amer. J. Anat. **68:**209-262, 1941.

Brooks, D. B., Heiple, K. G., Herndon, C. H., and Powell, A. E.: Immunological factors in homogenous bone transplantation: IV. The effect of various methods of preparation and irradiation on antigenicity, J. Bone Joint Surg. **45-A:**1617, 1963.

Brown, A.: Sculptured synthetic prosthesis as implants in plastic surgery, Arch. Otolaryng. (Chicago) **45:**339, 1947.

Brown, T.: Reazione imprevedibile agli impianti, Surgery **47:**987, 1960.

Bruch, H.: Obesity in relation to puberty, J. Pediat. **19:** 365-375, 1941.

Buchanan, G. M.: Preparation of tantalum plates for the repair of cranial defects, J. Canadian Dent. Ass. **15:** 137-141, 1947.

Budge, C. T.: Closure of an antraoral opening by use of the tantalum plate, J. Oral Surg. **10:**32-34, 1952.

Budrass, W.: Transplantation of preserved human and animal bone, Langenbeck. Arch. Klin. Chir. **298:**244, 1961.

Bugnot, G.: Contribution à l'étude de la greffe dentaire, Paris, 1886, J. B. Baillière & Fils.

Buniatov, N. N.: Comparative data on auto-, hetero-, and homoplastic bone grafts in the surgical treatment of patients with tuberculosis of the hip joint, Azerbaidzh. Med. Zh. **10:**16, 1962.

Burger, M., Sherman, B. S., and Sobel, A. E.: Acceleration of bone repair by chondroitin sulfate treatment of implants, School of Aerospace Medicine, U.S.A.F. Aerospace Medical Center, Brooks Air Force Base, Texas, Report 61-63, July, 1961.

Burrows, R. B.: Variations produced in bones of growing rats by parathyroid extract, Amer. J. Anat. **62:**237-290, 1938.

Burwell, R. G.: Studies of the primary and the secondary immune responses of lymph nodes draining homografts of fresh cancellous bone (with particular reference to mechanisms of lymph node activity), Ann. N. Y. Acad. Sci. **99:**821, 1962.

Burwell, R. G.: Studies in the transplantation of bone: IV. The immune responses of lymph nodes draining second-set homografts of fresh cancellous bone, J. Bone Joint Surg. **44-B:**688, 1962.

Burwell, R. G.: Studies in the transplantation of bone: V. The capacity of fresh and treated homografts of bone, J. Bone Joint Surg. **45-B:**386, 1963.

Burwell, R. G., and Gowland, G.: Studies in the transplantation of bone: I. Assessment of antigenicity, serological studies, J. Bone Joint Surg. **43-B:**814, 1961.

Burwell, R. G., and Gowland, G.: Studies in the transplantation of bone: II. The changes occurring in the lymphoid tissue after homografts and autografts of fresh cancellous bone, J. Bone Joint Surg. **43-B:** 820, 1961.

Burwell, R. G., and Gowland, G.: Studies in the transplantation of bone: III. The immune responses of lymph nodes draining components of fresh homologous bone treated by different methods, J. Bone Joint Surg. **44-B:**131, 1962.

Cahn, L. R.: Pathology of oral cavity, Baltimore, 1941, The Williams & Wilkins Co., p. 183.

Calhoun, N. R., and Blackledge, G. T.: Plaster of Paris implants in the mandible of dogs, Quart. Nat. Dent. Ass. **21:**13-15, 1962.

Calhoun, N. R., Greene, G. W., and Blackledge, G. T.: Effects of plaster of Paris implants on osteogenesis in the mandible of dogs, J. Dent. Res. **42:**1244, 1963.

Calhoun, N. R., Greene, G. W., and Blackledge, G. T.: Plaster: a bone substitute in the mandible of dogs, J. Dent. Res. **44:**940-946, 1965.

Calonius, B.: Biologiska aspekter pa effekten av tandproteser: Foredrag vid Svenska Tandlakare-Sallskapets Arsmote, Svensk. Tandlak. T. **55:**231, 1962.

Calve, J.: De l'emploi de tissu spongieux heterogene en chirurgie ossiuse, Bull. Mem. Soc. Nat. Chir. **61:**1170, 1935.

Cambell, E., Meirowsky, A., and Hyde, G.: Studies on use of metals in surgery, Ann. Surg. **114:**474-479, 1941.

Cameron, D. A.: The fine structure of osteoblasts in the metaphysis of the young rat, J. Biophys. Biochem. Cytol. **9:**583, 1961.

Camurati, C., and Parenti, G.: Homoplastic bone grafts (experimental research), Minerva Ortop. **13:**471, 1962.

Cane, P., and Sgobbi, S.: Bone grafts in the surgical treatment of fibrous dyplasia, Chir. Organi. Mor. **51:**494, 1963.

Capozzi, L., and Benagiano, L.: Complete lower denture with tantalum ligature anchorage, Dent. Abstracts **4:** 38-90, 1959.

Capozzi, L.: Evaluation of denture implants: a five year report, Dent. Abstracts **4:**3-5, 1959.

Carco, P., and Paterno, P.: Sulla natura di alcune alterazioni ellettrocardiografiche nei tonsillitici primi risultati delle prove da sforzo, Minerva Med. **31**(1):9, 1940.

Carlsson, G. E., Hedegard, B., and Koivumma, K. K.: Studies in partial denture prosthesis: II. An investigation of mandibular partial dentures with double extension saddles, Acta Odont. Scand. **19:**215-237, 1961.

Carlsson, G. E., Hedegard, B., and Koivumaa, K. K.: A longitudinal study of mandibular partial dentures with double extension saddles, Acta Odont. Scand. **20:**95-119, 1962.

Carlsson, G. E., Hedegard, B., and Koivumaa, K. K.: Final results of a 4-year longitudinal investigation of dentogingivally supported partial dentures, Acta Odont. Scand. **23:**443-472, 1965.

Carnesale, P. G.: The bone bank, Bull. Hosp. Spec. Surg. **5:**776, 1962.

Casotti, L.: Evoluzioni della protesi dentaria, Ann. Clin. Odont., Vol. 321, April, 1936.

Casotti, L.: L'arte dentaria del Maggiolo, Ann. Clin. Odont. **4:**228-235, 1947.

Casotti, L.: L'innesto dentario e la sua storia, Riv. Ital. Stomat. **4:**607-619, 1952.

Castleman, B., and Mallory, T. B.: Pathology of parathyroid gland in hyperparathyroidism, Amer. J. Path. **11:**1-72, 1935.

Casto, T. D.: Results of 3 iridio-platinum roots implanted, Dent. Cadmos **56:**493, 1914.

Catalano, L.: Studio perliminare per un impianto tatale endooseo, Inform. Ondontostomat., No. 2, 1967.

Cecchetto, E.: Contributo clinico all'oftalmia metastatica, Fracastoro **11:**105, 1915.

Cecconi: Notes et memoires pour servir à l'histoire de l'art dentaire en France, Parigi, 1959.

Cervia, G.: Valutazione critica dei successi e degli insuccessi della applicazione di impianti sotto periostei ed endossei, Comunicazione presentata al 2e Simposio Internazionale degli impianti alloplastici a scopo protetico, March, 1955.

Chaklin, V. D., Abal, I., Masova, E. A., and Lavrishcheva, G. I.: Regeneration processes during intra-extramedullary osteosynthesis, Ortop. Travm. Protez. **24:**10, 1963.

Chalmers, J.: Transplantation immunity in bone homografting, J. Bone Joint Surg. **41-B:**160-179, 1959.

Chalmers, J., and Ray, R. A.: The growth of transplanted foetal bones in different immunological environments, J. Bone Joint Surg. **44-B:**149, 1962.

Charad Nur, A.: Implantacion reparatrice immediata con dientes de acrilico, Rev. Dent. Chile **38:**397, 1946.

Charbonnier, C.: Confereneza e proiezioni, impianti endossei e iuxtaossei, Teheran, 1961.

Charney, J.: The closed treatment of common fractures, ed. 3, Baltimore, 1961, The Williams & Wilkins Co.

Cherchève, M., Hubert, J. P., and Bordon, R.: Les implants biologiques et "la banque des dents," Prom. Dent., No. 5, 1ᵉ trimestre, 1969.

Cherchève, R.: Nouveaux aperçus sur le problème des implants dentaires chez l'edente complète: implants en tuteurs, Rev. Franc. Odontostomat., Vol. 1, July, 1956.

Cherchève, R.: Impressioni sul Congreso degli Impianti, Inform. Dent., No. 9, 10, 12, 1958.

Cherchève, R.: Perfezionamento della tecnica degli impianti alloplastici endossei, Atti 2 Simposio Internazional, Pavia, 1959.

Cherchève, R.: Considerazioni fisiologiche e pratiche su una osservazione originale di un impianto endosseo, Inform. Dent. **24:**677-680, 1959.

Cherchève, R.: Report on implants into bone, Rev. Franc. Odontostomat. **9:**621-638, 1962.

Cherchève, R.: Report of the 13th session on implant dentures, Miami, Inform. Dent. **44:**4355-4360, 1962.

Cherchève, R.: Les implants endo-osseux, Paris, 1962, Librairie Maloine, pp. 127-138.

Cherchève, R.: Implantation technique, Inform. Dent. **45:**539-544, 1963; ibid., **45:**1477-1502, 1963.

Cherchève, R.: The "third week" of the course on dental implants of Lariboisière, Rev. Franc. Odontostomat. **10:**1007-1017, 1963.

Cherchève, R.: About implants, Inform. Dent. **10:**853-855, 1964.

Cherchève, R.: Etudes critiques des methodes implantaires, Rev. Franc. Odontostomat. **16**(8):1307-1315, 1965.

Cherchève, R.: Correction d'une sévère dysmorphose du maxillaire, consecutive à un trouble ostéomyelique mandibulaire, Rev. Franc. Odontostomat., Vol. 1, No. 2, February, 1965 (extract).

Cherchève, R.: Dental implantation and anatomy, Chir. Dent. France **36:**43-45, 1968.

Cherchève, R.: Implants endo-osseux: amelioration de la technique des implants alloplastiques endo-osseux, Communication du 2 Symposium International des Implants, 1958.

Cherchève, R., and Dott, Le Dinh: Sturio del controllo radiologico preliminaire nell'esexuzione degli impianti endo-mascellari, Inform. Dent. **14:**517-520, 1957.

Cherchève, R., and Cherchève, M.: Descrizione di una tecnica originale semplificata di impianti dentali misti, Inform. Dent. **15:**668-675, 1957.

Cherchève, R., and Cherchève, M.: Procedimento originale d'impianto unico intraosseo, Inform. Dent. **48:**1608-1610, 1957.

Chiarini, G. C.: Responsibility and liability of the dentist when inserting denture-supporting acrylic implants, Dent. Abstracts **3:**394-395, 1958.

Churchill, E. D., and Cope, O.: Parathyroid tumors associated with hyperparathyroidism: eleven cases treated by operation, Surg. Gynec. Obstet. **58:**255-271, 1934.

Ciriello, G.: Acrylic implants and dental grafts, Rev. Ital. Stomat. **9:**1087-1143, 1954.

Ciriello, G.: Gli impianti endomascellari a sostegne di protesi, Rev. Ital. Stomat. **10:**11-20, 1955.

Ciriello, G., and Toldo, V.: Biological experiments on materials used in alloplastic perimaxillary implants, Int. Dent. J. **8:**22, 1958.

Cislaghi, E.: Magnetic prosthesis for better retention, Int. Dent. J. **3:**66, 1952.

Clark, I., and Bassett, C. A. L.: The amelioration of hypervitaminosis D in rats with vitamin A, J. Exp. Med. **115:**147, 1962.

Cleland, H. N., and Sevastikoglov, J. A.: Experimental studies of embryonic bone transplantation, Acta Orthop. Scand. **32:**1, 1962.

Climesco, V., and Constantinesco, N.: On the treatment of pseudarthroses and great loss of bony substances from the leg, Lyon. Chir. **59:**84, 1963.

Cobb, J. R.: Subperiosteal Vitallium implants in dogs, Oral Surg. **13:**1153-1162, 1960.

Coffin, F.: Surgery for prosthetics, Brit. J. Oral Surg. **2:** 9-19, 1964.

Cohen, J.: The investigation of metallic failure in devices implanted in the body, Surg. Clin. N. Amer. **41** (6):1645, 1961.

Cohen, J.: Failure in performance of surgical implants, J. Bone Joint Surg. **46**(2):416-421, 1964.

Coiquad, A.: On a case of bone graft for pseudarthrosis of the femur by the use of a heteroplastic graft, Maroc Med. **40:**817, 1961.

Colico, G. L.: Long term control of juxta-osseous implants, Minerva Stomat. **12:**99-101, 1963.

Combatti, V., and Ducci L.: The clinico-radiographic course of the screw-fastened cortical graft in ununited fractures, Riv. Infort. Mal. Prof. **48:**555, 1961.

Combre, G. M.: The depressibility of the mucosa and nerve implants, Inform. Dent. **47:**3484-7, 1965.

Conrad, J. J.: Freeze dried homogenous bone transplants (resident thesis), Bull. Hosp. Joint Dis. **22:**153, 1961.

Continolo, C.: Problèmes prosthetiques en implantologie, Comunicazione presentata al 4 Seminario degli Impianti ad Ago., Parigi, November 10-13, 1967, Inform. Odontostomat. **2**(2):10-13, 1967.

Coronel, S., and Kerneis, J. P.: Le resine acriliche intra-tissulari, Rev. Stomat. **5**(6):281, 1948.

Covo, I. H.: Regarding risks in implantation, Inform. Dent. **44:**2294-2296, 1962.

Cranin, A. N.: Nomenclature submitted by Nomenclature Committee, American Academy of Implant Dentures, J. Implant Dent. **2:**41-43, 1956.

Cranin, A. N.: Polyvinyl resin sponge implants in rebuilding atrophic alveolar ridges, J. Implant Dent. **8:**33-49, 1962.

Cranin, A. N.: Implant dentures, J.A.D.A. **67:**441-442, 1963.

Cranin, A. N.: Simplifying the subperiosteal implant denture technique, Oral Surg. **22:**7-20, 1966.

Cranin, A. N., and Cranin, S. L.: Utilization of the partial denture in complete oral rehabilitation, J.A.D.A. **57:** 188-193, 1958.

Cross, W. G.: Heterogenous bone graft, Dent. Pract. (Bristol) **5:**429, 1955.

Cross, W. G.: Bone-grafts in periodontal disease, Dent. Pract. (Bristol) **6:**98, 1955.

Cross, W. G.: Maxillary subperiosteal chrome-cobalt implant, Dent. Pract. **5:**430, 1955.

Cross, W. G.: Bone implants in periodontal diseases— a further study, J. Periodont. **28:**184, 1957.

Cross, W. G.: The histology of a bone implant, Dent. Pract. (Bristol) **8:**26, 1957.

Cross, W. G.: The use of bone implants in the treatment of periodontal pockets, Dent. Clin. N. Amer., pp. 107-115, 1960.

Cruz, F., and Protzel, M. S.: Metallic implant in a totally edentulous patient, Dent. Abstracts **1:**415-416, 1956.

Cruz, F., and Protzel, M. S.: Method for the temporary fixation of a mandibular implant substructure, preliminary report, Dent. Dig. **63:**6-267, 1956.

Cserepfalvi, M.: Transplantation of teeth in humans. In Peer, L. A.: Transplantation of tissues, vol. II, Baltimore, 1959, The Williams & Wilkins Co., pp. 300-309.

Cserepfalvi, M.: Experimental homogenous transplantation of human teeth obtained from a human cadaver, J. Oral Implant Transplant Surg., Vol. 12, 1966.

Cserepfalvi, M.: Clinical report of homotransplantation of teeth, J.A.D.A., Vol. 66, 1963.

Culand, H.: A proposito della ritenzione delle protesi totali de parte degli impianti metallici e dei pilastri intra-muccosi, Inform. Dent., Vol. 27, 1955.

Cullen, R.: How do I begin endosseous implants? Dent. News, July, 1968.

Currie, F. V.: Full mandibular subperiosteal implant denture, J. Canadian Dent. Ass. **27:**559-566, 1961.

Currie, F. V.: Dental implants as viewed by a general practitioner, Dent. Dig. **68:**158-168, 1962.

Dahl, G. S. A.: Om mojligheten for inplantation i kaken av metallskelett som bas eller retention for fasta eller avtagbara proteser, Odont. T. **51:**440-446, 1943.

Dahl, G. S. A.: Ar det mojligt att mod frangang gora implantat av Vitallium i kakarna som bas for protes, Svensk. Tandlak. T., 1950.

Dahl, G. S. A.: Dental implants and superplants, Rass. Trim. Odont. **4:**25, 1956.

Dahl, G. S. A.: Impianti sottoperiostali "superplant," Rass. Trim. Odont. **37:**25-36, 1956.

Dahl, G. S. A.: Sopraimpianti et Impianti, XXXI Congr. Ital. Stomat. **28:**9, 1956.

Dahl, G. S. A.: Subperiosteal implants and superplants, Dent. Abstracts **2:**685, 1957.

Dahl, G. S. A.: Some aspects on the implant button technique, J. Implant Dent. **5:**49-53, 1958.

Dahl, G. S. A.: Superplants, J. Implant Dent. **7:**15-21, 1961.

Dahl, G. S. A.: Promoteur des implants juxta-osseux implants et suprastructures, Rev. Franc. Odontostomat., No. 9, 1961.

Dahl,, G. S. A.: Mechanical principles of superplants, Acta Odont. Scand. **21:**515-531, 1963.

Dahl, G. S. A.: Mechanics of superplants, Dent. Progr. **3:** 82-87, 1963.

Dahl, G. S. A.: Valeur de la selle fixé en implantologie, Implants Aiguille, October, 1963.

Dahl, G. S. A.: Some aspects on the use of mucosal inserts, Svensk. Tandlak. T. **58:**523-530, 1965.

Dahl, G. S. A.: Superplante Biomechanik und Klinische Anwendungs moglichkeiten, Quintessenz **16**(1):45-51, 1965.

Dahmen, G., and Koch, W.: Histological studies on the incorporation and alteration of heterologous malerated bone implants, Arch. Orthop. Unfallchir. **54:**139, 1962.

Dalise, R.: Ripiantamento trapiantamento ed impianta-mento dei denti, Napoli, 1910, Ed. Tip. Forense.

Danis, A.: L'osteogenine existe-t-elle? Etude experi-mentale, Acta Orthop. Belg. **22**:501-506, 1956.

Dassen, R., and Fustinoni, O.: Sistema nervoso, Rio de Janeiro, 1953, Editora Guanabara.

Day, B.: Bridge abutment screwed into the jaw, Dent. Items Int. **55**:316, 1933.

Daza, T.: Implantaciones dentarias subperiosticas, Rev. Soc. Odont. Atlantica **4**(3/4):5-17, 1963.

De Bella, A. T.: Contributo agli impianti alloplastici endoossei con dispositivo a telescopio, Minerva Stomat., 1959.

De Bow, M.: Premedication in implant surgery, Dent. Survey **32**:795, 1956.

De Grady, M.: Intraosseous implants with subperiosteal extensions: a new technic, Dent. Abstracts **4**:27-28, 1959.

De Grady, M.: Presentazione di una fissazione originale per impianti, Société Française d'Implantologie, 1960.

Delbart, G., and Vivent, R.: Les implants au Congrès de New York, Inform. Dent. **4**(28):1, 1960.

Delcoulx, P.: Segmentary sponge graft in diaphyseal pseudoarthrosis with loss of substance, Mem. Acad. Chir. (Paris) **89**:240, 1963.

Deleu, J.: Tetracycline localization in the early stages of isogenous bone graft, Nature **198**:194, 1963.

Delgado, J. B.: Los implantes metalicos dentarios y la otorinolaringologia, Rev. Esp. Estomat. **11**(4):297-310, 1963.

Delitala, F.: Endoprotesi in ortopedia, Riv. Ital. Stomat., January, 1955.

Delitala, F.: Endoprotesi in sostituzionedi parti interne del corpo umano, Bologna, 1956, Edizioni Cappelli.

Delitala, F.: L'inventeur de la traction directe sur le squelette, Alessandro Codivilla (1681-1912), Sci. Med. Ital., Vol. 4., 1956.

Delitala, F.: L'imponderabile in chirurgia, Chir. Organi Mov., Vol. 44, No. 3, 1957.

Delitala, F.: Difficolta pericoli errori nell'operare (dai ricordi di un ortopedico), Clin. Ortop., Vol. 13, November-December, 1961.

Demicheu, N. P.: Use of frozen bone homografts in closed fractures in experimental conditions, Ortop. Travm. Protez. **23**:19, 1962.

De Oliveira, V M..: Plastic implant in correction of alveolar depression, Dent. Dig. **65**:24-26, 1959.

De Palma, A. F., Sawyer, B., and Hoffman, J. B.: Fate of osteochondral grafts, Clin. Orthop. **22**:217, 1962.

De Palma, A. F., and Smythe, V. L.: Recurrent fibrous dysplasia in a cortical bone graft: a case report, Clin. Orthop. **26**:136, 1963.

De Rischy, S.: Impianti sottoperiostei parziali controllo dopo quattro anni, Rass. Trim. Odont. **1**:109-115, 1959.

De Rysky, S.: L'impronta nell intervento per impianto sotto-periosteo, Riv. Ital. Stomat. **10**:29-33, 1955.

De Souza, J. A., and Fonseca, D. M.: Consideracoes sobre dentaturas implantadas, Rev. Paul. Chir. Dent. **6**:337-344, 1958.

De Souza, J. A.: Biomecanica factor de sucesso na tera-peutica protetica implantada subperiostica total, J. Estomat., January, 1963.

Deway, K., and Zugsmith, R.: Experimental investigations of the tissue reaction in implantation of artificial teeth and foreign bodies, J. Dent. Res. **12**:435, 1932.

Digman, R. O.: Repair of facial and cranial defects with iliac bone, Plast. Reconstr. Surg. **6**:179, 1950.

Dineen, J. R., and Gresham, R. B.: Rib osteoperiosteal grafts: a preliminary report of their use in the treat-ment of fresh and united fractures of the long bones, J. Bone Joint Surg. **44-A**:1653, 1962.

Dingwall, J. A., Millonig, R. C., and Westcott, W. W.: Personal communication.

Djeledoff, I. T.: Method of constructing a metal implant for the maxilla, Int. Dent. J. **8**:31-32, 1958.

Djoric, L. N.: Contribution to the treatment of large bone defects, Srpsk. Arh. Celok. Lek. **90**:989, 1962.

Dolder, E. J.: The bar joint mandibular denture, J. Prosth. Dent. **11**(4):689, 1961.

Dom, F.: Considérations sur les implantations sous-peri-ostees, Rev. Belg. Stomat. **54**:637, 1957.

Donatelli, L., Sorrentino, L., and Di Rosa, M.: Pharma-cological research on the mineral metabolism of the bone under repair; methods and results, Arch. Int. Pharmacodyn. **139**:265, 1962.

Dondey, P. L.: Etude sur le magnetisme et les implants en chirurgie dentaire, Rev. Franc. Odontostomat., June-July, 1958.

Dondey, P. L.: Implants magnetiques, Inform. Dent. **103**:7-9, 1959.

Dondey, P. L.: Les implants magnetiques stabilisateurs, Voix Dent. **103**:7-9, 1959.

Doner, A. G.: Implant dentures: a panel discussion, J. Prosth. Dent. **10**:1116-1148, 1960.

Doner, J. M.: Surgical preparation of the edentulous mouth for subperiosteal mandibular implantation, Dent. Student Mag. **40**:380-384, 1962.

Donnelly, H. P., and Fox, S. A.: A successful lower im-plant denture technique, J. California Dent. Ass. **31**: 1, 1955.

Dora, J.: Uber Implantation von Vitallium Gerusten in cinen Sitzung zur Unterlage von fixen Brucken-prothesen, D.D.Z. **19**:1117, 1956.

Dora, J.: Insertion of Vitallium substructure in one ap-pointment, J. Implant Dent. **4**:37-39, 1957.

Dora, J.: Implant dentures with Vitallium substructure and abutments, Dent. Abstracts **2**:12, 1957.

Dora, J.: Technische Arbeiten bei der Doraschen Sub-periostaten implantation in fallen vollstandingen Zahnverlusten im Unterkeifer, D.D.Z. **12**:1660, 1957.

Dora, J.: Uber die einphasige Implantation zwecks Bruck-enprothesen-Grundlage, R.M.S.O. **8**:712-724, 1960.

Dorigny: Reimpianto dei denti, 1864.

Dorr, A. D., Moloney, W. C., Dowd, G., and Boschetti, A. E.: Bone and marrow transplants in the rat, Blood **18**:423, 1961.

Drago, J.: Penetrazione di corpi estranei nel seno mascellare, Rev. Odont. Conc. **5**:61-5, 1958.

Dresser, W. J., and Clark, H. B.: Study of polyvinyl resin sponge in jaws of dogs, J. Dent. Res. **37**:45-46, 1958.

Dresser, W. J., and Clark, H. B.: Study of tissue response to polyvinyl resin sponge implants in the jaws of dogs, J. Oral Surg. **17**:3-13, 1959.

Dubois, A.: Implantologie—aiguilles et doctorat en cirurgie dentaire, Rev. Odontoimplant., No. 3, September, 1966.

Dubois, A., and De Chemant: Dissertazione sui denti artificiali, 1797.

Duclos, J., Freidel, Dumas de Mourges, Vincent Merie-Beral: Greffes implantations, inclusions, Compte rendu au XVI Congrès Stomatologie, Paris, 1959, Masson et Cie., editeurs.

Duclos, J., Farouds, R., and Vincent, R.: A propos des implantations dentaires, Comun. Congresso Rhodan-ien Marsiglia, 1947.

Dudley, H. R., and Spiro, D.: The time structure of bone cells, J. Biophys. Biochem. Cytol. **11**:627, 1961.

Duijtjes, F.: Implantation tests with heterologous bone: comparative study, on the guinea pig, on tissue re-action to calf bone preserved in a deep-freeze and of calf bone treated by the Maatz Bauermeister method, Nederl. T. Geneesk. **107**:425, 1963.

Dumont, A.: Contribution à l'étude des implants endo-osseoux, Schweiz. Mschr. Zahnheilk. **70**:647-654, 1960.

Dumont, A.: Contribution à l'étude des implants endo-osseux: le guidage automatique de la trepanation osseuse, Rev. Suisse Odontostomat. **7**:647-653, 1960.

Dumont, A.: Presentation du Bureau International des Implants, Congrès Ass. Odontostomat. Implant., Paris, 1961.

Dumont, A.: International office for dental implants, Dent. Abstracts **7**:671, 1962.

Dumont, A.: Les implant spirales on Titane, Compte rendu des Journées Implantaires de Lausanne, Groupe Suisse d'Etude des Implants, 1965, p. 171.

Ebling, C. D.: History and physiologic aspects of implant dentures, Temple Dent. Rev. **25**:22-23, 34-35, 1955.

Ecke, H.: The transplantation of homologous and heterol-ogous chips of epiphysis in animal experiments, Langenbeck. Arch. Klin. Chir. **300**:39, 1962.

Edlan, A.: Complete dentures by fixed means of sub-periosteal metal implants, Cesk. Stomat. **13**:361-371, 1958.

Edwards, J. M.: Implantation, Dent. Cadmos **31**(5):371-550, 1889.

Edwards, J. W.: Implantation of metallic capsules, Dent. Off. Lab. **3**:84, 1889.

Ehricke, A.: Die Odontoplastik im Lichte der Plantations-lehre, Berlin, 1920, Sammlung Meusser.

Eisenring, R. T. J.: Mikroskopische Untersuchung der bedeckten Mundschleimhaut, Munich, 1955, Carl Hanser Verlag.

El'Berg, G. A., and Grigor'Ev, N. I.: Use of bone homo-grafts in surgical practice, Vestn. Khir. Grekov. **87**: 71, 1961.

Elfenbaum, A.: Roentgenographic evaluation in denture construction, J. Implant Dent. **3**:12, 1957.

Engel, M. B.: Roentgenographic cephalometric appraisal of untreated and treated hypothyroidism, Amer. J. Dis. Child. **61**:1193-1214, 1941.

Engstrom, B., and Frostell, G.: Bacteriological studies of the non-vital pulp in cases with intact pulp cavities, Acta Odont. Scand. **19**:23-39, 1961.

Enneking, W. F.: Immunologic aspects of bone trans-plantation, Southern Med. J. **55**:894, 1962.

Enneking, W. F., Webb, W. R., Kellum, H. E., and Jackson, J.: Aortic grafts of chelated bone, J. Surg. Res. **2**:293, 1962.

Entin, M. A., Alger, J. R., and Baird, R. M.: Ex-perimental and clinical transplantation of autogenous whole joints, J. Bone Joint Surg. **44-A**:1518, 1962.

Erdheim, J.: Tetania parathyreopriva, Mitt. Grenzgeb. Med. Chir. **16**:632-744, 1906.

Ehrich, J. B.: Implants of bone or cartilage for depres-sion defects of the nose, Proc. Mayo Clin. **33**:167, 1958.

Ericsson, S. G.: Broprotesens inverkan pa de marginala parodontala forhallandena i bettet, Svensk. Tand-lak. T. **46**:171-182, 1953.

Euler, H.: Ueber das Altern des menschlichen Zahn-systems, Deutsch. Zahn. Wschr. **43**:393-403, 1940.

Ewen, S. J.: Bone swaging, J. Periodont. **36**:1, 1965.

Ewen, S. J., and Glicksten, C.: Ultrasonic therapy in periodontics, Springfield, Illinois, 1968, Charles C Thomas, Publisher.

Ezra-Cohn, H. E., and Cook, S. F.: Blood-typing com-pact human bone tissue, Nature **191**:1267, 1961.

Fildermann, J.: A propos des implants, Rev. Franc. Odontostomat. **2**:183, 1955.

Fillippi, J.: Implantations dentaires en resine acrylique, No. 39, 1954.

Fiore-Donno, G.: Les implants partiels en prothèse fire, Rev. Men. Suisse Odontostomat. **12**:1090, 1960.

Fleming, H. S.: Homologous and heterologous intraocu-lar growth of transplanted tooth germs, J. Dent. Res. **31**:166, 1952.

Fleming, H. S.: Transplantation of teeth. In Peer, L. A., editor: Transplantation of tissues, vol. II, Balti-more, 1959, The Williams & Wilkins Co., pp. 271-299.

Fletcher, M. H.: Some notes on experimental implanta-tion of teeth, Ohio J. Dent. Soc. **11**:1, 1891.

Flinchbaugh, R. W.: Prosthodontic aspects of an implant

for hemi-mandible, J. Prosth. Dent. **8:**1039, 1942, 1958.

Flhor, W.: Impianti endossei per ponti e protesi amovi bili, Zb. Welt. **4:**75, 1953.

Flhor, W.: De la possibilité d'implants au niveau de la face et des maxillaires, Rev. Franc. Odont. **9:**1361, 1958.

Foldvari, I.: Type of prosthesis in implants, J. Implant Dent. **5:**39-40, 1959.

Foldvari, I.: Functional correlation of abutments of subperiosteal implant dentures, J. Prosth. Dent. **12:**796, 1962.

Foldvari, I.: Recording centric relation for implant dentures, J. Prosth. Dent. **12:**584-587, 1962.

Fontaine: Les implants sur leur aspect medico-legal, Société Française des Implants Séance, June, 1961, Librairie Maloine.

Forbes, D. B.: Subcortical iliac bone grafts in fracture of the tibia, J. Bone Joint Surg. **43-B:**672, 1961.

Formiggini, M.: Protesi dentaria a mezzo d'infibulazoine diretta endoalveolare, Riv. Ital. Stomat., March, 1947.

Formiggini, M.: Protesi fisse in brocche edentule a mezzo di infiblazioni dirette endomascellari, Riv. Ital. Stomat. **9:**814-822, 1954.

Formiggini, M.: Otto anni di practica col mio metodo d'infibulazione metallica endomascellare, risultati e considerazioni, Riv. Ital. Stomat., January, 1955.

Formiggini, M.: Impianti alloplastici endomascellari con viti metalliche cave, Atti Simp. Impianti Alloplastic **3:**19-20, 1955.

Formiggini, M. S.: Fixed prostheses in edentulous mouths by means of endomaxillary direct implantations, Dent. Abstracts **1:**416, 1956.

Formiggini, M. S.: Impianti alloplastici endossei a mezzo di infibulazione endomascellare, Lezione al corso di aggiornamento dell'Universita di Siena di Medicini Stomatologica, Siena, 1956, Tipografia Nouva.

Formiggini, M.: Methode personelle d'implants alloplastiques endoosseux a spiral metallique, R.M.S.O. **10:**906-911, 1958.

Forsberg, H.: Transplantation of os purum and bone chips in the surgical treatment of periodontal disease (preliminary report), Acta Odont. Scand. **13:**235, 1956.

Fouere, H.: Les implants metalliques sous-periostes, technique de laboratoire, Rev. Franc. Odontostomat. **10:**1231, 1956.

Fourteau, P.: L'implant bequille, moyen de contention des prosthèses completes inférieures, Rev. Franc. Odontostomat. **21:**167, 1966.

Frank, J.: Celluloid bei implantation kunstlicher Zahne, O.U.V.F.Z. **3:**233, 1891.

Frank, V. H.: Mandibular canal localization, Oral Surg., Vol. 21, 1966.

Frantzen, W.: Implantieren von Logan-Zahnkronen mit Lithoidwurzeln, Z. Wbl. **12:**2, 1899.

Freedman, H.: Magnets to stabilize dentures, J.A.D.A. **47:**288-297, 1954.

Friedenstein, A. J.: Humeral nature of osteogenic activity of transitional epithelium, Nature **194:**698, 1962.

Friez and Larouche: Nouveau procédé de blocage bi-maxillaire à l'aide d'implants metalliques intra-osseux, Rev. Stomat., Vol. 58, No. 3, March, 1957.

Fromaigeat: Revue sur les implants, Soc. Chir. Dent. Stomat. **8:**11, 1956.

Fromaigeat: A propos des implants metalliques sousperiostes, Rev. Franc. Odontostomat. **1:**23, 1957.

Frugoni, C.: La clinica delle infezioni focali, Atti Terapi. Med. **1:**276, 1937.

Fruth: Replantation with porcelain and part of root, Dent. Cosmos, 1905.

Fryfogle, F. J.: Surgical commentary of Vitallium implants, J. Implant Dent. **5:**23-24, 1958.

Galand, M.: Implants into bone for the partially edentulous, Cah. Odontostomat. **12:**17-30, 1962.

Galluzzo, F.: Su un caso di impianto endosseo secondo Formiggini, Boll. Metallografico **2-3:**77-82, 1959.

Gandin, J.: An observation on articular reconstruction by means of preserved homografts, Rev. Chir. Orthop. **46:**763, 1960.

Gans, B. J., and Sarnat, B. G.: Sutural facial growth of the Macaca Rhesus monkey: a gross and serial roentgenographic study by means of metallic implants, Amer. J. Orthodont. **37:**827-841, 1951.

Gans, B. J., and Sarnat, B. G.: Study of natural growth by means of metallic implants in the Macaca Rhesus monkey, Amer. J. Orthodont. **39:**227, 1953.

Gardner, A. F.: Use of anorganic bone in dentistry, J. Oral Surg. **22:**332-340, 1964.

Gay, A., Rialdi, G., and Gatto, E.: On the presence of some blood antigens in human osseous tissue, Arch. Maragliano Pat. Clin. **16:**771, 1960.

Gegenbaur, C.: Ueber die Bildung des Knochengewebes, Jenaische Z. Med. Naturw. **1:**343, 1864.

Genone, B.: Ricerche istologiche sugli impianti iuxaossei con una nouva tecnica di inclusione e di preparazione per usura, Rass. Trim. Odont. **4:**906-909, 1957.

Georgiade, N., and Dingwall, J.: Use of heterogenous bone implants and osteogenetic extract in maxillofacial surgery, Bull. Soc. Int. Chir., No. 1, 1965.

Georgiade, N., Van Lenvon, M. M., Dingwall, J. A., and Georgiade, R.: The uptake of strontium in experimental implants of fresh autogenous cancellous bone; processed heterogenous cancellous bone; processed heterogenous cancellous bone pretreated with an osteogenetic extract, Bull. Soc. Int. Chir. **24:**31-37, 1965.

Georgiade, N., Woolf, R., Richard, F., and Pickrell, K.: Use of bovine bone in reconstructive surgery, Plast. Reconstr. Surg. **24:**13, 1959.

Gerber: Les implants sous periostes, point de vue du prothetiste, Rev. Franc. Odontostomat., No. 8, 1958.

Gershkoff, A.: Fundamentals of the implant denture, J. Prosth. Dent. 2:40-50, 1952.

Gershkoff, A.: Implant dentures and public relations, J. Implant Dent. 4:20-21, 1958.

Gershkoff, A., and Goldberg, N. I.: Case histories and reports of mandibular implant inserted on half jaw and half rib graft, J. Implant Dent. 1:34-35, 1955.

Gershkoff, A., and Goldberg, N. I.: Implant dentures, Philadelphia, 1957, J. B. Lippincott Co.

Giambell, G., and Ruffoni, R.: Antimitotic antibiotic and the taking of experimental bone grafts, Minerva Ortop. 13:324, 1962.

Giedroyc, J.: Some observations on remote results of the transplantation of a boiled bone graft (5-years' observation), Chir. Narzad. Ruchu. Ortop. Pol. 26: 305, 1961.

Gilmer, W. S., Tooms, R. E., and Salvatore, J. E.: An experimental study of the influence on implanted polyurethane sponges upon subsequent bone formation, Surg. Gynec. Obstet. 113:144, 1961.

Gilmore, S. F.: A method of retention, J. Allied Dent. Soc. 8:113, 1913.

Ginestet, G.: Rapport au Congrès de 3e International des Implants, Faculté de Médecine, Paris, 1961, Librairie Maloine.

Ginestet, G.: Rev. Odontostomat. 8(5):666, 1962.

Ginestet, G., Dupuis, and Donedy: Aimants intra-osseux, Rev. Stomat., No. 7, 1957.

Girod, P.: Contribution à l'étude des infections focales, Paris, 1931, Pontarlier.

Giuffreda, G.: Communicazione istologica sugli impianti in acrilico, Clin. Odont. Prot., June, 1958.

Giuffreda, G.: Rapport histologique sur les implants d'acrylic, Clin. Odontostomat., 1958.

Gladkova, G. S.: Some comparative data on 2 methods of study of bone graft take by the use of radioactive indicators, Med. Radiol. (Moskva) 7:40, 1962.

Glickman, I.: Clinical periodontology: recognition, diagnosis and treatment of periodontal disease in the practice of general dentistry, Philadelphia, 1964, W. B. Saunders Co.

Globensky, L. M.: Implant denture, Int. Dent. J. 7: 540-542, 1957.

Gloss and Gold: Tolerance due Vitallium et de l'austanium dans l'implant sous periose chez le chien, Surg. Path., 1957.

Glowinski, Z.: Our observation on the treatment of post-inflammatory defects of long bones with porous bone chips, Chir. Narzad. Ruchu. Orthop. Pol. 26:427, 1961.

Gnone, B.: Ricerche istologiche sugli impianti iuxta-ossei con una nuova tecnica di inclusione e di preparazione per usura, Rass. Trim. Odont. 38:906, 1957.

Gola, L.: Impianti alloplastici endossei ammortizzati, Atti 2e Simposi Impianti Alloplastico, Pavia, 1959.

Goldbaum, J. C., and Marte, J. B.: Les implants-aiguilles à l'echelle animale, Rev. Odontoimplant., No. 2, June, 1966.

Goldberg, I.: Fundamentals of the implant denture, J. Prosth. Dent. 1:40, 1952.

Goldberg, N. I.: Problem of education in implant odontics, J. Implant Dent. 5:15-16, 1959.

Goldberg, N. I., and Gershkoff, A.: Further report on the full lower implant denture, Dent. Dig. 56:11, 1950.

Goldberg, N. I., and Gershkoff, A.: Implants: biologic or mechanical? New York J. Dent. 16:397, 1950.

Goldberg, N. I., and Gershkoff, A.: Fundamentals of the implant denture, J. Prosth. Dent. 2:1-40, 1952.

Goldberg, N. I., and Gershkoff, A.: Implant lower denture, Dent. Dig. 5:11, 1952.

Goldberg, N. I., and Gershkoff, A.: Scientific Communication Session, American Academy of Implant Dentists, Chicago, 1953.

Goldberg, N. I., and Gershkoff, A.: Six year progress report on full denture implants, J. Implant Dent. 1:13-16, 1954.

Goldberg, N. I., and Gershkoff, A.: Implant dentures, rationale of the mandibular implant denture, Dent. Clin. N. Amer., 567-578, Nov, 1960.

Goldhaber, P.: Behavior of bone tissue culture. In Sognnaes, R. F., editor: Calcification in biological systems, Washington, D. C., 1960, American Association of Advertising Science.

Goldhaber, P.: Calcification within diffusion chambers containing bone isografts, Clin. Orthop. 25:204, 1962.

Goldman, H. M.: Subgingival curettage, a rationale, J. Periodont. 19:54, 1948.

Goldman, H. M., and Cohen, D. W.: The infrabony pocket: classification and treatment, J. Periodont. 29: 272, 1958.

Goldman, H. M., Forrest, S. P., Byrd, D. L., and McDonald, R. E.: Current therapy in dentistry, ed. 3, St. Louis, 1968, The C. V. Mosby Co.

Goldzier, M.: Biochemical aspects of constitution. In Goldzier, M., editor: Biology of individual, Baltimore, 1934, The Williams & Wilkins Co.

Goldzier, M.: Diagnostic significance of cranial roentgenograms in pituitary disease, Endocrinology 27: 185-190, 1940.

Gomez, V. P.: Nueva techinica sobre implantes metallicos, Rev. Odont., No. 170, 1958.

Gonclaves, W. O., and Kanitz, W.: Upper implants; a modified technique, Dent. Dig. 61:353-355, 1955.

Goransson, P.: Kombination av fast och avtagbar protes, Goteborgs Tandlak.-Sallskaps Arsbok, pp. 19-37, 1963.

Gorlin, R. J., and Goldman, H. M.: Thoma's oral pathology, ed. 6, St. Louis, 1970, The C. V. Mosby Co.

Goslee, G. H.: Removable bridgework, Dent. Items 34: 731, 1912.

Gottardi, G., Veronese, V., and Nicolin: Implanti metallici sottoperioteali a sostegno di protesi fisse, Rev. Ital. Stomat. **9**:682-688, 1954.

Gottardi, G., Veronese, V., and Nicolin: Impianti metallici sottoperiostei: materiali usati, tecnica operatori e resultati, Riv. Ital. Stomat. **19**:48-49, 1959.

Gourley, I. M. G., and Arnold, J. P.: The experimental replacement of segmental defects in bone with plaster of Paris–epoxy resin mixture, Amer. J. Vet. Res. **21**: 1119-1122, 1960.

Gramm: Impianto di corpi estranei nei mascellari, Dent. Dig. p. 832, 1898.

Grandin, M.: Contribution à l'étude des inclusions pre-prosthétiques sous periostées, Rev. Franc. Odontostomat. **2**:279-287, 1955.

Grandin, M.: Technique operatoire des implants metalliques sous periostes, Rev. Franc. Odontostomat., No. 10, 1956.

Grandin, M.: Les implants sous periostes: valeur et avenir de la methode, Rev. Franc. Odontostomat., 1957.

Grant, A. R., and Melick, D. W.: Bone chip plastic repair of congenital chest deformities, Arch. Surg. **86**: 940, 1963.

Graulich, H. R.: Gli impianti endossei di Formiggini, Rev. Belg. Odont., No. 2, 1957.

Green, C. D.: Denture implants—yes or no? Lebanese Dent. J. **14**:27-28, 1963.

Greenfield, J.: Dental brief, November, 1910. In Gaillard et Noguet: Dentisterie technique operatoire, Paris, 1930, Editions Baillière.

Greenfield, J.: Una radice artificale, Lab. Progr. Dent. Rev., Vol. 15, 1911.

Greenfield, J.: Implantation of artificial crown and bridge abutments, Dent. Cosmos **55**:364-430, 1913.

Gregoire, A., and Macnab, I.: Polyurethane foam in the treatment of fractures, Canad. J. Surg. **5**:101, 1962.

Greisheimer, E. M.: Physiology and anatomy, ed. 5, Philadelphia, 1945, J. B. Lippincott Co.

Gresham, R. B., and Thomas, E. D.: A comparative histologic study of the early phases of transplanted bone autografts, freezed dried homografts, and processed calf heterografts, Surg. Forum **13**:452, 1962.

Grewe, J. M., and Felts, W. J.: Effects of prior chlortetracycline hydrochloride exposure on the behavior of subcutaneously implanted neonatal mouse humeri, Anat. Rec. **143**:363, 1962.

Gross, P. P., and Gold, L.: Compatibility of Vitallium and Austanium in completely buried implants in dogs, Oral Surg. **10**:769-780, 1957.

Grossman, L. I.: Tratamento dos canais rediculares, Trad. de Sylvio Belaqua, Livr. Atheneu, p. 407, 1956.

Gruber, I. E., and Elkins, L.: Vitallium implantation, New York Dent. J. **23**:9-14, 1957.

Gubelman, O.: Methods and criteria of intraosseous and subperiosteal implants, Dent. Abstracts **2**:428-429.

Guentert, G.: Implantation Prothese feur den Unterckister, Dent. Reform **53**:23-24, 1942.

Guergue, A.: Present status of implantation, Dent. Abstracts **1**:551, 1956.

Guichardiere, A.: Le reazioni del tessuto congiuntivo a contatto del metacrilato, Lyon Med. **186**(2):17, 1952.

Guilleminet, M., and others: Osteosynthesis with grafts of lyophilized calf bone in the treatment of fractures and pseudarthrosis of the leg, Lyon Chir. **51**:371, 1961.

Guilleminet, M., Stagnara, P., Michel, C. R., and Lapras, A.: Heterogenous bone from a bone bank in diaphysical osteosynthesis of the leg; indications and results, Presse Med. **70**:257, 1962.

Gungerich: Implantation Zahne, Deutsch. Mschr., 1891.

Gunn, D. R.: Bridging large defects in bone, Med J. Malaya **16**:267, 1962.

Haas, E.: On the use of body substance and homoplastic substance and homoplastic substances as implant material in facial area, Med. Welt. **19**:1051, 1963.

Haas, S. I.: A study of the viability of bone after removal from the body, Arch. Surg. **7**:213, 1923.

Haas, S. I.: Further observations of the survival of bone after removal from the body, Arch. Surg. **10**:196, 1925.

Haasch, K.: Clinical experiences with the carinated graft, Chirurgie **34**:21, 1963.

Habib, R.: Considerations concernant les implantations aiguilles, Rev. Trim. Implant., No. 3, April, 1968.

Hacpille, P.: Les implants-aiguilles et les accidents de la route: cas d'une racine artificielle transfixée, Rev. Odontoimplant., No. 1., March, 1966.

Haderup, V.: Stenographie and Stenophonie der Zahne, Deutsch. Mschr. Zahnheilk. **12**:223-232, 1894.

Hahn, W. E.: Capacity of developing tooth germ elements for self-differentiation when transplanted, J. Dent. Res. **20**:5, 1941.

Haike, J.: Experiences with bone preservation in palacos, Langenbeck. Arch. Klin. Chir. **298**:254, 1961.

Hale, M. I.: Autogenous transplants, Oral Surg. **1**:96, 1956.

Hammer, H.: Der histologische Vorgang bei der Zahnreplantation, Deutsch. Zahn. Mund. Kieferchir. **1**:H2, 1934.

Hammer, H.: Der histologische Vorgang bei der Zahnreplantation nach Vernichtung der Wurzelhaut, Deutsch. Zahn. Mund. Kieferheilk. **4**:H3, 1937.

Hammer, H.: Der gegenwartige Stand der Zahnreplantation, Deutsch. Zahn. Mund. Keiferheilk. **5**:H8, 1938.

Hammer, H.: Die Zahnruckpflanzung, 1950, Arbeitsgemeinschaft Medicine Verlag.

Hammer, H.: Die Zahnruckpflanzung, Deutsch. Zahnaerztl. Z. **5**:H12, 1950.

Hammer, H.: Die Replantation des devitalen Zahnes, Munchen, 1951, Hanser-Verlag.

Hammer, H.: Indikation und Kontraindikation zur subperiostalen Gerusteinpflanzung, Deutsch. Zahnaerztl. Z. **10**:1101-1114, 1955.

Hammer, H.: Indicazioni e controindicazioni degli impianti alloplastici, Simposio di Pavia, 1955.

Hammer, H.: Replantation and implantation of teeth, Int. Dent. J. 5:449, 1955.

Hammer, H.: Zahnreplantation und Implantation korperfremder Stoffe, Autoreferat, Oest. Z. Stomat. 52:357, 1955.

Hammer, H.: Zum Problem der operativen Verbesserung ungunstiger Prosthesenlager im Unterkieferbereich im besonderen, durch subperiostale Gerustimplanationen, Deutsch. Zahnaerztl. Z. 10:416, 1955.

Hammer, H.: Il reimpianto dei denti, Mondo Odontostomat., Vol. 3, 1967.

Handelsman, M. B., and Gordon, E. F.: Growth and bone changes in rats injected with anterior pituitary extract, J. Pharmacol Exp. Ther. 38:349-362, 1930.

Hansen, J.: Alloplastiske implantater i odontologisk kirurgi, Nord. Klin. Odont. 4:1-18, 1958.

Harndt, E.: Die Erfolgsaussichten der subgingivalen Curettage paradentaler Taschen, Zahn. Zahn. Z. 8:899, 1953.

Harris, S. M.: An artificial tooth-crown on a leaden root, Dent. Cosmos 55:433, 1887.

Harrisson: Reimpianto, J. Brit. Dent. Ass., 1895.

Hary, M.: Conception of a bar of solidarization of implant needles, with the effect of conjunction with the removable prosthesis above, Inform. Dent. 47:2455-2468, 1966.

Hassan, A. A., and Ahmed, S. S.: Case report of an implant lower denture, Lebanese Dent. Mag. 5(9):15, 1955.

Hedegard, B.: Cold-polymerizing resins (dissertation), Acta Odont. Scand. 13:17, 1955.

Hedegard, B.: Nagra problem inom amnesomradet proteslara, Odont. Foren. T. 27:65-77, 1963.

Hedegard, B.: Recent improvements in clinical dental prosthesis arising out of developments in dental materials, Int. Dent. J. 15:381-384, 1965.

Hegedus, Z., and Inke, G.: Impianto di radici artificiali in resina, Inform. Dent., Vol. 12, 1957.

Hegedus, Z., and Inke, G.: Erfahrungen mit der Implantation von Kunstlichen Zahnwurzeln aus Methylmetakryrat, Schweiz. Mschr. Zahnheilk. 67:29, 1957.

Hegedus, Z., and Inke, G.: Implantation of tooth roots made of methyl methacrylate, Dent. Abstracts 2:428-429, 1957.

Hejna, W. J., and Ray, R. D.: Comparative study of bone implants, Surg. Forum 14:448, 1963.

Held, A. J.: Endosseous implants for the reinforcement of teeth, Oral Surg. 15:227-237, 1962.

Held, A. J.: Chirurgie preprosthetique et implantologie, Rev. Men. Suisse Odontostomat., Vol. 76, 1966.

Held, A. J., Held, D., Spirgi, M., and Charbon, R.: Reazioni ossee a contatto dei diversi tipi di impianto, Soc. Odontostomat. 68:891-892, 1958.

Held, A. J.: Risultati a distanza ottenuti con l'impianto di radici in porcellana, Rev. Soc. Odontostomat., 1939.

Hellman, M.: Changes in human face brought about by development, Int. J. Orthodont. 13:475, 1937.

Henndon, C. H.: Principles of bone graft surgery: different methods of operative procedure and indications for each in instructional course lectures, American Academy of Orthopedic Surgery, vol. 17, St. Louis, 1960, The C. V. Mosby Co., pp. 149-164.

Hersch, J. G.: Implant dentistry, Dent. Student Mag. 33:24-28, 1955.

Herschfus, L.: Further pathologic studies of implants in dogs, J. Implant Dent. 2:20, 1955.

Herschfus, L.: Histopathologic findings on Vitallium implants in dogs, J. Prosth. Dent. 4:413-419, 1954.

Herschfus, L.: Progress report of implants: histopathologic findings in dogs and a clinical report in a human, J. Implant Dent. 1:19-25, 1955.

Herschfus, L.: Tips on techniques, J. Implant Dent. 2:52-53, 1955.

Herschfus, L.: Histopathologic studies of five-year implants in dogs, J. Implant Dent. 4:12-21, 1957.

Herschfus, L.: Histopathology in animal implantodontics, J. Implant Dent. 5:12-23, 1958.

Herschfus, L.: Evaluation of the present status of implantodontics, Oral Surg. 12:800-813, 1959.

Herschfus, L.: Implants: accusations by an American (comment on article), Probe (London), September 27-28, 1959.

Herschfus, L.: Use of ostamer in implant odontics, J. Implant Dent. 6:2-29, 1959.

Herschfus, L.: Refresh your interest in implant dentures, intraperiosteal mandibular implant, Detroit Dent. Bull. 30:11, 1961.

Herschfus, L.: Use of tantalum powder with Vitallium intraperiosteal implants, J. Implant Dent. 7:51-56, 1961.

Herschfus, L.: A thought provoking appraisal, J. Implant Dent. 8:17, 1962.

Herschfus, L.: A perspective appraisal of the mandibular intraperiosteal implant, J. Oral Implant Transplant Surg. 10:3-14, 1964.

Herschfus, L.: Mandibular intraperiosteal denture implant, Chron. Omaha Dent. Soc. 27:276, 1964.

Herschfus, L.: An experimental evaluation of ostamer and tantalum powder in intra-periosteal implant dog surgery, J. Oral Implant Transplant Surg. 11:12-17, 1965.

Herschfus, L.: Use of self-curing resins for direct implant impressions, J. Implant Dent. 2:22-25, 1966.

Hertz, J.: Kirurgi for Tandleger og Tandlegestuderende, Stockholm, 1957, Almqvist and Wiksell.

Hertz, J.: Pre-prosthetic surgery, Brit. J. Oral Surg. 2:1-8, 1964.

Herzberg, F., and Schour, I.: Effects of thyroxine on rate of eruption and dentin apposition, J. Dent. Res. 20:276, 1941.

Hewitz, U.: Unilateral free end implant, J. Implant Dent. 5:54, 1958.

Heyden, E.: Vorschlag zu einer nuen Methode, um kunstliche Zahne in der Alveole zu retenieren, Korr. Z., p. 193, 1891.

Hildebrand, G. Y.: Studies in dental prosthetics, Svensk. Tandlak. T., Vol. 30, 1937.

Hildebrand, G. Y.: Om axialbelastningens kliniska betydelse, Svensk. Tandlak. T. 49:749-762, 1956.

Hill, R. T.: Anatomy of the head and neck, Philadelphia, 1946, Lea & Febiger.

Hillischer, H. T.: Implantation kunstlicher Zahne, Deutsch. Mschr. Zahnhk. 9:439, 1891.

Hinds, E. C.: Use of tantalum trays in mandibular surgery in twenty patients, Dent. Abstracts 9:178-183, 1964.

Hinman: Del reimpianto dei denti, Progr. Dent., 1895.

Hipple, A. H.: Implantation to teeth, Dom. Dent. J. 2: 143, 1890.

Hiroky, K.: Studi sperimentali sui vari metalli usati negli impianti, J. Osaka Univ. Dent. Soc., Vol. 2, 1957.

Hodosh, M.: Implantation of plastic teeth, Dent. Student Mag. 44:660-663, 1966.

Hodosh, M.: Implants of acrylic teeth in human beings and experimental animals; clinical and microscopic studies, Oral Surg. 18:596-599, 1964.

Hodosh, M.: Periodontal acceptance of plastic tooth implants in primates, J.A.D.A. 70:362-371, 1965.

Hoffer, O.: Elementi di clinica odontoiatrica: Lezioni raccolte dal Dott, Guastamacchia C. 2, Milan, 1958, Edizione Cortina.

Hoglund, N.: Ospurums anvandining inom odontologien, Odont. T. 50:43, 1943.

Holden, M. H.: Surgery and the flat lower ridge, Leeds Dent. J. 5:76-82, 1966.

Holland, D. J.: Alveoplasty with tantalum mesh, J. Prosth. Dent. 3:354-357, 1953.

Holst, Ostly, Osvald, and Benagiano: Trattato di odontostomatologia e protesi, Rome, 1960, Edizone Russo.

Holtzer, H., Abbott, J., Lash, J., and Holtzer, S.: The loss of phenotypic traits by differentiated cells in vitro: I. Dedifferentiation of cartilage cells, Proc. Nat. Acad. Sci. U.S.A. 46:1533, 1960.

Hopkins, J. A., and Jolson, J. R.: Experiences with unilateral implants, J. Implant Dent. 3:43-46, 1957.

Hoppe, W., and Bremer, H.: Experimenteller Beitrag zur enossalen Implantation alloplastischen Materials im Kieferbereich, Deutsch. Zahnaerztl. Z. 11:H10, 1956.

Hoppe, W., and Bremer, H.: Contributo sperimentale al problema degli impianti endossei in materiale alloplastico nella regione dei mascellari, Dent. Zahn. Zeit. 10:551, 1956.

Hoskins, M. M.: Effect of acetyl thyroxin on teeth of new born rats, Proc. Soc. Exp. Med. Biol. 25:55, 1927.

Houssay, B. A.: Fisiologia humana, Buenos Aires, 1951, El Ateneo.

Hruska, A., Jr.: Reimpiantamento di denti e impiantamento di radici di porcellana secondo, Brill. Zahn. Rund. 11:1939.

Hruska, A., Jr.: Reimplantation von Zahnen und Implantation von Brillschen Porzellanwurzelin, Zahnaerztl. Rundsch. 48:434, 1939.

Hruska, A., Jr.: Commento allo studio del Dott. L. Marziani su "Le radici artificiali come ancoraggio di protesi mobili inferiori," Clin. Odont. 111:2, 1959.

Huggins: Transplantation of tooth germ elements, J. Exp. Med. 60:199, 1934.

Huggins: The formation of bone under the influence of epithelium of the urinary tract, Arch. Surg. 22:203, 1931.

Humphreys, H. F.: Teeth from case of hypoparathyroidism, Proc. Roy. Soc. London 23:633-634, 1939.

Hunter, J.: Observation on the teeth, London, 1775.

Hunter, J.: Natural history of human teeth, London, 1775.

Hurley, L. A.: The role of soft tissues in osteogenesis: an experimental study of canine spine fusions, J. Bone Joint Surg. 41-A:1243, 1959.

Hutchinsin, G.: Repair of skull defects by tantalum, Brit. Dent. J. 90:312-315, 1951.

Iliovici, E., and Benillouz: Homéopathie et art dentaire, Inform. Dent., No. 657, 1960.

Imesch, J.: Réimplantations et transplantations dentaires, Rev. Men. Suisse Odontostomat., Vol. 76, 1966.

Iorio, P. A., and Carneiro: Contribuicao ao estudo dos implantes dentarios, Rev. Farm. Odont., January, 1968.

Izikowitz, L.: Implantationsprotesens historia och dess utveckling under 50-talet, Svensk. Tandlak. T. 54: 51-67, 1961.

Izikowitz, L.: Report on superplants, J. Implant Dent. 7: 22-30, 1961.

Izikowitz, L.: Superplants: eine klinische Nachuntersuchung, Zahnaerztl. Prax. 12:249-252, 1961.

Izikowitz, L.: Suprastructures, bridges fixés avec ou sans selles sur implants sous periostes, Association Européens pour Implants, Faculté de Médecine, Paris, 1961, Librairie Maloine.

Izikowitz, L.: Superplants: preliminary report of a follow-up histologic examination, Oral Surg. 14:1290-1299, 1961.

Izikowitz, L.: Superplants: en introduktion i teknik och klinik, Svensk. Tandlak. T. 17:2-11, 1962.

Izikowitz, L.: Superplants: follow-up roentgenologic examination, Dent. Dig. 69:27-31, 1963.

Izikowitz, L.: Superplants: a longitudinal study, Acta Odont. Scand. 23:1-70, 1965.

Izikowitz, L.: Temporary fixed saddle bridges, J. Oral Implant Transplant Surg. 11:38-43, 1965.

Izikowitz, L.: The superlant: a clinical, radiologic, histologic and bacteriologic follow-up investigation of a type of fixed saddlebridge (dissertation), Acta Odont. Scand. 24(Suppl. 47):5-159, 1966.

Izikowitz, L., and Nilzen, A.: Allergies in implant odontics, J. Implant Dent. 6:32-36, 1959.

Izikowitz, L., and Nilzen, A.: Nomenclature (Submitted by Nomenclature Committee Of the American

Academy of Implant Denture), J. Implant Dent. 6: 32-36, 1959.

Izikowitz, L., and Wedendal, P.: Sattlextensionbrucken (SE-Brucken), Schweiz., Mschr. Zahnheilk. 78:850-868, 1968.

Jablonsky, Simaljakt, and Keemon: Determination de la potential "in vitro" à un certain pH dans les metaux employés en stomatologie, Rev. Franc. Odontostomat., No. 7, 1959.

Jack, L.: Impianto di denti, Dent. Cosmos, 1897.

Jacquet, A.: Les implants metallique sous-periostes: complications, Rev. Odontostomat. 8:1281, 1961.

Jaffe, H. L.: Hyperparathyroidism (Recklinghausen's disease of bone), Arch. Path. 16:63-112, 1933.

Janecek, M., and Horn, V.: Use of frozen homoplastic bone grafts in clinical practice, Acta Chir. Orthop. Travm. Cech. 29:119, 1962.

Janeck, M., and Horn, V.: Use of homoplastic bone grafts in orthopedics, Chir. Narzad. Ruchu. Ortop. Pol. 27: 249, 1962.

Jaskarcek, B.: Le problème des prosthèses mobiles, Inform. Dent. 30:1464, 1948.

Jaskarzec, B.: Implantation de piliers et armatures dans les restaurations prothetiques, Inform. Dent. 32:14-618, 1950.

Jaskarcek, B.: Les implants metalliques sous periostes, Rev. Franc. Odontostomat., p. 577, 1956.

Jeanneret, C.: Impianti endoossei, Ann. Stomat. 6:753, 1960.

Jeanneret, M.: Nuova tecnica di impianti endossei, Baden, 1960, R. Rohrer.

Jeanneret, M.: Sviluppo dell'impianto endosseo, Rev. Men. Soc. Odontostomat., 1961.

Jeanneret, M.: Modified Formiggini implant, Rev. Franc. Odontostomat. 9:639-649, 1962.

Jensen, G. R., and Viikari, S. J.: Om inplantationsproteser, Suomen Hammaslaak. Toim. 48:67, 1952.

Jermyn, A. C.: Reflections of the editor, J. Implant Dent. 1:10-12, 1955.

Jermyn, A. C.: Ball-point balanced occlusion in the implant denture, J. Implant Dent. 2:26-35, 1955.

Jermyn, A. C.: Correction of prognathism by the implant denture, J. Implant Dent. 2:26-35, 1956.

Jermyn, A. C.: Technique and problems of placing implant screws, J. Implant Dent. 2:36-40, 1956.

Jermyn, A. C.: Peri-implantoclasia: cause and treatment, J. Implant Dent. 5:25-48, 1958.

Jermyn, A. C.: Anterior implant with center-poise balanced superstructure, J. Implant Dent. 7:57-65, 1961.

Jermyn, A. C.: Implant dentures, Dent. Radiog. Photog. 3:34, 1961.

Jimenez, C. A.: Problems caused by bone grafts, Med. Esp. 46:96, 1961.

Johnson, N. W.: Implant studies in rats, J. Dent. Res. 42:9-10, 1963.

Johnson, N. W.: Method for assessing the reactions of the oral tissues of the rat to implant materials, Brit. Dent. J. 114:441, 1963.

Johnston, J. P., Philipps, R. W., and Dykema, R. W.: Modern practice in crown and bridge prosthodontics, Philadelphia, 1960, W. B. Saunders Co.

Jones, J. R., and Bassett, C. A.: An experimental study of cortical "matchstick" grafts to reinforce immature callus, Surg. Gynec. Obstet. 117:611, 1963.

Jones, P. M.: Implant dentures: a case report and evaluation, J. U. M. K. C. School Dent. 14:16-20, 1956.

Jourdan and Maggiolo: Le manuel de l'art du dentiste, Nancy, 1807.

Kaketa, T.: A case report of implant denture, Nippon Acta Radiol. 1:62-67, 1957.

Kaketa, T.: Improved method of endo-osseous implant dentures, Nippon Acta Radiol. 12:186, 1963.

Kaketa, T.: Clinical investigations of endosseous implants, Nippon Acta Radiol.10:195-199, 1966.

Kaketa, T.: Histopathological findings on endo-osseous implants in dogs, Bull. Tokyo Dent. Coll. 2:61-70, 1969.

Kallenberg, K., and Maeglin, B.: Contributo alla conoscenza dei processi di guarigione susseguenti ad inserzione di una structura metallica sottoperiostea, Schweiz. Mschr. Zahnheilk. 4:300, 1947.

Kallenberg, K., and Maeglin, B.: Comportamento dell muccosa a conatto di impianti metallici, Inform. Dent., Vol. 52, 1957.

Kallenberg, K., and Maeglin, B.: Healing process after insertion of subperiosteal implants, Dent. Abstracts 2:737-738, 1957.

Kallenberg, K., and Maeglin, B.: Zur Frage der Einheilungstorgaenge bei Geruestimplanten: Processo di guarigone dopo l'applicazione di impianti subperiostei, Schweiz. Mschr. Zahnheilk 67:300-307, 1957.

Kallenberg, K., and Maeglin, B.: Le problème des implants sous periostes, Schweiz. Mschr. Zahnheilk. 10: 892, 1958.

Kammer, S.: Implantation of steel framework for dental prostheses, Dent. Stomat. 5:349-355, 1955.

Kammer, S.: Experiences with subperiosteal implantation of cast structures, Int. Dent. J. 8:25-26, 1958.

Kammer, S.: Complete and partial implant dentures, Dent. Abstracts 4:37, 1959.

Kanitz, W., and Gonclaves, W. O.: Upper implants a modified technique, Dent. Dig. 61:353, 1955.

Karges, D. E., Anderson, K. J., Dingwell, J. A., and Jowsey, J.: Experimental evaluation of processed heterogenous bone transplants, Clin. Orthop. 29:230, 1963.

Karlstrom, S.: Pontostruktormetodiken; dess principer samt dess broframstallning tillampade teknik belyst av behandlade fall, Svensk. Tandlak. T. 40:613-704, 1947.

Karlstrom, S.: Ponostruktorsmetodiken sedd i kasuistikens belysning, Svensk. Tandlak. T. 45:439-465, 1952.

Karlstrom, S.: Efterkontroll av brofall framstallda enligt den sk Pontostruktorsmetodiken, Sevensk. Tandlak. T. **53:**957-972, 1960.

Karnofsky, D., and Cronkite, E. P.: Effect of thyroxine on eruption of teeth in newborn rats, Proc. Soc. Exp. Biol. Med. **40:**568-570, 1939.

Kauffer, H. J.: Fisiologia e meccanica di unimpianto radioclare [Root implantation: physiologic and mechanical], Dent. Items **37:**1-33, 1915.

Keech, M. K.: The formation of fibrils from collagen solutions: the effect of mucopolysaccharides and nucleic acids: an electron microscope study, J. Biophys. Biochem. Cytol. **9:**193, 1961.

Keith, A., and Campion, G. G.: Enquiry into nature of skeletal changes in acromegaly, Lancet **1:**933, 1911.

Keith, A., and Campion, G. G.: Contribution to mechanism of growth in human face, Dent. Rec. **42:**61-88, 1922.

Kells, C. E.: Textbook of operative dentistry, Philadelphia, 1918, The Blakiston Co., pp. 473-485.

Kelly, K. B.: Replacement of an upper incisor by acrylic implantation, 11th Aust. Dent. Congr. Proc., Vol. 33, 1948.

Kendall, E. G.: Hormones, Ann. Rev. Biochem. **10:**285-336, 1941.

Kennedy, E.: Partial denture construction, Dent. Items, 1928.

Key, A. J.: Stainless steel and Vitallium in internal fixation of bone, Arch. Surg. **43:**614-626, 1941.

Killebrew, R. H.: Mandibular implant denture, J. Prosth. Dent. **2:**618-624, 1952.

Killebrew, R. H.: Decade of implant dentures, J. Prosth. Dent. **11:**1156-1165, 1962.

Kincade, R. G.: Implant dentistry, Contact Point **35:**228-234, 1957.

Kinricks, E. R., and Beck, V. L.: Implant in mandibular resection, case report, J. Implant Dent. **5:**21-24, 1959.

Kleinschmidt, J.: One year Vitallium implants, Refuat Hashinaim. **8:**3-6, 1954.

Kleinschmidt, J.: Method to replace single teeth, J. Implant Dent. **1:**26-33, 1955.

Klewamsy, P.: The value of intraosseous acrylic implants in the treatment of mandibular fractures in edentulous patients, Rev. Franc. Odontostomat. **13:**191-194, 1966.

Klotz, M.: Sinus et implants d'odontostomatologie, October, 1965.

Knowlton, J. P.: Masticatory pressures exerted with implant dentures as compared with soft-tissue borne dentures, J. Prosth. Dent. **3:**721-726, 1953.

Knowlton, J. P.: Implant denture progress, Washington Dent. J. **23:**9-10, 1954.

Knowlton, J. P.: Rationale of design of mandibular implants, J. Prosth. Dent. **6:**412-420, 1956.

Koenig, H., and Heller, J. H.: Affect the dynamics of bone healing by administration of a bone extract, Surg. Gynec. Obstet. **3:**203, 1960.

Koivumaa, K. K.: Changes in periodontal tissues and supporting structures connected with partial dentures, Suom. Hammaslaak. Toim., Vol. 52, Suppl. 1, 1956.

Koivumaa, K. K.: A histological investigation of the changes in gingival margins adjacent to gold crowns, Odont. T. **68:**373-385, 1960.

Koivumaa, K. K.: Studies in partial dental prothesis, I, Suom. Hammaslaak. Toim. **56:**248, 1960.

Komari, G.: Viti endossee coniche e viti a due parti, Inform. Odontostomat., No. 3-4, 1966.

Komari, J., and Horvath, L.: Die Schliessung von Frontzahnlucken mittels Vittalium-Gerust-Implantaten, Deutsch. Zahnaerztl. Z. **18:**442-447, 1963.

Kono, H.: Experimental studies and clinical observation of the implantation used: zirconium, Bull. Tokyo Med. Dent. Univ. **8:**253, 1961.

Korkhaus, G.: Changes in form of jaws and in position of teeth produced by acromegaly, Int. J. Orthodont. **19:**160-174, 1933.

Kotch, R. L.: Surgical treatment of osteomyelitis with metal implant: report of a case, New York Dent. J. **16:**499-503, 1950.

Kotiza, F.: Corps étrangers chroniques des sinus paranasaux, Cesk. Otolaryng. **8:**269-277, 1959.

Kovacs, D. G.: Consideration of growth and quality of connective tissue capsule around subperiosteal implants, Fogorv. Szemle **57:**102-111, 1964.

Kovacs, D. G.: Survey of sub-periosteal implant using panoramic roentgenography, Deutsch. Zahnaerztl. Z. **20:**1077-1084, 1965.

Kovalenko, P. P.: Homotransplantation of lyophilized bone in pseudarthroses in experimental conditions, Eksp. Khir. Anest. **8:**46, 1963.

Kowolton, J. P.: Masticatory pressures exerted with implant dentures as compared with soft-tissue–borne dentures, J. Prosth. Dent. **5:**721, 1953.

Kowolton, J. P.: Linee direttive per il disegno di impianti mandibolari sottoperiostei, J. Prosth. Dent. **3:**412, 1956.

Kraft, E.: Ueber die steigerung der funktion lerausnehmharer prothesen durch implantatverankerung, Deutsch. Zahn. Z. **12:** 1957.

Kranz, P.: Innere Sekretion in Beziehung zur Kieferbildung und Zahnentwicklung, Deutsch. Zahnheilk. Vortragen. **32:**1-104, 1914.

Krebs, A. A.: Expansion of the mid-palatal suture studied by means of metallic implants, Europ. Orthodont. Soc. Trans. **34:**163-171, 1958.

Kresse, E. J.: Patient education in the dental office, Proceedings of the first Scientific Session of the American Academy of Implant Dentistry, Vol. 14, 1953.

Krippaehne, W. W., Hunt, T. K., Jackson, D. S., and Dunphy, J. E.: Studies on the effect of strees on transplants of autologous and homologous connective tissue, Ann. J. Surg. **104:**267, 1962.

Krogh-Poulsen, W.: Moderne odontologisk Protetik, Tandlaegebladet **64:**147-166, 1960.

Kromer, H.: Bone homografts in the surgical treatment of cysts of the jaws and periodontal pockets, Oslo, Norway, Oslo University Press.

Krueger, E.: Comparative experimental studies on autoplastic bone transplanted with and without periosteum, Langenbeck. Arch. Klin. Chir. 299:150, 1961.

Kruger, V.: Erfahrungen mit der Oral Rehabilitation auf Grund eigner, Studien in den U.S.A., D.D.Z. 16:256-259, 1961.

Ksoki, K., Laaksonen, A. L., and Luostarinen, E.: Fate of foetal human bone xenografts in rats, Nature 193:1092, 1962.

Kueppermann, W.: Experiences with heteroplastic bone in the treatment of fractures, Langenbeck. Arch. Klin. Chir. 298:246, 1961.

Kutnovskii, S. I.: Formation of a leg stump with free bone transplant from spongiosa, Ortop. Travm. Protez. 21:24, 1960.

Kutzueb, H. J.: Erkankungen des Zahnfleisches: Einfluss von Pubertat, Menstruation, Schwangerschaft und Klimakterium, Umschau 57:371-372, 1957.

Lachard, J., and Sinibaldi, F.: A propos du traitement des lesions inflammatoires du plancher sinusien, Rev. Stomat. 61:431-433, 1960.

Lacour, G.: Considerazioni sui denti artificiali per la base dei porti fissi, Riv. Suizzena Odont., No. 2, 1947.

La Croix, P.: The organization of bones, Philadelphia, 1951, The Blakiston Co.

La Forgia, P. D.: Alcuni impianti dentali in svedion-resina acrilica, Riv. Ital. Stomat. 5:488, 1953.

La Forgia, P. D.: Il reimpianto dentario della pratica stomato logica, Riv. Ital. Stomat. 41:48, 1955.

Lager, H.: Orthodontic treatment analysed by aid of metallic implants: report of a class II case, Europ. Orthodont. Soc. Trans. 34:396-403, 1958.

Lakner, L.: Implantation of artificial crown and bridge abutments, Dent. Cosmos 55:364-430, 1913.

Lakner, L.: Experimental work on a method for the replacement of missing teeth by direct implantation of a metal support into the alveolus, Amer. J. Orthodont. Oral Surg. 25:467-472, 1939.

Lakner, L.: Three years' experience with Vitallium in bone surgery, Amer. J. Surg. 114:2, 1941.

Lakner, L.: The chirurgical retention of full dentures, Dent. Rec. 12:277, 1944.

Lakner, L.: Surgical retention of full dentures, Dent. Dig. 51:373-375, 1945.

Lakner, L.: Retencion quirurgica de dentaturas completas, Oral Hyg. 5:361, 1947.

Lange, D.: Studies on intraosseous "biological implantation" in therapeutic and posttraumatic reimplantations, Deutsch. Zahnaerztl. Z. 20:1157-1164, 1965.

Langer, C., and Wagner J. E.: Implantacoa de pecas fundidas: baseadas em trabalhos experimentais feitos em caes (comportamento de tecidos), Rev. Farm. Odont. 29:263, 1963.

Lansberg, I.: Metallic implant for full dentures, Refuat Hashinaim. 9:1-9, 1955.

Lansberg, I.: Full metallic implants for full dentures, Int. Dent. J. 7:556, 1957.

Lanzella, A.: Relations between phosphoric esters and homoplastic bone graft, Arch. Orthop. 74:551, 1961.

Lapchinsky, A. G., and Malinowsky, A. A.: An attempt at experimental homoplastic transplantation of teeth in the dog, Acad. Sci. U.R.S.S. 29:750, 1940.

La Rosa Werner, L.: Recopilacion de trabajos cientificos, Caracas, 1958.

La Rosa Werner, L.: Report of stresses exerted by complete lower implants on bony structures, J. Oral Implant Transplant Surg. 11:7-11, 1965.

Laskiewica, A.: Clinical considerations on the traumatic injuries and foreign bodies of the paranasal sinuses, Prac. Otorhinolaryng. 21:499-516, 1959.

Laurin, C. A., Sison, V., and Roque, N.: Mechanical investigation of experimental fractures, Canadian. J. Surg. 6:218-228, 1963.

Lavine, L. S., Warren, R. F., and Murray, J. W.: A study of the site of action of parathyroid hormone, Bull. N. Y. Acad. Med. 39:269.

Lavrishcheva, G. L.: Homoplasty of defects of tubular bones with bone fragments, Eksp. Khir. Anest. 6:35, 1961.

Lebourg, L., and Biou, C.: The imbedding of plaster of Paris in surgical cavities of the maxilla, Sem. Hôp. Paris 37:1195-1197, 1961.

Le Dinh, Bourselet, M., and Tridon: Technique radiologique en vue d'implants, radiographie standard tomographie et logegrammes, Rev. Franc. Odontostomat. 10:1017-1030, 1963.

Lee, T. C.: Present day evaluation of implant dentures, J. California Dent. Ass. Nevada Dent. Soc. 35:168-172, 1959.

Lee, T. C.: Materials used in implants, J. Implant Dent. 6:26-32, 1960.

Lee, T. C., and Lattig, E. J.: Mandibular subperiosteal implant technique, J. Philippine Dent. Ass. 11:21-24, 1958; ibid., Pakistan Dent. Rev. 8:25-29, 1958; ibid., J. California Dent. Ass. Nevada Dent. Soc. 34:400-405, 1958.

Lefoulon: Nouveau traité théorique et pratique de l'art du dentiste, Parigi, 1841.

Leger-Dorez, H.: Implantation de racines extensibles, Traité de prosthèse dentaire, Paris, 1920, Editions Ash, Sons & Co.

Lehmans, I.: Risultati ottenuti in due anni di esperimento con l'impianto ad arco, Riv. Ital. Stomat. 4:409-416, 1946.

Lehmans, J.: Contributo allo studio degli impianti endossei: impianto ad arco estensibile, Rev. Stomat. 415:224, 1959.

Lehmans, J.: Resultats obtenus au cours des deux années d'experimentation de l'implant à arceau, Rev. Stomat. 61(4-5):231-238, 1960.

Lehmans, J.: Implant à arceau endo-osseux, Rev. Odontostomat., 1961.

Lehmans, J.: Resultat de trois années d'experimentation des implants endoosseux, Rev. Odontostomat., 1961.

Lelkes, K.: Neuere Beitrage zur Moniliasis der Mundohle, Ost. Z. Stomat. 5:243-249, 1956.

Le Nart, V., and Lenart, I. F.: Implant in the maxilla, Rev. Stomat. 63:1046-1051, 1962.

Lentulo: Implants, Ann. Odontostomat., No. 4, 1959.

Levander, G.: A study of bone regeneration, Surg. Gynec. Obstet. 67:706-714, 1938.

Levignac, J.: Traitement chirurgical des fractures de la mandibule: les osteosynthesis, Ann. Chir., No. 8, August, 1955.

Levignac, J.: Evolution actuelle de la chirurgie maxillofaciale, Rev. Franc. Odontostomat., December, 1957.

Levignac, J.: Rev. Franc. Odontostomat., 1959-1960.

Levignac, J.: Mandibules senescence et implants, 3e Congrès International, Faculté de Médecine, Paris, 1961, Librairie Maloine.

Levy, A. T.: Mandibular implant denture: a case history, J. California Dent. Ass. Nevada Dent. Soc. 29:96-98, 1953.

Levy, A. T.: Vitallium implant closure of an oral-antral opening, J. California Dent. Ass. Nevada Dent. Soc. 29:373-374, 1953.

Levy, A. T.: Anterior replacement by subperiosteal implantation, J. California Dent. Ass. Nevada Dent. Soc. 30:161-162, 1954.

Levy, A. T.: Fracture of the mandible reduced by implant denture technique, J. California Dent. Ass. Nevada Dent. Soc. 30:11-12, 1954.

Lew, I.: Implant denture—a simplified upper technique using immediate prosthesis, Dent. Dig. 58:10-15, 1952.

Lew, I.: Full upper and lower denture implant, Dent. Concepts 4:17, 1952.

Lew, I.: Implant denture: a simplified upper technique using immediate prosthesis, Dent. Dig. 1:10, 1952.

Lew, I.: Progress report on full implant dentures, J. Prosth. Dent. 3:571, 1953.

Lew, I.: Case histories and reports: upper and lower implant dentures—fixation with surgical prosthetic splint, J. Implant Dent. 1:36-38, 1955.

Lew, I.: Acrylic implants, New York J. Dent. 25:228, 1955.

Lew, I.: Implant denture, J. Dent. Med. 10:126-129, 132-135, 1955.

Lew, I.: Implant concepts from abroad, J. Implant Dent. 2:16-21, 1956.

Lew, I.: Free-end saddle prosthesis, Dent. Dig. 63:24-26, 1957; ibid., 63:456-460, 1957.

Lew, I.: Mucosal inserts—a progress report, J. Prosth. Dent. 7:798-803, 1957.

Lew, I.: Study of edentulous mandibles in implant procedures, J. Implant Dent. 5:25-32, 1959.

Lew, I.: Progress in implant dentistry—an evaluation, J.A.D.A. 59:478-492, 1959.

Lew, I.: Implant denture case study of twelve years' duration, J. Implant Dent. 8:41-43, 1962.

Lew, I., and Kestenbaum, I.: An implant button technique for denture prosthesis, Dent. Dig. 59:298, 1953.

Lew, I., and Kestenbaum, I.: Le tecnica dell'impianto per le dentiere totali, Rass. Letter. Clin. Odont., 1954.

Lewark, N.: The effects of acrylic implants on oral tissues, Chron. Omaha Dent. Soc. 29(20): 9-11, 1966.

Lewin, A.: Bilateral mandibular implants in an occlusal reconstruction: a case report, J. Dent. Ass. S. Afr. 15: 47-52, 1960.

Lewin Epstein, J.: Use of polyvinyl alcohol sponge in alveoplasty; a preliminary report, J. Oral Surg. 18: 453-460, 1960.

Lewis, F. W.: Implantation of an artificial tooth, Dent. Cosmos 5:384, 1889.

Lewis, F. W.: Oral manifestations of endocrine disturbances—myxedema, Dent. Cosmos 77:47-49, 1935.

Lhotsky, B.: Bio-materielle beziehungen in der implantodontologie, Blatter F. Zhk. 11:12, 1960.

Lhotsky, B.: Uber Gewebeumbauvorgange in Bieziehung zuenossalen Spiralgerusten nach Formiggini, D.D.Z. 18:475, 1963.

Lhotsky, B.: Vakuum und injektionprothetik, Blatter Zhk., No. 4, 1960.

Lhotsky, B.: Entsehung und Bedeutung des Bindegewebslagers bei Enosalen Implantaten, Zahnaerztl. Prax. 15: 19-22, 33-34, 1964.

Lhotsky, B.: Implantate in biochemiscren Dezeinuzen Sonderdruck aus Zahnarzil, 1964.

Lhotsky, B.: Information and importance of the connective tissue base and the endosseal implants, Zahnaerztl. Prax. 15:19-23, 1964.

Lhotsky, B.: Zur Ventraglichkeit Alloplastischer Implante Sonderdruck, D.D.Z., 1965.

Lichtblau, S.: Dislocation of the sacro-iliac joint: a complication of bone-grafting, J. Bone Joint Surg. 44-A: 192, 1962.

Lima Verde, J. G.: Processos psicogenicos em odontologia, Rev. Farm. Odont. 317:332, 1967.

Limoge, A.: Psychology of dental implantation, Inform. Dent. 48:2042-2045, 1966.

Lindahl, Bengt-Martensson, and Kjell: Reimplantation of a tooth.: a case report, Odont. Rev. 11:325-330, 1960.

Linkow, L. I.: The unilateral implant, Dent. Dig. 60:302-306, 1954.

Linkow, L. I.: Implantation unilateral, Oral Hyg., June-July, 1957.

Linkow, L. I.: An evaluation of the unilateral implant, a five year report, Dent. Dig. 14:383-387, 1958.

Linkow, L. I.: Abutments for full mouth splinting, J. Prosth. Dent. 11(5):920-924, 1961.

Linkow, L. I.: Full arch splint, J. Prosth. Dent. 11(6): 1117-1121, 1961.

Linkow, L. I.: Contact areas in natural dentitions and

fixed prosthodontics, J. Prosth. Dent. **12**(1):132-137, 1962.

Linkow, L. I.: Mesially tipped mandibular molars, J. Prosth. Dent. **12**(3):554-558, 1962.

Linkow, L. I.: Reconstruction of anterior teeth with extreme vertical and horizontal overlap, J. Prosth. Dent. **12**(5):947-950, 1962.

Linkow, L. I.: Full arch oral reconstruction—simplified, New York, 1962, Springer Publishing Co.

Linkow, L. I.: Evaluation of the unilateral implant, eight year report, Dent. Dig. **68**:158-168, 1962.

Linkow, L. I.: Intra-osseous implants utilized as fixed bridge abutments, J. Oral Implant Transplant Surg. **10**(2):17-23, 1964.

Linkow, L. I.: Importance of axial inclinations of teeth in attainment of parallelism, J. Prosth. Dent. **15**(3):517-524, 1965.

Linkow, L. I.: Metal implants assessed, Dent. Times **9**(9):6, 7, 1965.

Linkow, L. I.: Clinical evaluation of the various designed endosseous implants, J. Oral Implant Transplant Surg. **12**:35-46, 1966.

Linkow, L. I.: The age of endosseous implants, Dent. Concepts **18**(3):4-10, 1966.

Linkow, L. I.: The radiographic role in endosseous implant interventions, Chron. Omaha Dent. Soc. **29**(10):304-311, 1966.

Linkow, L. I.: Maxillary endosseous implants, Dent. Concepts **10**:14-23, 1966.

Linkow, L. I.: The versatility of implant interventions, Dent. Concepts **10**(2):5-17, 1966.

Linkow, L. I.: L'era degli impianti ossei, Inform. Odontostomat. **8**:14-15, 1966.

Linkow, L. I.: The era of endosseous implants, J. D. C. Dent. Soc. **42**(2):47, 1967.

Linkow, L. I.: Prefabricated endosseous implant prostheses, Dent. Concepts **10**:3-11, 1967.

Linkow, L. I.: Re-evaluation of mandibular unilateral subperiosteal implants, a 12 year report, J. Prosth. Dent. **17**(5):509-514, 1967.

Linkow, L. I.: Internally threaded endosseous implants, Dent. Concepts **10**:16-20, 1967.

Linkow, L. I.: Atypical implantations for anatomically contraindicated situations, Dent. Concepts **11**(5):11-17, 1967.

Linkow, L. I.: Pin implants, Prom. Dent. **3**:4-10, 1968.

Linkow, L. I.: The blade vent—a new dimension in endosseous implants, Dent. Concepts **11**:3-18, 1968.

Linkow, L. I.: Histopathologic and radiologic studies on endosseous implants, Dent. Concepts **11**(3):3-13, 1968.

Linkow, L. I.: Prefabricated mandibular prostheses for intraosseous implants, J. Prosth. Dent. **20**(4):367-375, 1968.

Linkow, L. I.: The endosseous blade: a new dimension in oral implantology, Rev. Trim. Implant. **5**:13-24, 1968.

Linkow, L. I., and Martini, J.: Case report of the month —the value of dental tisssues in the reconstruction of a cleft palate-lip-anodontic case with the aid of endosseous implants, New York J. Dent. **39**(1):15-19, 1969.

Linkow, L. I.: The status of oral implants, Inform. Odontostomat., No. 1, 1969.

Linkow, L. I.: The endosseous blade—a progress report, Prom. Dent. **5**:6-17, 1969.

Linkow, L. I.: Mouth reconstruction for the edentulous maxilla using endosseous blades, Dent. Concepts **12**(1):3-21, 1969.

Linkow, L. I.: The endosseous blade implant and its use in orthodontics, Int. J. Orthodont. **18**(4):149-154, 1969.

Linkow, L. I.: Endosseous oral implantology; a 7 year progress report, Dent. Clin. N. Amer. **14**:185-200, 1970.

Linkow, L. I.: Prefabricated maxillary endosteal implant prosthesis, J. Prosth. Dent. **23**(3):327-336, 1970.

Linkow, L. I.: Endosseous blade-vent implants: a two year report, J. Prosth. Dent. **23**:441-449, 1970.

Linkow, L. I.: Alloplastic implants. In Goldman, H. M., Forrest, S. P., Byrd, D. L., and McDonald, R. E.: Current therapy in dentistry, St. Louis, 1968, The C. V. Mosby Co.

Lirot, R. E.: Implantation and esthetics, Inform. Dent. **47**:613-620, 1965.

Lirot, R. E.: Coordination of clinical and laboratory technics in subperiosteal dental implants, Rev. Franc. Odontostomat. **10**:364-389, 1968.

Lisitsyn, K. M.: Clinical use of embryonic bone heterografts preserved in parallin, Vestn. Khir. Grekov. **89**:24, 1962.

LoBianco, F.: Spiral intraosseous implants according to Perron: preliminary study of the case, Dent. Cosmos **33**:973-980, 1965.

Loechler, P. S., and Mueller, M. W.: Successful implant denture, Northwest Dent. **31**:134, 1952.

Loechler, P. S., and Mueller, M. W.: Implant denture construction, J. Missouri Dent. Ass. **33**:18-21, 1953.

Loechler, P. S., and Mueller, M. W.: Surgical, clinical, and histopathologic notes on the human implant denture, J. Implant Dent. **1**:23-31, 1954.

Lopez, A.: Articular grafts, Med. Esp. **47**:501, 1962.

Lubit, E. C., and Rappaport, E.: Vitallium implantation, New York Dent. J. **15**:217-223, 1949.

Lukashenko, A. A.: Utilization of auto-osteoblastic tissue in the surgical treatment of the bone cavities in children, Nov. Khir. Atkn., 1962.

Lusena, M., and Chini, V.: Le infezioni focali, Riforma Med., Vol. 49, 1933.

Lyght, C. E., and others: The Merck manual of diagnosis and therapy, ed. 40, Rahway, New Jersey, 1966, Merck & Co., Inc.

Lyon, H. W., Boyne, P. J., and Losee, F. L.: Response of oral tissues to grafts of heterologous anorganic bone: II. Host response to implants of anorganic bovine spongy bone, J. Dent. Res. **37**:44-45, 1958.

Lyons: Replantation of teeth, Lancet, September, 1873.

Maatz, R., and Bauermeister, A.: A method of bone maceration, J. Bone Joint Surg. 36-A:721, 1957.

Maatz, R., and Bauermeister, A.: Clinical experiences with the Keil graft, Langenbeck. Arch. Klin. Chir. 298:239, 1961.

Mack, A.: Implant dentures, Brit. Dent. J. 96:151, 1954.

Mack, A.: Symposium question: Do you think that implant dentures are satisfactory from a biological standpoint? Oral Health 44:216-217, 1954.

Mack, A.: Subperiosteal dental implants, Brit. Dent. J. 99:287-293, 1955; discussion, 99:293-295, 1955; reply, 99:295, 1955.

Maeglin, B.: Processi di guarigione susseguenti ad inserzione di una struttura metallica sottoperiostea, Schweiz. Mshr. Zahnheilk. 4:300, 1947.

Maeglin, B.: Contact d'implants metalliques, Inform. Dent., No. 52, 1957.

Maeglin, B.: Knochen im Bereiche subperiostaler gerustimplante, Schweiz. Mschr. Zahnheilk. 10:885, 1958.

Maestre, H. J.: Indications and problems of bone grafts in pathology of the locomotor system, Med. Esp. 47:508, 1962.

Maggiolo: Manuel de l'art dentaire, Nancy, 1809, Editions C. Leseure.

Magnusson, R., and Oldfelt, C. O.: An operated case of enchondroma tibiae in which the course of healing was followed with SR-85, Acta Orthop. Scand. 32:290, 1962.

Mahe, G.: Reimplantation, transplantation, implantation, Arch. Stomat., September, 1911; ibid., February, 1912.

Mankin, M.: Osteogenesis induced by vesical mucosal transplant in the guinea pig, J. Bone Joint Surg. 44-B:165, 1962.

Malingre: Complications des implants endo-osseux: leurs causes et leurs traitements, Congrès International du Faculté de Médecine, Paris, 1961.

Mandl, F.: Klinisches und Experimentelles zur Frage der lokalisierten und generalisierten Ostisfibrosa B. Diegeneralisierte Formder Ostitis Fibrosa, Arch. Klin. Chir. 143:245-284, 1926.

Marco, C. J., and Bonet, S. E.: Various osteopathies treated with ossopan, Med. Esp. 45:121, 1961.

Marken, K. E.: Studies of deviations between observers in clinicoodontologica recording, Umea Research Library Series 2:8, 1962.

Marquit, B., and Harrison, G. I.: A new method of utilizing homografts, Arch. Otolaryng. 73:50, 1961.

Martin, H. C.: Implant dentures, J. Tennessee Dent. Ass. 37:220-222, 1957.

Martin Du Grady: Implants mixés, technique et instrumentation, Rev. Franc. Odontostomat., Vol. 8, 1958.

Martin Du Grady: Esame comparativo dei metodi en doiuxta-ossei, Ass. Odontostomat. Implant., 1961.

Marziani, L.: Co-report: tantalum implant dentures, Int. Dent. J. 8:255-257, 1958; discussion, 8:257-260, 1958.

Marziani, L.: Radici artificiali come ancoraggio di protesi complete mobili inferiori, Clin. Odont. 10:244, 1947.

Marziani, L.: Use of tantalum in reconstructive surgery with special regard to oral subperiosteal implants, Int. Dent. J. 3:13, 1952; correction, 4:627, 1953.

Marziani, L.: Dental implants and implant dentures, their theory, history and practice, Int. Dent. J. 4:459, 1954.

Marziani, L.: Implants dentaires: théorie, histologie et applications techniques, Inform. Dent., Vol. 38, 1954.

Marziani, L.: Impianti metallici, acrilici e innesti dentari nei tessuti mascellari a sostegno di protesi, Riv. Ital. Stomat. 9:1211, 1955.

Marziani, L.: Implantaciones subperiosticas en los maxilares para sosten de protesis, Riv. Ital. Stomat. 9:1211, 1955.

Marziani, L.: Les implants alloplastiques en chirurgie et en particulier les implants comme solutien de prosthèse dentaire, Rev. Franc. Odontostomat. 5:757, 1957.

Marziani, L.: Les implants sous periostes en tantale, Schweiz. Mschr. Zahnheilk. 10:903, 1958.

Marziani, L.: Methode de laboratoire dans les implants en tantare, Belg. T. Tandheelk., 1959.

Marziani, L.: Endosseous implants by trans-radicular root, Riv. Ital. Stomat. 20:1162-1178, 1965.

Marziani, L.: Implantation of a tantalum screw for consolidation of a fractured root, Riv. Ital. Stomat. 20:1209-1214, 1965.

Massler, M., and Schour, I.: The P-M-A index of gingivitis, J. Dent. Res. 28:63, 1949.

Mattila, K.: A roentgenological study of internal defects in chrome-coba implants and partial dentures, Acta Odont. Scand. 22:215-228, 1964.

Mattila, K.: Roentgenologinen tutkimus kromi-kobolttisten osaproteesi ja implantaatirunkojen sisaisista raken nevirheista, Soum. Hammaslaak Toim. 59:436-448, 1968.

Maurel, G.: A propos de plusiers cas d'implants sousperiostes, Rev. Franc. Odontostomat., Vol. 2, 1958.

Maurel, G.: Les implants metalliques sous-periostes en pratique courante, Semaine Edentologique Internationale à Paris, April, 1947.

Maurel, G.: Gli impianti e le inclusioni acriliche nella pratica odonto-stomatologica e maxillo-faciale, Inform. Dent., Vol. 24, 1953.

Maurel, G.: Les implants et les inclusions d'acrylique dans la pratique odontostomatologique et maxillo-faciale, Rev. Stomat. 75:21, 1953.

Maurel, G.: Etat actuel de l'utilisation des inclusions d'acrylique en chirurgie maxillo-faciale et en pratique odontostomatologique, Rev. Franc. Odontostomat. 2:295-308, 1955.

Maurel, G.: Etat actuel des inclusions d'acryliques en chirurgie maxillofaciale et en pratique odontostomatologie, Rev. Franc. Odontostomat., Vol. 10, 1956.

Maurel, G.: Implants metalicos en desdentadoe totales, Clin. Cir. Max. 8:941, 1959.

Maurel, G.: Les implants sous periostes en prosthèse dentaire, Paris, 1960, Librairie Maloine.

Mayer, R.: Treatment of recurrent luxation of the mandible with a Vitallium pin, Acta Stomat. Belg. 62:381-391, 1965.

Mazzotto, F., and Sabras, P.: Prosthèses fixés chez les edentés par l'inclusion sous muqueuse d'un double arc à inlays dans le tissu osseux, Rev. Odont. 7-8:359, 1952.

McCall, J. O.: Vitallium implant and a bridge abutment, Dent. Items 63:15-17, 1946.

McCall, J. O.: Textbook of periodontia, Philadelphia, 1953, McGraw-Hill Book Company.

McCall, J. O.: Clinical dental roentgenology, ed. 4, Philadelphia, 1957, W. B. Saunders Co.

McCullagh, E. P., and Resch, C. A.: Some endocrine factors in dental development and maintenance, J.A.D.A. 28:1436-1446, 1941.

McEvoy, L. L.: Removal of foreign body in the maxillary sinus, Dent. Ass. 58:126, 1959.

McGrannahan, W. W.: Implant denture following mandibular resection, Dent. Dig. 72:300-306, 1966.

Melcher, A. H.: Use of heterogenous anorganic bone in periodontal bone grafting: a preliminary report, J. Dent. Ass. S. Afr. 13:80, 1958.

Mendelson, M.: Implant denture: a case report, J. Florida Dent. Soc. 34:5-8, 1963.

Menegaux, O. D.: Action cytotoxique de certains metaux sur des osteoblastes humains cultives in vitro, Presse Med., October, 1935.

Merle-Beral, V.: Impianti dentari e innesti o inclusioni di denti artificiali, XIII Congrès Français Stomatologie, Paris, 1953.

Merville, L.: Implants metalliques sous-periostes: indications et contre-indications de technique, Rev. Franc. Odontostomat. 9:1287-1288, 1961.

Merville, L.: Indications and contraindications of subperiosteal implants, Rev. Franc. Odontostomat. 10: 744-752, 1963.

Meyer, J.: Les travaux pratiques du cours post-universitaire d'implantologie-aigulle, Rev. Odontoimplant., Vol. 2, June, 1966.

Meyer, W.: Histologie der Zahne und des Geb isses-Zahn-Mund und Kiefer, Monaco, 1943, Urban Schwarzenberg.

Meylan, P.: Simple idée, Inform. Dent. 29:1437, 1947.

Meylan, P.: Cheville alveolaire, Rev. Suisse Odont. 61: 317, 1951.

Milteer, A. D.: Surgical impression techniques, J. Implant Dent. 1:13-18, 1955.

Milton, H.: Impianti di denti in plastica, J.A.D.A. 60: 123, 1960.

Miranda, C. E. R., Cruz, E. O., and Carvalho, A. P.: Manual de biofisica, Universidade do Brasil, 1960.

Mitscherlich, A.: Die Replantation und die Transplantation der Zahne, Langenbeck. Arch. Klin. Chir. 4: 375, 1863.

Mitscherlich, A.: Replantation and transplantation of teeth, Arch. Dent., pp. 169-184, 1865.

Moore, G., and Haman, H.: Removal of metal foreign body from antral floor, Brit. Dent. J. 12:405-406, 1959.

Morel-Maillard, J.: Radicular extensor, Inform. Dent. 47(44):90-91, 1965.

Morozov, A. I.: On the regeneration of the bone and on the fate of the tubular homografts in osteoplasty of large defects of the diaphysis of the hip in experimental conditions, Ortop. Travm. Protez. 23:52, 1962.

Morris, E. O.: The bacteriology of the oral cavity, Brit. Dent. J. 95:77-82, 1953.

Mortimer, H.: Pituitary and associated hormone factors in cranial growth and differentiation in white rat: roentgenological study, Radiology 28:5-39, 1937.

Mosk, S.: Plastic tooth implants, dental survey, J. Dent. Pract., August, 1967.

Moss, M. L.: Extraction of an osteogenic inductor factor from bone, Science 127:755, 1958.

Moss, M. L.: Studies of the acellular bone of teleost fish: three intraskeletal grafts in the rat, Acta Anat. 49: 266, 1962.

Mossdorf, H.: Implantations and implant magnetprosthese, Zahnaertzl. Prax. 17:794, 1952.

Mowlem, R.: Iliac bone and cartilage transplants: use and behavior, Brit. J. Surg. 29:182, 1941.

Mueller, H., and Pitzke, K. F.: Ertl and conversion graft: a contribution to graft plastic surgery in fracture of the leg with delayed callus formation and pseudarthrosis, Bruns Beitr. Klin. Chir. 202:399, 1961.

Mueller, M. E.: Zum Vortrag Dr. Issel—Bericht der 74 Tagung der Btsch Gesell F. Zahn—Mundund Kiefer hail Kunde, Monaco, 1953.

Mueller, M. E.: Technik der operativen Frakturenbehandlung, Berlin, 1953, Springer-Verlag.

Mueller, M. W.: Implant dentures, Texas Dent. J. 75: 9-16, 1957.

Mueller, M. W.: Ten year evaluation of implant dentistry: introduction to the panel discussion, J. Prosth. Dent. 10:1116-1117, 1960.

Mueller, M. E.: Internal fixation for fresh fractures and for non-union, Proc. Roy. Soc. Med. 56:455-459, 1963.

Muhleman, H. R., and Boitel, R. H. Quoted by Stieger, A. A.: Progress in partial denture prostheses, Int. Dent. J. 2:568, 1952.

Muratori, G.: Storia ed evoluzione degli inn esti e trapianti dentari dall'antichità ad oggi, Atti del XVI Congresso Nazionale di Storia della Medicina, Bologna-Ravenna, 1959.

Muratori, G.: Quelques cas d'implants endo-osseux, Rev. Franc. Odontostomat., 1961.

Muratori, G.: Evoluzione storica della vite da impianto Formiggini, Arti Sanitarie Ausiliarie, No. 19, April, 1962.

Muratori, G.: Esame isotologico di un impianto endoosseo estratto dopo 5 ani, Riv. Ital. Stomat., Vol. 3, March, 1963.

Muratori, G.: Evoluzione storica degli impianti allo-plastici in stomatologia, Arcisped. S. Anna Ferrara **17**(6):15-20, 1964.

Muratori, G.: L'insufficienza masticatoria come causa di gastroen teropatie: evoluzione storica della tecnica implamare preprostescia, Clinica **24**:4, 1964.

Muratori, G.: Sistema personale di impianto endoosseo a travata suitabile, Dent. Cadmos **32**:6, 1964.

Muratori, G.: Metado personale di impianto endoosseo a barra di fissazione rimovibile, Minerva Stomat. **14**:95-102, 1965.

Muratori, G.: Histological examination of an implant after five years, Newsletter Amer. Acad. Implant Dent., No. 3, July, 1967.

Muratori, G.: Infezioni focali ed implantologia, Minerva Stomat. **16**:476-481, 1967.

Muratori, G.: L'impianto endoosseo: dall'intervento alla protesi, Dent. Cadmos, January-March, 1967.

Muratori, G.: Parallelismo e disparallelismo in implan-tologia, Inform. Odontostomat. **3**:3, 1967.

Muratori, G.: Stato attuale dell'implantologia endoossea nel mondo, Riv. Ital. Stomat., Vol. 7, 1967.

Muratori, G.: Deux implants endo-osseux (examen his-tologique après 5 et 6 ans), Inform. Dent., Vol. 36, 1967.

Muratori, G.: Impianti endo-ossei alloplastici nei mascel-lari: istologia e radiologia dai 5 ai 7 anni di distanza, Minerva Chir. **22**(11):687-688, 1967.

Muratori, G.: Indicazioni e contreindicazioni, errori e loro prevenzione in implantologia endo-ossea: rimovi-bilità della sovrastruttura, Communication presented to the XXXIX Italian Congress of Stomatology, Catania-Taormina, September 27 to 30, 1967.

Muratori, G.: Semplicità, razionalità e sicurezza nell'-esecuzione di un impianto endoosseo, Inform. Odonto-stomat., No. 1, 1967.

Muratori, G.: L'impianto endo-osseo, Dent. Cadmos, No. 1-7, 1967-1968.

Muratori, G.: Histologie reabsorbtion osteo muqueuse et regeneration osseuse in implantologie endoosseuse, Prom. Dent, Vol. 1, 1968.

Muratori, G.: Importance de l'amovibilite en implantol-ogie endoosseuse, Inform. Dent. **2**(24):6-13, 1968

Muratori, G.: Histologie, reabsorption ostéo-muqueuse et regénération osseuse en implantologie endo-osseuse, Prom. Dent., 1 trimestre, 1968.

Muratori, G.: Importance de l'amovibilité en implanto-logie endo-osseuse, Inform. Dent. No. 2-24, June, 1968.

Muratori, G.: L'impianto endosseo a sovrastruttura rimovibile e fissa (dall'intervento alla protesi), Milan, 1969, Edizioni Cadmos.

Muratori, G.: L'implantologo: una nuova figura in odon-tostomatologia, Inform. Odontostomat., No. 1, 1969.

Muratori, G.: Una nuova dimensione in odontotecnica; la

protesi su impianto, Dent. Cadmos, anno XXXVII, No. 3, March, 1969.

Muratori, G.: L'impianto-appoggio: nuovo elemento im-plantare di appoggio da affiancare alle normali viti da impianto nella pratica endo-ossea, Minerva Stomat. **18**(6):299-305, 1969.

Muratori, G.: Impianti e trapianti in stomatologia (tecni-ca chirurgica e protesica), Rassegna Med. Culturale, Vol. 46, No. 5, 1969.

Muratori, G.: Classificazione, razionalità, sicurezza ed igiene degli impianti endo-ossei con protesi rimovi-bile, Boll. Soc. Ital. Parondont., No. 19, January-February, 1969.

Muratori, G.: Trapianti e impianti: scienza e psicologia, Inform. Attualita Mondiali, Vol. 16, October, 1969.

Muratori, G.: The endosseous implant with removable and fixed superstructure, Parma, 1969, Tip. Gia Cooperativa.

Muriloo, C.: Implantes dentarios en acrilico, Rev. Esp. Stomat. **2**:3, 1954.

Nabers, C. L., and O'Leary, T. J.: Autogenous bone transplants in the treatment of osseous defects, J. Periodont. **36**:1, 1965.

Nadasid, M.: Inhibition of experimental arthritis by athermic pulsating short waves in rats, Orthopedics **2**:105-107, 1960.

Nakazawa, I., and Kobayashi, S.: Case report of im-plant denture, Bull. Tokyo Med. Dent. Univ. **5**:13-17, 1958.

Nally-Berta: Essai de classification des attachements pre-fabriqués en Suisse, Rev. Mens. Suisse Odont., 1959.

Neugebauer, P.: Implantation des dents en porcelain ou resine acrylique, Inform. Dent. **31**:1143, 1949.

Neuner, O.: Relazione circa un nuovo metodo per im-pianti metallici sottoperiostei, Rev. Ital. Stomat. **14**:32-54, 1959.

Nevin, M.: A resumé of local anesthesia, Mod. Dent., April, 1947.

Nevins, L. M., Stahl, S. S., and Sorrin, S.: The response of experimentally injured alveolar bone to cultured calf bone implantation in dogs, Oral Surg. **14**:1256, 1961.

Newman, C., and Van Huisen, B.: Reazioni di tessuti agli impianti in vitallium, J. Prosth. Dent. **6**:721, 1954.

Newman, C., and Van Huysen, G.: Tissue reaction to Vitallium implantation, J. Prosth. Dent. **4**:850-854, 1954.

Nichols, F. C.: Semi-buried denture implants: review of literature and experimental study, J. Oral Surg. **12**:217-231, 1954.

Nikoforova, E. K.: Evaluation of autografts and homo-grafts in the surgical therapy of scolioses in children and adolescents, Acta Chir. Orthop. Traum. Cech. **29**:380, 1962.

Nilson, E.: Avlastningsbarens anvandning vid fasta och

avtagbara broar, Svensk. Tandlak. T. **49**:129-165, 1956.

Nilson, E.: Hur skola vi konstruera vara broar med hansyn till framtida forandringar i bettet? Norske Tannlaegeforen. Tid. **68**:49-62, 1958.

Nilson, E.: Speciella Brokonstruktioner, Nord. Klin. Odont. **21**(IV):1-25, 1959.

Nishimura, K. K., Yaeger, J. A., and Sabet, T. Y.: Fate of osteocytes in adult mouse whole bone isografts and homografts, Anat. Rec. **144**:85, 1962.

Nix, D. F., and Nye, L. E.: Upper implant dentures, J. California Dent. Ass. **20**:318, 1953.

Nockemann, P. F., and Schilling, H.: Preservation of heteroplastic bone, Bruns Beitr. Klin. Chir. **203**: 67, 1961.

Nockeman, P. F., and Schilling, H.: On the use of heteroplastic bone transplants, Deutsch. Med. J. **13**: 219, 1962.

Novis, R. H.: Design and construction of subperiosteal implant dentures, Dent. Tech. **12**:141-145, 1955.

Nyquist, G.: Audiatur et altera pars', Odont. T. **52**:202, 1944.

Obwegeser, H. J.: Experiences with subperiosteal implants, Oral Surg. **12**:777-786, 1959.

Ogus, W. I.: Impianto di radice in Vitallium (The Vitallium root implant), Conference of the Northeastern Dental Society, 1942.

Ogus, W. I.: The planning of incision, Dent. Dig. **54**:7, 1948.

Ogus, W. I.: Upper implant for an immediate partial denture, Dent. Dig. **58**:538-539, 1952.

Ogus, W. I.: Research report on the replant implant of individual teeth, Dent. Dig. **60**:358, 1954.

Orell, S.: Surgical bone grafting with "os purum," "os novum," and boiled bone, J. Bone Joint Surg. **19**: 873, 1937.

Orlay, H. G.: Splinting with endodontic implant stabilizers, Dent. Pract. **14**:481-498, 1964.

Orlay, H. G.: Endodontic implants, J. Oral Implant Transplant Surg. **11**:44-53, 1965.

Orlay, H. G.: A new universal prosthetic implant technique: the pin implants of Scialom, J. Oral Implant Transplant Surg. **11**:24-34, 1965.

Orlay, H. G.: Contention par implantation de stabilisateurs transradiculaires, Inform. Dent., Vol. 43, 1966.

Ostlund, S. G.: The effect of complete dentures on the gum tissues, Malmo, 1958.

Ostlund, S. G.: Den totala plattprotesen, Nord. Klin. Odont. **21**(VII):1-43, 1959.

Ostrom, C. A., and Lyon, H. W.: Pulpar response to chemically treated heterogenous bone in pulp-capping sites, Oral Surg. **15**:362, 1962.

Osvald, O.: Odontologisk kirurgi I, Nord. Klin. Odont. **20**:1-38, 1958.

Oursland, L. E.: Implant denture: a preliminary report, Bull. San Diego Dent. Soc. **21**:6-8, 1951.

Overby, G. E.: Esthetic splinting of teeth by vertical pinning, J. Prosth. Dent. **1**:112-118, 1961.

Overby, G. E.: Intracoronary splinting of mobile teeth by use of screws and sleeves, J. Periodont., July, 1962.

Oven, J.: The origin of new bone around heterografts transplanted to the chick embryo chorioallantois, Exp. Cell Res. **28**:441, 1962.

Page, H. L.: A new implant material for use in reconstructive surgical procedures: Surgibone (Boplant), Dent. Dig., Vol. 72, 1966.

Pajne, R. E.: Implantations of tooth by silver capsule method, Dent. Cosmos **43**:1401, 1901.

Palazzi, S.: Trattato di odontologia, Milan, 1950, Hoepli.

Palazzi, S.: Atti del simposio degli impianti alloplastici, Compte rendu du Congrès, March, 1955.

Palazzi, S.: Mete ragguante negli impianti alloplastici iuxtaperiostei, Med. Stomat., Vol. 1, 1956.

Palazzi, S.: Qualche precisazione sugli impianti alloplastici, Rass. Trim. Odont., Vol. 2, 1963.

Palfer-Sollier, M.: Les gouttières vissées en durallium dans la chirurgie mandibulare, Paris, 1958, Expansion Sciéntifique Française.

Palfer-Sollier, M.: Demonstrations pratiques aux cours de semaines implantaires: anesthèse, premédication, prevention des accidents, Paris, 1960.

Palfer-Sollier, M.: Pre- and post-operative therapeutics applied to implantology, Rev. Franc. Odontostomat. **12**:1201-1208, 1965.

Palmer, J. F.: Works of John Hunter, London, 1835.

Pampas, F., and Kahl, R. J.: Experiences with heteroplastic grafts of the spine, Langenbeck. Arch. Klin. Chir. **298**:266, 1961.

Pampas, F., and Kahl, R. J.: Indications for plastic operations on the spine in diseases and traumatic lesions of the spinal nervous system and our experiences with heteroplastic grafts, Zbl. Neurochir. **23**:50, 1962.

Panzoni, E., and Orlando, S.: Experimental subcutaneous implants of methacrylate plastic, Riv. Ital. Stomat. **18**:1672-1686, 1963.

Panzoni, E., and Orlando, S.: Experimental use of Teflon for investment of subcutaneous methacrylate implants, Riv. Ital. Stomat. **19**:29-38, 1964.

Pappas, G. W.: Surgical phase of the lower implant denture: an evolution of implant dentures, Dent. Student. Mag. **32**:18-23, 1954.

Parant, M.: Implant metallique mentonnier, Inform. Dent., Vol. 49, 1953.

Parant, M.: Les problèmes des implants, Actualites Odontostomat. **46**:151, 1959.

Parant, M.: Les implants, Rev. Odontostomat. **7**(5): 702, 1960.

Parant, M.: Assessment of implant dentures in 1961, Int. Dent. J. **11**:427-442, 1961.

Parant, M., and Jaskarzec, B.: De l'evolution du problème des implants metalliques sous periostes, Rev. Franc. Odontostomat. 2:295-308, 1955.

Parant, M., Jaskarzec, B., and Deschamps, Y.: Les implants metalliques sous-periostes dans les restauration prothetiques fixés, Int. Dent. 6:606, 1952.

Parker, G. D.: Apical implant as a monotooth splint, Dent. Dig. 62:58-62, 1956.

Pasqualini, V.: Perno momcone a cerchiaggio intraradicolare (tecnica personale), G. Odont. Dic., pp. 78-82, 1961.

Pasqualini, V.: Reperti anatomopatologici e deduzioni clinico-chirurgiche di 91 impianti alloplastici in 28 animali do esperimento, Riv. Ital. Stomat. 17:46-92, 1962.

Patterson, F. P.: Autogenous cortical bone grafts for delayed and nonunion of fractures of the tibial shaft, Canad. J. Surg. 5:53, 1962.

Paturet, G.: Traité d'anatomie humaine, I, Paris, 1951.

Paullus, W. S.: Surgical procedure for the lower implant denture, Dent. Dig. 59:56-61, 1953.

Paullus, W. S.: Histological report on unilateral implant, J. Implant Dent. 2:46, 1956.

Paumgartner: Reimplantation, transplantation und implantation, Z. Stomat. 31:226, 1933.

Payne, C.: Gold capsule implantation, Pacific Dent. Gaz. 8:653, 1900.

Payne, R.: Textbook of operative dentistry, Philadelphia, 1917, The Blakiston Co., pp. 810-831.

Pejrone, G.: Considerazioni sugli impianti sottoperiostei, Rev. Ital. Stomat. 10:20-25, 1955.

Pelletier, M.: Croquis d'infrastructure metallique sous perioste pour la restoration prosthetique des edentes complets, Communication à la Société Française d'Implantologie, 1952.

Pelletier, M.: Problèmes posés par les implants sous periostes les prosthèses sus jacentes et leur mode de réunion, communication à la Société Française d'Implantologie, 1956.

Pelletier, M.: Metallographie appliquée aux implants, Inform. Dent., Vol. 26, 1958.

Pelletier, M.: Implants stillite sous-periostes en odontostomatologie, Paris, 1960, Prelat.

Pelletier, M.: Subperiosteal implants into bone, Chir. Dent. France 22:37-47, 1962; ibid., 22:43-49, 1962; ibid., 22:75-78, 1962.

Pelletier, M., Maurel, G., and Esatoglu, J.: La dysostose cleidocranienne: étude clinique et pathogenique à propos d'un cas avec traitement maxillodentaire grâce aux implants sous periostes, Rev. Franc. Odontostomat., Vol. 1, 1959.

Pendleton, E. C.: Changes in the denture supporting tissues, J.A.D.A. 4:1-15, 1951.

Prereira: Urbano—curso de fisica, Sao Paulo, 1944, Livaria Academica.

Pernek, W. E., and Pafford, E. M.: Implant dentures versus conventional dentures, J. Implant Dent. 6:10-21, 1959.

Pernell, W. E.: History of implant work and a report on mandibular implants by the district impression method, J. Prosth. Dent. 2:51-54, 1952.

Pernell, W. E.: History and histology report of implant cast covering three and one half years, Arizona Dent. J. 1:8-10, 1955.

Pernell, W. E.: Implantation—its use and abuse, New York Dent. J. 21:150, 1955.

Perreten, F. M.: Confection d'un implant juxtaosseux, Rev. Trim. Implant., April, 1968.

Perron, A. C.: Impianti eteroplastici endomaxillari con la vite di Formiggini, Prot. Dent. 2:8, 1957.

Perron, A. C.: Confeccion de espirales Formiggini para implantes intraosseos, Prot. Dent., 1958.

Perron, A. C.: Emplantes introoseos aloplasticos con espirales Formiggini, An. Med., Vol. 45, February, 1958.

Perron, A. C.: Biopsia di un impianto endosseo Formiggini, Prot. Dent., 1959.

Perron, A. C.: Condiciones que deben reunir los implantos intraosseos, An. Esp. Odontostomat. 20:681-688, 1961.

Perron, A. C.: Fissazione e ritenzione degli impianti endossei, complicanze minori nell'impianto endosseo unitario, 3 Congr. Int. degli Impianti, July, 1961.

Perron, A.C.: Fiyacion y retencion de los implantes intraoseos del sistema Formiggini, An. Esp. Odontostomat. 20:782-799, 1961.

Perron, A. C.: Technique personnelle d'implants endoosseux et resultats, Odontostomat., December, 1961.

Perron, A. C.: Biodinamica de los implantes endo-ossos en espiral, Rev. Esp. Estomat., Vol. 11, No. 3, May-June, 1963.

Perron, A. C.: El paralelismo en los implantes endooseos, Prot. Dent. Coll. Sespar., Vol. 27, 1963.

Perron, A. C.: I fondamenti dell'implantologia endosea, Dent. Cadmos, 1965.

Person, P.: Biology of the mouth, Pub. 89, Washington D. C., 1968, American Association for the Advancement of Science.

Peyrone G., Zerosi C., and Sebastiani E.: Impianto parziale su cane e controllo istopatologici, Rass. Trim. Odont. 4:101, 1956.

Pfaff, P.: Abhandlung von Zahnen des menschlichen Korpers, Berlin, 1756.

Philippeaux, J. M.: Greffe d'une dent incisive de cochon dans le crête d'un coque, Compt. Rend. Soc. Biol. 1:336, 1870.

Piazzini, E., and Licata, G.: Considerazioni sugli impianti alloplastici intraossei in stomatologia, Clin. Trim. Odont. 3:1003, 1958.

Pierson: Metallotechmie, Paris, 1950, Baillière.

Pindborg, J. J.: Odontologisk medicin, Nord. Klin. Odont. 1(22):1-22, 1958.

Plischka, G.: Impianti sottoperiostei in tantalio, Communicaz Sull Relaz. Marziani, 39 Congr. Ital. Stomat., Venice, 1954.

Poletti, I. H., and Batt: De re dentaire aput veteres, Bologna, 1935, Cappelli.

Popkirov, S.: Clinical use of bone heterografts, Nauch. Tr. Vissh. Med. Inst. Sofia 40:51, 1961.

Portmann, M., Fortunato, G., and Ceresia, G.: Apropos of stapes substitution by autoplastic and homoplastic grafts, Rev. Laryng. 83:673, 1962.

Posselt, U.: Bettlara och bettanalys, Copenhagen, 1955, Dansk Videnskabs Forlag.

Posselt, U.: Physiology of occlusion and rehabilitation, Oxford, 1962, Blackwell Scientific Publications.

Priorov, N. N., and others: Replacement of bone defects with osteografts after the excision of benign tumors, Eksp. Khir. Anest. 6:3, 1961.

Pritchard, J. J.: The osteoblast. In Bourne, G. H., editor: The biochemistry and physiology of bone, New York, 1956, Academic Press, Inc., p. 179.

Protzel, M. S.: Method for the temporary fixation of a mandibular implant substructure: preliminary report, Dent. Dig. 62:66-267, 1956.

Pullus, W.: Histological report on unilateral implant, J. Implant Dent. 2:46, 1956.

Purdam, R. B.: Simplified fabrication of a tantalum four by five inch skull plate, Oral Surg. 6:1274-1280, 1953.

Quintin: Reimpianti, trapianti, impianti, Odontologie, 1906.

Raciti, S., and Mascali, F.: The development of experimental homoplastic transplants under the action nor-androstenolone decanoate, Minerva Ortop. 13:384, 1962.

Radentz, W. H., and Collings, C. K.: The implantation of plaster of Paris in the alveolar process of the dog, J. Periodont. 36:357-364, 1965.

Ramzy, I.: The implant lower denture, J. Royal Egyptian Med. Ass. 36:6-394, 1952.

Ray, R. D., and Sabet, T. Y.: Bone grafts; cellular survival versus induction: an experimental study in mice, J. Bone Joint Surg. 45-A:337, 1963.

Reichenbach, E.: Prosthetic treatment of maxillofacial defects, Int. J. Dent., June, 1958.

Reichenbach, E.: Histologische Untersuchung über die Reaktion des Knochen lagers auf Gerustimplantate, Deutsch. Zahn. Mund. Kieferheilk. 37:302-311, 1962.

Reichenbach, E., and Kirchner, I.: Ein weiterer Beitrag zur partiellen Prothese in der Sozialpraxis, Deutsch. Zahnaerztl. Z. 7:521-524, 1952.

Reiger, H. G.: Tantalum as a replacement for bone in oral surgery, Oral Surg. 3:727-731, 1950.

Reylly, J.: L'irritation neuro-vegetative et son rôl en pathologie, Med. Hyg. 275:351, 1954.

Rheinwald, U.: Epithelial reactions to subperiosteal implants, Dent. Abstracts 4:37, 1959.

Rialland, R.: Acryliques et tissus alveolares, Rev. Odont. 72:468, 1950.

Rialland, R.: Bridges a piliers artificiels (bridges bequilles), Rev. Odont. 75:134, 1953.

Richany, S. F., Blast, T. H., and Sprinz, H.: The repair of bone and fate of autogenous bone grafts in the skull, Acta Neurochir. 11:61, 1963.

Richardson, R. L., and Jones, M.: A bacteriologic census of human saliva, J. Dent. Res. 37:697-709, 1958.

Ricker, G.: Enticurf einer Relationspathologie, Stuttgart, 1905, G. B. Fischer and Co., Verlagsgesellschaft.

Rigal, R.: Implants sous-periostes unilateraux, Inform. Dent., Vol. 11, 1955.

Rispa, F.: Le problème prothetique et les metamorphoses biologiques des machoires edentées, Rev. Franc. Odontostomat., Vol. 5, 1959.

Ritacco, A., and Ritacco, N.: Implantes endodonticos intraosseos, Buenos Aires, 1967, Mundi Primeira Edicão.

Roaf, R., and Hancox, N.: Fate of heterogenous deproteinized bone implants, J. Bone Joint Surg. 45-B:617, 1963.

Robinson, I. B.: Experimental production of sarcomas by methyl methacrylate implants, J. Dent. Res. 34:721, 1955.

Robinson, J. E.: Magnets for the retention of a sectional intraoral prosthesis: a case history, J. Prosth. Dent. 13:1167-1171, 1963.

Robinson, M.: Silver implant instituted fifty-one years after resection of mandible, Dent. Abstracts 5:209, 1960.

Robinson, R. A.: An electron-microscopic study of the crystalline inorganic component of bone and its relationship to the organic matrix, J. Bone Joint Surg. 34-A:389, 1952.

Roccia, B.: Qualche risultato negli impianti metallici sotto periostei, Comunicazione presentata al 2 Simposio internazionale degli impianti alloplastici a scopo protetico, 1955.

Roccia, B.: Gli impianti metallici nella riparazione delle perdite di sostanza della mandibola, Comunicazione Congr. Ital. Stomatologie, Bologna, 1959.

Rode, H. M.: Implant dentures: a plea for caution and research, Dent. Clin. N. Amer., pp. 579-582, 1960.

Rodier: Esito di 60 denti impiantati, Rev. Stomat., 1902.

Roger, J.: Reverse pin technic, Rev. Esp. Estomat. 13: 483-8, 1965.

Rogosa, M., and others: Improved medium for selective isolation of veillonella, J. Bact. 76:455-456, 1958.

Rogosa, M., Mitchell, J. A., and Wiseman, R. F.: A selective medium for the isolation and enumeration of oral lactobacilli, J. Dent. Res. 30:682-689, 1951.

Roques, J. F.: Original method of metallography of a metallic implant, Rev. Franc. Odontostomat. 12: 1065-1070, 1965.

Rosin, A., Freiberg, H., and Zajicek, G.: The fate of rat

bone marrow, spleen and periosteum cultivated in vivo in the diffusion chamber with special reference to bone formation, Exp. Cell. Res. **29:**176, 1963.

Rossi, A.: Implantation de racines en acrylique utilisées comme piliers de bridge, Inform. Dent. **31:**917, 1949.

Rothchild, H.: Implant denture for a diabetic patient, J.A.D.A. **66:**217-221, 1963.

Rottenberg, A.: Implant de dents en acrylique, Rev. Odont. Stomat. Max. **8:**89, 1952.

Rottenberg, A.: Implant d'organes dentaires en acrylique, Rev. Belg. Stomat. **49:**283, 1953.

Rottenberg, A.: Current practice of implantation, Inform. Dent. **48:**798-801, 1966.

Roux: Technique simplified d'implant mandibulaire pour edente complet, Rev. Franc. Odontostomat., 1961.

Ruffoni, R.: The bone graft in the filling of skeletal cavernous lesions, Arch. Ortop. **73:**413, 1960.

Rusconi, L.: Nuovo procedimento per l'immobilizzazione della protesi competa inferiore, Riv. Ital. Stomat. **2:**137, 1954.

Rush, B.: Medical inquiries and observation, 1809.

Rushton, M. A.: Cases of accelerated and retarded dentition, Brit. Dent. J. **71:**277-279, 1941.

Rutledge, C. E.: Oral and roentgenographic aspects of teeth and jaws of juvenile diabetics, J.A.D.A. **27:**1740-1759, 1940.

Ryan, E. J.: Intraosseous metal implants for stabilization, Dent. Dig. **52:**485, 1946.

Salagaray, F., Sol, B., and Baldomero: Implantes subperiosticos de Vitallium en una sola sesion, Prot. Dent., No. 2, 1957.

Sandhaus, S.: Nouveaux aspects de l'implantologie, Compte rendu des journées implantaires de Lausanne, Med. Hygiene, pp. 17-21, February, 1965.

Sandhaus, S.: Actualités, Rev. Trim. Implant., No. 7, May, 1969.

Sandhaus, S.: Considerations implantologiques: l'implant CBS, Rev. Trim. Implant., No. 7, May, 1969.

Sandhaus, S.: Neve Aspekte der Implantologie, Rev. Trim. Implant., No. 7, May, 1969.

Sandhaus, S.: Transplantation cardiaque, Rev. Trim. Implant., No. 7, May, 1969.

Sato, T.: Parotid gland extract and calcification of dentin of rabbit, Gonma J. Med. Sci. **2:**183, 1953.

Schaffer, E. M.: Cementum and denture implants in a dog and a Rhesus monkey, J. Periodont. **28:**125-131, 1957.

Schafter, O., and Wein, M.: Impianti iuxta ossei in tantalio, Rev. Franc. Odontostomat. **5:**780, 1957.

Schel, O., and others: Alveolar bone loss as related to oral hygiene and age, J. Periodont. **30:**7-16, 1959.

Schermer, R.: Implant dentures, Dent. Items **72:**806-814, 1950.

Schermer, R.: Upper and lower implant denture, J. Implant Dent. **1:**17-22, 1954.

Schermer, R.: Mandibular single abutment implant, J. Implant Dent. **2:**28-30, 1955.

Schermer, R.: Report on removal of maxillary implant, J. Implant Dent. **7:**43-47, 1961.

Schiller, A.: Mastoid osteoplasty using autogenous cancellous bone, progress report and modified technique, J. Laryng. **75:**647, 1961.

Schilling, H., and Nockemann, P.: Histological observations on animal experiment and clinical experiences with a heteroplastic bone material, Mschr. Unfallheilk. **65:**227, 1962.

Schilling, H., and Nockemann, P.: Clinical trials with heteroplastic bone material, Bruns Beitr. Klin. Chir. **205:**89, 1962.

Schmidt, A. S.: Dass Satellimplant, Deutsch. Zahnaerztl. Z., 1958.

Schmidt, H. J.: Implantation of steel frames; from Anglo-American literature and the author's experience, Deutsch. Zahnaerztl. Z. **9:**933-936, 1954.

Schmidt, H. J.: Zur implantation von stahlgerusten, Deutsch. Zahnaerztl. Z. **9:**937-939, 1954.

Schmidt, H. J.: Die Geschichte einer Sattelimplantabrucke, D.D.Z. **16:**1267-1269, 1961.

Schmidt, H. J.: The fate of a saddle-implant bridge: 14 years of wear, Deutsch. Zahnaerztl. Z. **20:**1133-1135, 1965.

Schmidt, H. R.: Gravitat und Zahnfleischblutung und Kalkstoffwecksel. In Kantorowitz: Handworterbuch der gesamten Zahnheilkunde, Berlin, 1930, Herman Meusser.

Schmitt, A.: Uber Osteoplastik in klinischer und experimenteller Beziehung, Arch. Klin. Chir. **45:**401, 1893.

Schmuziger, P., and Obwegeser: Recherches sur les implants à l'Institut Dentaire de Zurich, Rev. Odont., 1958.

Schmuziger, P.: Besondere implantationskonstruktion, Schweiz. Mschr. Zahnheilk. **10:**919, 1958.

Schneider, H.: Die aseptische Implantation einer neuen kunstlichen Zahnwurzel, Z. Stomat. **12:**806, 1937.

Schour, I.: Changes in incisor of thirteen-lined ground squirrel (citellus tride-cemlineatus) following bilateral gonadectomy, Anat. Rec. **65:**177-199, 1936.

Schour, I.: Changes in teeth following parathyroidectomy: effect of parathyroid extract and calciferol on incisor of rat, Amer. J. Path. **13:**971-984, 1937.

Schour, I.: Tooth development. In Dental science and dental art, Philadelphia, 1938, Lea & Febiger.

Schour, I.: Calcium metabolism and teeth, J.A.M.A. **110:**870-877, 1938.

Schour, I.: Experimental dental histophysiology. In Dental science and dental art, Philadelphia, 1938, Lea & Febiger.

Schour, I., Brodie, A. G., and King, E. Q.: Hypophysis and teeth: IV. Case report of hypopituitary patient, Angle Orthodont. **4:**265-304, 1934.

Schour, I., Chandler, S. B., and Tweedy, W. R.: Changes in teeth following parathyroidectomy: effects of dif-

ferent periods of survival, fasting and repeated preg-
nancies and lactations on incisor of rat, Amer. J.
Path. **13**:945-970, 1937.

Schour, I., and Massler, M.: Studies in tooth development, growth pattern of human teeth, J.A.D.A. **27:**
1778-1793, 1940.

Schour, I., and Massler, M.: Studies in tooth development: growth pattern of human teeth (Part II),
J.A.D.A. **27:**1918-1931, 1940.

Schour, I., and Massler, M.: Prevalence of gingivitis in
young adults, J. Dent. Res. **27:**733-734, 1948.

Schour, I., and Rogoff, J. M.: Changes in rat incisor
following bilateral adrenalectomy, Amer. J. Physiol.
115:334-344, 1936.

Schour, I., Tweedy, W. R., and McJunkin, F. A.: Effect
of single and multiple doses of parathyroid hormone
on calcification of dentin of rat incisor, Amer. J.
Path. **10:**321-342, 1934.

Schour, I., and Van Dyke, H. B.: Effect of replacement
therapy on eruption of incisor of hypophysectomized
rat, Proc. Soc. Exp. Biol. Med. **29:**378-382, 1932.

Schour, I., and Van Dyke, H. B.: Changes in teeth following hypophysectomy: I. Changes in incisor of
white rat, Amer. J. Anat. **50:**397-433, 1932.

Schour, I., and Van Dyke, H. B.: Changes in teeth
following hypophysectomy: II. Changes in molar of
white rat, J. Dent. Res. **14:**69-91, 1934.

Schroeder, A.: Subperiosteal gold-mesh implantation completed in one appointment, Dent. Abstracts **2:**472-473,
1957.

Schroeder, F.: Raising of the alveolar ridge in the maxilla
using homologous material—compared to alloplastic
implantation, Deutsch. Zahnaerztl. Z. **21:**422, 1966.

Schuetze, E.: Twelve years' experiences with sterilized
homoplastic bone graft, Langenbeck. Arch. Klin.
Chir. **298:**251, 1961.

Schule, H.: Plastic reconstruction of vestibular alveolar
crest, Rev. Stomat. **63:**582-588, 1962.

Schurman, P., and Pfluger, H.: Die Histogenese Ecto-
Meso-Dermaler Mischgeschwulste der Mundhole,
Leipzig, 1931, Georg Thieme Verlag.

Schwier, V.: Sul problema della osteosintesi negli impianti, Chirurg., May 31, 1960, pp. 220-236.

Schwind, J. V.: Homotransplantation of extremities of
rats, Radiology **78:**806, 1962.

Schwindling, R.: Insertion of an implant within eight
hours, J. Implant Dent. **5:**55, 1958.

Schwindling, R.: Alloplastische Implantate in der Zahn-
ersatzkunde, Munich, 1960, Carl-Hanser Verlag.

Scialom, J.: Plea for implants, Inform. Dent. **44:**2739-
2744, 1962.

Scialom, J.: A new look at implants: a fortunate discovery;
needle implants, Inform. Dent. **44:**737-742, 1962.

Scialom, J.: Immediate needle-implants, Inform. Dent.
44:1606-1616, 1962.

Scialom, J.: Rappel scientifique et technique sur les implants-aiguilles, Implants Aiguilles, October, 1963.

Scialom, J.: Needle implants, Inform. Dent. **45:**253-266,
1963.

Scialom, J.: La selle fixé et les risques d'infiltration,
Evolution Odontoimplant. **1:**3, 7-10, 1963.

Scialom, J.: Interventions implantaires televisées à l'in-
térieur de l'abbaye, Implants Aiguilles, October, 1963.

Scialom, J.: Etre ou ne pas être implantologiste, Rev.
Odontoimplant., No. 1, March, 1966.

Scialom, J.: Editorial, Rev. Odontoimplant., p. 10, April,
1968.

Scialom, J.: Comunicacao em conferencia—segundo simposio internacional sobre implantes, reimplantes y
transplantes, Caracas, Venezuela, August 11-17, 1968.

Sebastiani, C.: Histological aspects of human autoplastic
bone transplants, Arch. Putti **14:**1, 1960.

Sebastiani, E.: Relievo dell'impronta nell'impianto sot-
toperiosteo, Rev. Ital. Stomat. **10:**26-28, 1955.

Seidenberg, M.: Alloplastic intraosseous implants as precursors to individual tooth replacements, J. Prosth.
Dent. **13:**963, 1963.

Seidenberg, M., and Lord, G. H.: Alloplastic intraosseous implants as precursors to individual tooth replacements, J. Prosth. Dent. **13:**963-971, 1963.

Senn, N.: Healing of aseptic bone cavities with decalcified chips, Amer. J. Med. Sci. **98:**219, 1889.

Serre, L.: Praktische Darstellung aller Operationen der
Zahnarztneikunst, Berlin, 1804, p. 321.

Sevastikoglon, J. A.: Morphological studies of fracture
healing tissue culture, Acta Orthop. Scand. **32:**109,
1962.

Shapiro, H. A., and MacLean, B. L.: Transplantation
of developing tooth germ in the mandible of the
cat, J. Dent. Res. **29:**93, 1945.

Shapiro, M.: The scientific bases of dentistry, Philadelphia, 1966, W. B. Saunders Co.

Sharrard, W. J., and Collins, D. H.: The fate of human
decalcified bone grafts, Proc. Roy. Soc. Med. **54:**
1101, 1961.

Sharry, J. J.: Complete denture prosthodontics, New
York, 1962, McGraw-Hill Book Co.

Shaykin, J. B.: Endodontic implant, J.A.D.A **68:**704-707,
1964.

Sherief, H. A.: An implant technique for full lower denture, J. Egyptian Med. Ass. **8:**590, 1952.

Shevick, B. B.: Precision formed polyethylene implants
for correction of mandibular contour, J. Southern
Calif. Dent. Ass. **25:**34-40, 1957.

Shklair, I. L., and Mazzarella, M. A.: Microbial changes
as a result of full-mouth extraction, J. Dent. Res. **39:**
653, 1960.

Shklar, G.: Tissue reactions to the plastic tooth implant:
current status of animal investigation, Oral Surg. **22:**
349-57, 1966.

Sholl, C. R.: Implantation of a porcelain tooth, Dent.
Cosmos **47**(1):157, 1905.

Shuey, J. M.: Selection of patients for implant dentistry

through medical evaluation, J. Implant Dent. 7: 43-47, 1961.

Sicard, A., Gerard, Y., and Bordjian, R.: Osteosynthesis by means of a preserved homogenous graft (bone bank), Ann. Chir. 16:851, 1962.

Sicher, H., editor: Orban's oral histology and embryology, ed. 6, St. Louis, 1966, The C. V. Mosby Co.

Sidky, E.: Implant dentures, Egyptian Dent. J. 2:18-42, 1956.

Siegrist, W. H., and Enneking, W. F.: Histological aspects of heterogenous bone transplantation, Transplant. Bull. 27:437, 1960.

Silvello, L., and Borelli, G.: The outcome of heteroplastic massive bone implants in patients after resection and grafting by Zanoli's method for knee neoplasms, Arch. Ortop. 75:914, 1962.

Sinclair-Hall, A. H.: Repair of bony and dentinal defects following implantation of polyvinyl alcohol sponge, J. Dent. Res. 43:476-94, 1964.

Skaloud, F.: Erfahrungen mit subperiostalen implantationen, Zahnaerztl. Prax., December, 1957.

Skaloud, F.: Notre experience resultant de 130 implants, Zahnaertzl. Prax., March, 1959.

Skaloud, F.: Experiences with subperiosteal implants, J. Implant Dent. 5:42, 1959.

Skinner, P. R.: Impianti metallici endossei per la stabiliz zazione della protesi, Dent. Dig. 9:485, 1946.

Skinner, P. R.: Intraosseous metal implants for denture stabilization, Dent. Dig. 52:427-430, 1946.

Skinner, P. R.: Intraosseous implant for stabilizing and retention of upper dentures, Dent. Dig. 57:202-207, 1951.

Skoblin, A. P.: Copper content in various segments of the osseous system in bone autoplasty, Vestn. Khir. Grekov. 87:59, 1961.

Slager, U. T., and Zucker, M. J.: The occurrence of electron spin resonance signals in bone grafts sterilized with high voltage electron beams, Transplant. Bull. 30:146, 1962.

Snedecor, G. W.: Statistical methods applied to experiment in agriculture and biology, ed. 5, Ames, Iowa, 1956, The Iowa State College Press.

Snyder, C. C., Wardlaw, E., and Kelly, N.: Gas sterilization of cartilage and bone implants, Plast. Reconstr. Surg. 28:568, 1961.

Soder, P. O., and Larje, O.: Fragamne i tablettform for demonstration ay tandbelaggningar, Svensk. Tandlak. T. 55:563-568, 1963.

Sol, B.: Comparative study of endo-osseoux and juxta-osseux implants, Rev. Franc. Odontostomat. 9:650-658, 1962.

Sol, B.: Periodontology and implantation, Parodontopathies, pp. 318-317, 1963.

Sol, B.: Osseous implantology in the practice of the dental clinic, Rev. Esp. Estomat. 13:455-474, 1965.

Sol, B., and Salagaray, F.: New type of implants, Rev. Franc. Odontostomat. 10:1106-1124, 1963.

Sol, B., and Salagaray, F.: Sens peristasique de l'anatomie stomatognathique, Rev. Trim. Implant., No. 3, April, 1968.

Sollier, W.: Problems concerning the relationship between the implant laboratory, the oral surgeon and the prosthodontist, Scientific Session American Academy of Implant Dentistry, Chicago, 1953.

Soskin, S.: Diabetes: disturbance in endocrine regulation of blood sugar, Northwest Med. 40:356, 1941.

Souza, J. A.: Fatores biomecanicos nos implantes, J. Estomat., November-December, 1963.

Souza, J. A.: Implantes sub-periosticos totals dos maxillares, Sao Paulo, 1964, Edicoes Iguacu.

Spira, E.: Bridging of bone defects in the forearm, J. Hosp. Joint Dis. 23:170, 1962.

Spirgi, M.: Implant in modern dentistry (endontics and periodontics), J. Conn. Dent. Ass. 36:17-20, 1962.

Spirgi, M., Cimasoni, G., and Pfister, E.: Les incrustations metalliques endo-osseuses en prosthèse fixe et amovible, Geneva, 1960, Institut de Medicine Dentaire.

Spreng, M.: Die Prothese und die lebenden Gewbe, Basel, 1945, Apollonia-Verlag.

Staegemann, G.: Der Prothesenschaden der Schleimhaut im histologischen Bild, D.D.Z. 15:1061-1065, 1960.

Staegemann, G.: Vorlaufige mitteilung über die Verwendung einer Kunstoff elfenbein: Kombination als alloplastiches—Implantationsmaterial, Deutsch. Stomat. 8:225, 1953.

Stamm, T. T.: Developments in orthopaedic operative procedures, Guy Hosp. Rep. 112:1, 1963.

Stanton, H.: Reaction of edentulous mandible to trauma, Implant Dent. J. 4:40, 1958.

Stanziola, F.: Bone transplantation: its use at the Hospital Santo Thomas, Arch. Med. Panama, Vol. 11, 1962.

Stassart, P. C., and Lhoest, J.: Establishment of a lyophilized bone bank: preliminary technical study, Rev. Med. Liege 18:86, 1963.

Stevens, J., and Ray, R. D.: An experimental comparison of living and dead bone in rats, physical properties, J. Bone Joint Surg. 44-B:412, 1962.

Stewart, M. J., and Bland, W. G.: Compression in arthrodesis: a comparative study of methods of fusion of the knee in ninety-three cases, J. Bone Joint. Surg. 40-A:585-606, 1958.

Stolman, J. M.: Role of ascorbic acid in the maintenance of blood vessel walls studied in polyvinyl sponge implants: preliminary report, J. Dent. Res. 38:680, 1959.

Strain, J. C.: Tooth socket implants, a preliminary report, J. Prosth. Dent. 4:116-119, 1954.

Strake, F. A., and Chase, R. L.: Second stage surgery; insertion of the implant substructure and subsequent prosthodontics, Dent. Dig. 66:420-427, 1960.

Stringa, G.: Studies of the vascularization of bone grafts, J. Bone Joint Surg. **39-B:**395, 1957.

Stringa, G., and Mizzau, M.: Autoplastic bone grafts in pseudarthrosis of the forearm, Arch. Putti **16:**364, 1962.

Strock, A. E.: Experimental work on a method for the replacement of missing teeth by the direct implantation of a metal support into the alveolus, Amer. J. Orthodont. Oral Surg. **25**(5):467-472, 1939.

Strock, A., and Strock, M. S.: Method of reinforcement for pulpless anterior teeth, J. Oral Surg. **1:**252-255, 1943.

Strock, A., and Strock, M. S.: Ulteriori studi sull'impianto di metalli inerti per la sostituzione de denti, Alpha Omegan **43:**107-110, 1949.

Strock, M. S.: Significance to dentists of recent developments in the study of diseases of the parathyroid glands: a paper read before H. N. Lowell Research Society and Harvard Dental School, November 9, 1933.

Strock, M. S.: Fractures of the mandible, Surg. Gynec. Obstet. **72:**1047-1051, 1941.

Strock, M. S.: Mouth in hyperparathyroidism, New Eng. J. Med. **224:**1019-1023, 1941.

Suh, K. R.: Transplantation of bone, J. Korea Surg. Soc. **5:**3, 1963.

Sulamaa, M.: The treatment of some skeletal deformities, Postgrad. Med. J. **39:**67, 1963.

Sullivan, E. J.: Discussion of implant denture, J. Prosth. Dent. **1:**49, 1952.

Sutro, C. J.: Transplantation of tooth germ elements to marrow cavities of tibias of kittens, Arch. Path. **28:**199, 1939.

Suzuki, H. K.: Some studies on the role of mucopolysaccharides in ossification, J. Arkansas Med. Soc. **59:**376, 1963.

Svetlova, M. L.: Complement activity of the serum in plastic surgery of bone under experimental conditions, Ortop. Travm. Protez. **24:**62, 1963.

Swanson, A. B., and others: Seven years' experience with irradiated bone graft material, Surg. Gynec. Obstet. **117:**573, 1963.

Takagi, T.: Experimental study on replacement of the vertebral body, J. Jap. Ortop. Ass. **35:**667, 1961.

Tam, J. C.: Two-state surgical process for a lower implant denture, J. Southern Calif. Dent. Ass. **23:**22-28, 1955.

Tandler, J., and Grosz, S.: Ueber den Einfluss der Kastration auf den Organismus, Arch. Ent. Organ. **27:**35-61, 1909.

Tarsoly, E.: Filling of bone cavities with egg shell-plaster mixture, Acta Chir. Acad. Sci. Hung. **4:**63-72, 1963.

Taylor, G. L., and Appelton, J. L. T.: Dental aspect of case of dwarfism (cretinism?), Dent. Cosmos **71:**124, 1929.

Tempestini, E.: Sulle infissioni transalveolari per la ritenzione e stabilita dell protesi mandibolari, Comunicazioni presentate al 2 Simposio internazionale degli impianti alloplastici a scopo protetico, Pavia, 1955.

Terry, J. M., and Boucher, L. J.: Epithelial reaction to plastic implants, J. Wisconsin Dent. Soc. **39:**263-266, 1963.

Terkla, L. G., and Laney, W. R.: Partial dentures, ed. 3, St. Louis, 1963, The C. V. Mosby Co.

Thierry, A.: Pilier de bridge visse dans le maxillaire, Inform. Dent. **32:**618, 1950.

Thilander, H.: Subperiosteal implants of polyvinyl sponge (Ivalon), Svensk. Lakartidn. **55:**563-574, 1962.

Thoma, K. H.: Trattato di chirurgia orale, Pavia, 1959, Edizioni Cortina.

Timme, W.: Endocrine aspects of constitution. In Timme, W.: Biology of individual, Baltimore, 1934, The Williams & Wilkins Co.

Tobonwhite, A.: Implantation of acrylic teeth in the jaws, Int. Dent. J. **8:**15-16, 1958.

Tomlin, A. J.: Reimplantation of four impacted second premolars, Oral Surg., Vol. 21, 1966.

Tonna, E. A., and Cronkite, E. P.: Cellular response to fracture studied with tritiated thymidine, J. Bone Joint Surg. **43-A:**352, 1961.

Toth, K.: Lower face-end prosthesis using immediate implantation of a pillar tooth with metal root, Fogorv. Szemle **58:**272-6, 1965.

Toto, P. D.: Reaction of bone and mucosa to implanted magnets, J. Dent. Res. **41:**1438-1449, 1962.

Toto, P. D.: Reaction of bone to magnetic implant, J. Dent. Res. **42:**643-652, 1963.

Touyon: Utilisation d'implant juxta osseux en reimplacement d'une incisive centrale, Ass. Odontostoma. Implant., 1961.

Trachenko, S. S.: On the problem of bone homoplasty, Ortop. Travm. Protez. **22:**6, 1961.

Trainin, F. B.: Sub-periosteal dental implants, Lebanese Dent. Mag. **6:**1-16, 1956.

Trainin, F. B.: Dental implants in theory and practice, Brit. Dent. J. **10:**389-398, 1956.

Trainin, F. B.: Implant materials and the gingival trough, Dent. Pract. **8:**2-7, 1957.

Trainin, F. B.: Design of subperiosteal dental implants, Lebanese Dent. Mag. **4:**5-6, 1959.

Trainin, F. B.: Implant dentures in Great Britain, J. Implant Dent. **6:**18-25, 1960.

Trainin, F. B.: Subperiosteal implants, J. Dent. Belg. **51:**31-40, 1960.

Trainin, F. B.: Les implants dentaires en Grande-Bretagne, Congrès Internationale des Implants, Paris, 1961.

Trainin, F. B.: Mucosal inserts: a technique for stabilizing the difficult upper denture, Dent. Pract. Dent. Rec. **12**:196-204, 1962.

Trainin, F. B.: Evolution of an original implant design, Dent. Delineator **17**:15, 1966.

Tramonte, S.: Concerning an important modification in endosseous implants, Rass. Trim. Odont. **44**:129-136, 1963.

Tramonte, S.: L'impianto endosseo con vite autofilettante, Film presentato al VI Seminario Internazional dell'-Accademia Americana degli Impianti, Atlantic City, October, 1963.

Tramonte, S.: L'implanto endosseo razionale, Milan, 1963, Editria Lusy.

Tramonte, S.: Intraosseous implantation, prejudices and fears, Inform. Dent. **48**:790-798, 1966.

Tramonte, S.: Su alcuni casi particolarmente interessanti di implanto endosseo con vite autofilettante, Ann. Stomat., Vol. 4, December, 1966.

Trapozzano, V. R., and Grant, F. C.: Acrylic cranioplasty, Oral Surg. **1**:815-826, 1948.

Trattner, G.: Table clinic presentation, Meeting of American Academy of Implant Dentures, Las Vegas, 1965.

Trauner, R.: What can be said today about the technique of subperiosteal implants? J. Implant Dent. **5**:40-41, 1959.

Treacher, F.: Technique for casting the superstructure of a dental implant, Dent. Tech. **14**:13-15, 1961.

Trueta, J.: A theory of bone formation, Acta Orthop. Scand. **32**:190, 1962.

Tsaltas, T. T.: Metaplasia of aortic connective tissue to cartilage and bone induced by the injection of papain, Nature **196**:1006, 1962.

Tullio, G., and Sgarzini, L.: Sull'applicazione contemporanea degli impianti subperiostei superiori e inferiori, Rass. Trim. Odont. **10-12**:40-49, 1956.

Turner, T. C., and others: Sterilization of preserved bone grafts by high voltage cathode irradiation, J. Bone Joint Surg. **38-A**:862-884, 1956.

Uhlig, H.: Principles, technics and applicability of implant denture construction, Dent. Abstracts **5**:590-592, 1960.

Uhlig, H.: Implants, J. Dent. Ass. S. Afr. **18**:515-522, 1963.

Ukai, H.: Functional teeth, Bull. Tokyo Dent. Coll. **7**:73, 1966.

Uris, M. R., MacDonald, N. S., and Jowsey, J.: The function of the donor tissue in experimental operations with radioactive bone grafts, Ann. Surg. **147**:129, 1958.

Urist, M. R.: Processed cortical bone for internal fixation in lumbosacral arthrodesis, Acta Orthop. Scand. **32**:357, 1962.

Urist, M. R., and McClean, F. C.: Osteogenetic potency and new bone formation by induction in transplants to the anterior chamber of the eye, J. Bone Joint Surg. **34-A**:443, 1952.

Urist, M. R., Moss, M. J., and Adams, J. M.: Calcification of tendon: a triphastic local mechanism. In press.

Vaes, G. M., and Nichols, G.: Oxygen tension and the control of bone cell metabolism, Nature **193**:374, 1962.

Valauri, A. J.: Correcting maxillofacial deformities: use of surgical prosthesis and epithelial inlays, New York J. Dent. **33**:55-57, 1963.

Van Varenbergh: Implantations dentaires: quelques mises au point necessaires, Inform. Dent., Vol. 37, 1949.

Vasey, C.: On the supposed influence of the cementum in sustaining the vitality of transplanted teeth, Lancet **1**:557, 1861.

Veloudakis, G.: Implant dentures, Egyptian Dent. J. **3**:56-63, 1957.

Venable, C. S., and Stuck, W. G.: Three years' experience with Vitallium in bone surgery, Amer. Surg. **114**:2, 1941.

Venable, C. S., and Stuck, W. G.: The internal fixation of fractures, Springfield, Illinois, 1947, Charles C Thomas, Publisher.

Veno, T.: Use of zirconium metal plate in arthroplasty of temporomandibular ankylosis, Bull. Tokyo Med. Dent. Univ. **2**:137-139, 1955.

Vernes, J.: Discours inaugural, Ass. Odontostomat. Implant Fac. Med., 1961.

Vernes, J.: Preface. In Maurel, G.: Les implants en prothèse dentaire, Paris, Librairie Maloine.

Vernes-Menegaux, V., and Magnant: De la tolerance de certains aciers utilisés en prothèse perdue, Rev. Med., 1941.

Vinditti, D., Forcella, G., and Pellegrino, G.: Osteosynthesis of recent diaphysial fractures with autoplastic implant, Arch. Putti **17**:529, 1962.

Vivent, R.: Implant techniques in America, Inform. Dent. **46**:357-360, 1964.

Volkov, M. V., and Panova, M. I.: Some problems of preservation and transplantation of homologous tissues, Ortop. Travm. Protez. **23**:11, 1962.

Waerhaug, J.: Implantation of acrylic roots in tooth sockets, Oral Surg. **9**:46-54, 1956.

Waerhaug, J.: Tissue reaction around acrylic root tips, J. Dent. Res. **36**:27-38, 1957.

Waerhaug, J.: Tissue reaction to self-curing acrylic resin implants, Dent. Pract. **8**:234-240, 1958.

Waerhug, J.: Gingivas og det marginale periodontiums histopatologi, Nord. Klin. Odont. **3**:1-17, 1958.

Waerhaug, J.: Hvilke krav ma det stilles til vare brokonstruksjoner sett fra en biologisk synvinkel, Norkse Tannlaegeforen. Tid. **68**:205, 1958.

Waerhaug, J.: Lokala reaktioner i brostodets marginala parodontium och darav betlingade indikationer:

symposium: Broprotes, Svensk. Tandlak. Sallskapets Kongress, August, 1960.

Wagner, J., and Langer, C.: Implantacao de pecus fundidas baseadas en trabalhos experimentais feitos en caes, Rev. Farm. Odont., January, 1963.

Walfane, I. A., Lascana, V., and Gonzales, I. C.: Transplantation of the dental follicle in various mediums, Rev. Ass. Med. Argentina 56:71, 1942.

Weber, S. P.: Implants as an aid to the periodontium, Dent. Dig. 71:16-19, 1965.

Weigele, E. B.: Ueber die resezierten Zahnwurzeipitze verschraubten Stifzahne, Deutsch. Mschr. Zahnheilk., 40, 1922.

Weigele, E. B.: Über die chirurgische Verankerung von Prothesen am zahnlosen Unterkeifer, Vjschr. Zahnheilk. 2:254, 1928.

Weigele, E. B.: Implantat-Technik fur totale untere Prothesen, Zahnaerztl. Welt. 7:529, 1952.

Weinberg, B. D.: Subperiosteal implantation of a Vitallium (cobalt-chromium alloy) artificial abutment, J.A.D.A. 40:549-554, 1950.

Weinmann, J. P.: Biological factors influencing implant denture success, J. Implant Dent. 2:12, 1956.

Weinmann, J. P., and Sicher, H.: Bone and bones, ed. 2, St. Louis, 1955, The C. V. Mosby Co.

Weinreb, M. M., and Bogen, M.: One-day procedure for complete lower Vitallium implants, J. Prosth. Dent. 9:1056-1065, 1959.

Weinreb, M. M., and Bogen, M.: One-day procedure for full lower implants, J. Implant Dent. 6:33-42, 1960.

Weiskopf, J.: Erfahrungen mit 65 subperiostalen Metallgerust-Implantationen, Deutsch. Zahnaerztl. 15:1129-1144, 1960.

Weiss, M.: Total upper juxta-osseous implant with tantalum, Int. Dent. J. 8:29, 1958.

Weiss, M.: Etude statistique sur les diverses methodes d'implantation, Rev. Franc. Odontostomat., No. 8, 1958.

Weiss, M.: Techniques des implantations inferieures juxta-osseuses en tantale, Actualites Odontostomat., No. 46, 1959.

Weiss, M.: The superstructures in dental implantation, Rev. Ass. Dent. Mex. 22:335-339, 1965.

Weiss, M.: Modification de la methode des "blades" du Dr. Linkow, Rev. Trim. Implant., No. 7, May, 1969.

Weiss, M.: Reunions et congrès, Rev. Trim. Implant., No. 7, May, 1969.

Weiss, M.: Simplified juxtaosseus implantology for total restoration of a maxillary, Rev. Trim. Implant., No. 6, February, 1969.

Weiss, M.: Symposium d'implantologie, Rev. Trim. Implant., No. 7, 1969.

Weiss, M., and Skaffter: Le point de vue medical en matière d'implant, Communication à la Société Française d'Implantologie, June, 1959.

Weiss, M., Weitz, F., and Shapiro, A. J.: A procedure for successful upper and lower implant dentures, J. Prosth. Dent. 1:105, 1954.

Weiss, M., Weitz, F., and Shapiro, A. J.: Indications et contre indications des differentes méthodes d'implantation, Ass. Odontostomat. Implant., 1960.

Weiss, P. A.: Molecular reorientation as unifying principle underlying cellular selectivity, Proc. Nat. Acad. Sci. U.S.A. 46:993, 1960.

Weiss, P. A.: Cells and their environment, including other cells. In Brenan, M. J., editor: Biological interactions in normal and neoplastic growth, Boston, 1962, Little, Brown and Co.

Weitz, F., and Shapiro: Full upper implant denture, J.A.D.A. 46:80, 1953.

Weitz, F., and Shapiro: Implant denture: principles, description and function, Dent. Survey 29:757-759, 1953.

Weitz, F., and Shapiro: Procedure for successful upper and lower implant denture, J. Prosth. Dent. 4:105-115, 1954.

Welti, H.: Maladie de Basedow chez l'enfant, Trans. Amer. Ass. Study Goiter, pp. 101-107, 1938.

Werner, L. A.: Full upper implant denture, Caracas, Venezuela.

West, W. K., and Frank, G. R.: Use of the strut bone graft, Amer. Surg. 29:186, 1963.

Westerberger, M. L., and Clark, H. B.: Implant dentures, J. Oral Surg. 13:5-65, 1955.

White, R. G.: Studies in the transplantations of bone: a new approach, J. Bone Joint Surg. 44-B:3, 1962.

Wiart, M.: Les implants metalliques sous periostes: indications et contre-indications, Rev. Franc. Odontostomat. 1:222, 1956.

Wiart, M.: Indications et contre-indications des implants sous periostes, Ass. Odontostomat. Implant., 1960.

Wiart, M.: Indications des implants sous-periostes, Rev. Odontostomat., 1961.

Wiederkehr, H. A.: Über die Gewbsfreundlichkeit einiger neuren alloplastichen Stoffe unter besonderer Berucksichtigung ihrer Verwendungsmoglichkeit in der Kieferchirurgie, Med. Dent. Dissertation, Kiel, 1953.

Wiley, A. M.: Tissue responses to polyurethane foam, Canad. J. Surg. 5:97, 1962.

Willfane, I. Z., and Lascano, G.: Transplantation of the dental follicle in various mediums, Rev. Ass. Med. Argentina 56:71, 1942.

Williams, J. B., and Irvine, J. W.: Preparation of inorganic matrix of bone, Science 119:771, 1954.

Williams, R. G.: Comparison of living autogenous and homogenous grafts of cancellous bone heterotopically placed in rabbits, Anat. Rec. 143:93, 1962.

Willstaedt, H., Levander, G., and Hult, L.: Studies in osteogenesis, Acta Orthop. Scand. 19:417-432, 1950.

Wilson, J. H.: Partial dentures, Sydney, 1955, Angus and Robertson.

Wise, R. A.: Histological study of transcervical fracture

of femur after internal fixation, J. Bone Joint Surg. **23:**941-947, 1941.

Wolf and Williams: Endocrinology in modern practice, ed. 2, Philadelphia, 1939, W. B. Saunders Co.

Wolfe, M. M.: Technic of the ivory implant for correction of saddle nose, Arch. Surg. **37:**800, 1938.

Wolff, J.: Das Gesetz der Transformation der innern Architektur der Knochen bei pathologischen Veranderungen der ausseren Knochenform, Sitzungsb. Preuss. Akad. Wissensch. Phys.-Math. Kl., 1884.

Wolff, J.: Die Lehre von den funktionellen Knochengestalt, Virchow. Arch. **155:**256, 1899.

Wolff, J.: Ueber die Theorie des Knochenschwundes durch vermehrten Druck und der Knochenanbildung durch Druckentlastung, Arch. Klin. Chir. **42:**302, 1891.

Wolfram, R. S.: Implant dentures, Ann. Dent. **20:**31-33, 1961.

Woodhall, B., and Spurling, R.: Tantalum cranioplasty for war wounds of the skull, Ann. Surg. **121:**649, 1945.

Woodhouse, C. F., Idriss, F. S., and French, D.: The transplantation of living bone grafts, J. Int. Coll. Surg. **38:**329, 1962.

Wooffendale, P.: Practical observation of the human teeth, London, 1783.

Wuellenweber, R.: On plastic closure of combined defects of the vault of the cranium and the scalp, Chirurg. **33:**101, 1962.

Wuhrman, H.: Ueber Implantation versuche, Zahnaerztl. Stomat. **35**(12):804, 1937.

Wulff, J., and Uhlig, H. H.: Nature of passivity in stainless steel and other alloys, Met. Tech., June, 1939; ibid., October, 1939.

Wunderer, S.: Quattro anni di impianti sottoperiostei nella clinica di chirurgia mascellare dell'Universita di Vienna, Riv. Ital. Stomat., Vol. 12, 1958.

Wyburn, M. B.: Tissue grafts, Glasgow Med. J. **30:**345, 1949.

Xresse, E. J.: Rehabilitating the edentulous with implantation, J. Implant Dent. **4:**32-36, 1957.

Young, R. W.: Nucleic acids, protein synthesis and bone, Clin. Orthop. **26:**147, 1963.

Young, R. W., Resca, H. G., and Sullivan, M. T.: The yeasts of the normal mouth and their relation to salivary acidity, J. Dent. Res. **30:**426-430, 1951.

Younger, W. J.: Transplantation of teeth into artificial socket, Pacific Med. Surg. J. **29:**17, 1886.

Younger, W. J.: Implantation of teeth, Dent. Cosmos, 1887.

Younger, W. J.: Some of the latest phases in implantations and other operations, Dent. Cosmos **35:**102, 1893.

Younger, W. J.: In Brophy, T. W., editor: Oral surgery, Philadelphia, 1917, P. Blakiston, pp. 810-831.

Zaborszky, Z.: Experiences with bone screws in osteosynthesis, Orv. Hetil. **103:**1615, 1962.

Zang, C.: Darstellung Blutiger Heilkundiger Operationen, Vienna, 1814.

Zaremba, J., and Urbanska, G.: On the use and osteogenic role of maternal bone homografts in the treatment of congenital pseudoarthrosis of the tibia in children, Chir. Narzad. Ruchu. Ortop. Pol. **27:**43, 1962.

Zawadzki, H.: Maxillary sinus diseases and treatment, New York, 1969, Vantage Press.

Zeller, O.: Zur Verankerung kunstlicher Gebisse im zahnlosen Ober-und Unterkiefer, Deutsch. Mschr. Zahnheilk. **37:**4, 1919.

Zemla, J.: Development of views regarding the problem of bone transplantation, Czas. Stomat. **15:**29, 1962.

Zenkevich, G. D.: Glycoproteins in the blood serum during the process of bone tissue regeneration after fractures and transplantation, Vop. Med. Klin. **7:**592, 1961.

Zepponi, F.: Protesi fisse a mezzo di infibulazioni endomascalari, Riv. Ital. Stomat. **1:**45-47, 1955.

Zepponi, F.: Impianti metallici endossei nella protesi parziale fissa, Rass. Trim. Odont., 1956.

Zepponi, F.: Controllo radiografico degli impianti endossei, Rev. Franc. Odontostomat., No. 3, 1958.

Zepponi, F.: Osservazioni istologiche sull'impianto endosseo, Atti 2 Simposio Impianti Alloplastico, Pavia, 1959.

Zepponi, F.: Interventions, Discussions, Ass. Odontostomat. Implant., 1961.

Zepponi, F., and Santoro, O.: L'impianto endosseo in protesi dentale: contributo clinico, radiografico, istologico, Ann. Stomat., Vol. 42, 1959.

Zepponi, F., Santoro, O., and Abruzzese: Considerazioni e risultati sugli impianti endossei in stomatologia dopo dieci anni di esperienza personale, Ass. Odontostomat. Implant., 3, Congr. Internaz., Parigi, 1961.

Zerosi, C.: Complete lower subperiosteal implant denture inserted in a dog: histopathologic findings, Dent. Abstracts **2:**684-685, 1957.

Zerosi, C., and Baratieri, A.: Les reactions epithelioconjonctivales au contact d'implants sousperiostes, Schweiz. Mschr. Zahnheilk. **10:**878, 1958.

Zerosi, C., and Baratieri, A.: Visione panoramica dei reperti isopatologici di tessuti sottoposti ad impianti iuxtaossei: nuovi rilievi istologici da ricerche personali sperimentali e da rilievi biotici, Atti 2ᵉ Simposio Impianti Alloplastico, Pavia, 1959.

Zerosi, C., Perone, G., and Sebastiani, B.: Impianto parziale sperimentato su cane e controlli istopatologici, Rass. Trim., pp. 101-111, 1956.

Zimmerman, I. E.: Implant in case of mandibular tremor, J. Implant Dent. **4:**28-30, 1958.

Ziskin, D. E.: Gingivae during pregnancy, Surg. Gynec. Obstet. **57**:719, 1933.

Ziskin, D. E.: Roentgenological and histological studies of teeth and gingivae of diabetes, J. Dent. Res. **21**:296, 1942.

Znamenski, M. N.: Implantation kunstlicher Zahne, Deutsch. Mschr. Zahnheilk. **9**:87, 1891.

Zonden, H.: Diseases of endocrine glands, ed. 3, Baltimore, 1936, William and Wood Co.

Zvonkov, N. A.: Experience with the use of bone homotransplants preserved by refrigeration in clinical conditions, Khirurgiia **37**:87, 1961.

Zvonkov, N. A., and Beliakova, T. N.: Morphological characteristics of the changes in homoplasty with refrigeration-preserved bone (experimental research), Ortop. Travm. Protez. **24**:3, 1963.

Index

1